FSFNM
LIBRARY

WOMEN IN MIDLIFE

WOMEN IN CONTEXT: Development and Stresses

Editorial Board:
Matina Horner, *Radcliffe College*
Martha Kirkpatrick, *University of California at Los Angeles*
Claire B. Kopp, *University of California at Los Angeles*
Carol C. Nadelson, *New England Medical Center*
        Tufts University School of Medicine
Malkah T. Notman, *New England Medical Center*
        Tufts University School of Medicine
Carolyn B. Robinowitz, *American Psychiatric Association*
Jeanne Spurlock, *American Psychiatric Association*

THE WOMAN PATIENT

Volume 1: *Sexual and Reproductive Aspects of Women's Health Care*
Edited by Malkah T. Notman and Carol C. Nadelson

Volume 2: *Concepts of Femininity and the Life Cycle*
Edited by Carol C. Nadelson and Malkah T. Notman

Volume 3: *Aggression, Adaptations, and Psychotherapy*
Edited by Malkah T. Notman and Carol C. Nadelson

BECOMING FEMALE: PERSPECTIVES ON DEVELOPMENT
Edited by Claire B. Kopp

WOMEN'S SEXUAL DEVELOPMENT: EXPLORATIONS OF INNER SPACE
Edited by Martha Kirkpatrick

WOMEN'S SEXUAL EXPERIENCE: EXPLORATIONS OF THE DARK CONTINENT
Edited by Martha Kirkpatrick

THE CHALLENGE OF CHANGE: PERSPECTIVES ON FAMILY, WORK, AND EDUCATION
Edited by Matina Horner, Carol C. Nadelson, and Malkah T. Notman

WOMEN IN MIDLIFE
Edited by Grace Baruch and Jeanne Brooks-Gunn

WOMEN IN MIDLIFE

EDITED BY
GRACE BARUCH
Wellesley College
Wellesley, Massachusetts

AND

JEANNE BROOKS-GUNN
Educational Testing Service
Princeton, New Jersey

PLENUM PRESS · NEW YORK AND LONDON

HQ
1233 Women in midlife
W872
1984

91

Library of Congress Cataloging in Publication Data

Main entry under title:

Women in midlife.

  (Women in context)
  Includes bibliographies and index.
  1. Middle aged women—United States—Addresses, essays, lectures. 2. Middle aged women—Addresses, essays, lectures. 3. Middle aged women—Psychology—Addresses, essays, lectures. 4. Sex role—Addresses, essays, lectures. 5. Middle aged women—Mental health—Addresses, essays, lectures. I. Baruch, Grace K. II. Brooks-Gunn, Jeanne. III. Title: Women in mid-life. IV. Series. [DNLM: 1. Women—Psychology. 2. Middle age—Psychology. HQ 1233 W872]
  HQ1059.5.U5W65 1984   305.4   84-3374
  ISBN 0-306-41444-9

©1984 Plenum Press, New York
A Division of Plenum Publishing Corporation
233 Spring Street, New York, N.Y. 10013

All rights reserved

No part of this book may be reproduced, stored in a retrieval system, or transmitted, in any form or by any means, electronic, mechanical, photocopying, microfilming, recording, or otherwise, without written permission from the Publisher

Printed in the United States of America

To Susannah
G.K.B.

To Rebecca
J.B.-G.

Contributors

Diane E. Alington • Centenary College, Hackettstown, New Jersey

Rosalind C. Barnett • Wellesley College Center for Research on Women, Wellesley, Massachusetts

Debra Barnewolt • Center for the Comparative Study of Social Roles, Department of Sociology, Loyola University, Chicago, Illinois

Grace K. Baruch • Wellesley College Center for Research on Women, Wellesley, Massachusetts

Jeanne Brooks-Gunn • Educational Testing Service, Rosedale Road, Princeton, New Jersey

Catherine DeLorey • Women's Health Research Institute, Boston, Massachusetts

Julia Hay • Wisconsin Family Studies Institute, University of Wisconsin, Madison, Wisconsin

Carolyn G. Heilbrun • Department of English, Columbia University, New York, New York

Barbara Kirsh • Educational Testing Service, Rosedale Road, Princeton, New Jersey

Margie E. Lachman • Department of Psychology, Brandeis University, Waltham, Massachusetts

Judy Long • Department of Sociology, Syracuse University, Syracuse, New York

Helena Z. Lopata • Department of Sociology, Loyola University, Chicago, Illinois

Zella Luria • Department of Psychology, Tufts University, Medford, Massachusetts

Robert G. Meade • Department of Psychology, Tufts University, Medford, Massachusetts

Malkah T. Notman • Department of Psychiatry, Tufts–New England Medical Center, Boston, Massachusetts

Lydia O'Donnell • Wellesley College Center for Research on Women, Wellesley, Massachusetts

Mary Brown Parlee • Graduate Center, City University of New York; Center for the Study of Women and Society, New York, New York

Karen L. Porter • Maxwell School, Health Studies Program, Syracuse, New York

Nancy K. Schlossberg • Department of Education, University of Maryland, College Park, Maryland

Jeanne Spurlock • American Psychiatric Association, Washington, D.C.

Ann Stueve • 23 Hamilton Avenue, Ossining, New York

Jane Traupmann • Family Development Center, Cambridge, Massachusetts

Lillian E. Troll • Department of Psychology, Rutgers University, New Brunswick, New Jersey

Beatrice Blyth Whiting • Graduate School of Education, Laboratory of Human Development, Harvard University, Cambridge, Massachusetts

Vivian Wood • School of Social Work, University of Wisconsin, Madison, Wisconsin

Acknowledgments

Hilary Evans, senior editor of the Women in Context series, and Claire Kopp, editor of the series volume, *Becoming Female*, originally proposed this book on midlife women and invited us to co-edit it. Their enthusiasm was infectious, and we have profited greatly from many lively discussions.

As co-editors, we have each relied on our individual support systems while the book was in progress. For Jeanne Brooks-Gunn, Rosemary Deibler and Lorraine Luciano at the Educational Testing Service in Princeton provided assistance on all aspects of manuscript preparation and offered much-needed support and encouragement during editing. Margaret Mahoney and Tom Moloney of the Commonwealth Fund deserve a special thanks for their support during the last year; their thoughts on the special problems of disadvantaged midlife women who are unemployed and/or heads of households were particularly stimulating. Orville Brim and Richard Lerner were partially responsible for the decision to include midlife women in conceptualizations of the timing of female reproductive events and psychological adaptation.

Grace Baruch relied relentlessly on the skills and good will of Kathie DeMarco, who managed the innumerable tasks of a two-city project with patience and precision. The intellectual companionship of Rosalind Barnett is reflected throughout the book. Finally, we are grateful for the patience of our families, especially our husbands, whose support survived lengthy late-night telephone calls that too often occurred on holiday weekends.

Contents

Introduction • The Study of Women in Midlife   1
         GRACE K. BARUCH AND JEANNE BROOKS-GUNN

PART I • Conceptual Approaches to Midlife   9

Chapter 1 • Life Events and the Boundaries of Midlife for Women   11
         JEANNE BROOKS-GUNN AND BARBARA KIRSH

Chapter 2 • Methods for a Life-Span Developmental Approach to Women in the Middle Years   31
         MARGIE E. LACHMAN

Chapter 3 • Middle-Aged Women in Literature   69
         CAROLYN G. HEILBRUN

PART II • Roles and Relationships   81

Chapter 4 • The Middle Years: Changes and Variations in Social-Role Commitments   83
         HELENA Z. LOPATA AND DEBRA BARNEWOLT

Chapter 5 • *Multiple Roles of Midlife Women: A Case for New Directions in Theory, Research, and Policy* JUDY LONG AND KAREN L. PORTER	109
Chapter 6 • *The Psychological Well-Being of Women in the Middle Years* GRACE K. BARUCH	161
Chapter 7 • *Social Change and Equality: The Roles of Women and Economics* DIANE E. ALINGTON AND LILLIAN E. TROLL	181
Chapter 8 • *The Daughter of Aging Parents* ANN STUEVE AND LYDIA O'DONNELL	203
Chapter 9 • *Motherhood in the Middle Years: Women and Their Adult Children* VIVIAN WOOD, JANE TRAUPMANN, AND JULIA HAY	227
Chapter 10 • *Black Women in the Middle Years* JEANNE SPURLOCK	245
Chapter 11 • *Problems of American Middle-Class Women in their Middle Years: A Comparative Approach* BEATRICE BLYTH WHITING	261

PART III • Enhancing Well-Being   275

Chapter 12 • *Health Care and Midlife Women* CATHERINE DELOREY	277
Chapter 13 • *Reproductive Issues, Including Menopause* MARY BROWN PARLEE	303

Chapter 14 • *The Midlife Woman as Student* 315
NANCY K. SCHLOSSBERG

Chapter 15 • *The Anxiety of the Unknown—Choice, Risk, Responsibility: Therapeutic Issues for Today's Adult Women* 341
ROSALIND C. BARNETT

Chapter 16 • *Reflections and Perspectives on 'Therapeutic Issues for Today's Adult Women'* 359
MALKAH T. NOTMAN

Chapter 17 • *Sexuality and the Middle-Aged Woman* 371
ZELLA LURIA AND ROBERT G. MEADE

Index 399

Introduction

The Study of Women in Midlife

GRACE K. BARUCH AND JEANNE BROOKS-GUNN

To describe the middle years—that relatively long span when one is neither young nor old—as a neglected period may no longer be accurate, given current scientific and popular interest in adult development and aging. But midlife is still too often seen merely as a kind of staging area on the way to old age, when one gathers one's forces and tries to stock up on assets—health, money, relationships—that will be needed for the rigors of the last phase of life. The middle years have been characterized more as a transition period than as a time of growth, satisfaction, and creativity. As this volume will show, although midlife is not without its difficulties, it is, for many women, a time of unexpected pleasure, even power.

MAJOR THEMES

A central theme of this volume is the impact of social change. The influence of economic conditions, of ideology, of the normative timing of such life events as age of marriage and childbearing, are addressed in many chapters from many different perspectives. Social changes are shown to have both negative and positive consequences. On the negative side, for example, the sex differential in life expectancy is a biosocial phenomenon that greatly restricts the availability of sexual partners—or, more precisely, heterosexual partners—for older women. On the positive side, the postponement of marriage and childbearing is related to women's increased commitment to the labor force, which in turn may serve to reduce their poverty in old age. Related to the theme of social change, then, is the question of the extent to which future cohorts of

---

GRACE K. BARUCH • Wellesley College Center for Research on Women, Wellesley, Massachusetts 02181. JEANNE BROOKS-GUNN • Educational Testing Service, Rosedale Road, Princeton, New Jersey 08541.

middle-aged women will resemble their counterparts of today, given the myriad changes over time.

A second theme of the book is the question of the extent, permanence, and even the reality of improvement in the condition of midlife women. There is convincing evidence of improved mental health—less depression, greater self-esteem—than was so in the 1950s. (Veroff, Douvan, and Kulka, 1981). At the same time, the economy is shrinking, discouraging women's employment and increasing the possibility of poverty. It may be that, as life expectancy increases, the penalties of aging are being postponed rather than abolished.

A third theme is that of diversity. In the past, women have too often been treated in research and theory as one homogeneous group. This has been especially true for middle aged women. The authors of many chapters emphasize the diversity of experience of midlife women—not only across groups (culture, race, cohort) but within groups. We see the heterogeneity of black women, of women who are returning to school, of daughters who are caring for aging parents, of those who enter therapy.

Finally, the need for reassessment and improvement of both therapy and of research design and measurement is emphasized. Assumptions and stereotypes that permeate conceptual models and empirical work perpetuate inaccuracies and gaps in our knowledge. From rigorous studies employing the latest insights of life-span development methodologies to works of fiction portraying patterns not yet discussed by social scientists, new models are being proposed.

Topics and Approaches to the Study of Midlife

This volume is organized into three sections: Conceptual Approaches to Midlife, Roles and Relationships, and Enhancing Well-Being.

CONCEPTUAL APPROACHES TO MIDLIFE. In this section, authors address such questions as: What is midlife? How can it be studied? How is it changing?

Jeanne Brooks-Gunn and Barbara Kirsch discuss current perspectives on the boundaries and events of the middle years, placing these in the context of social and historical changes. The fluidity of boundaries and changes in the timing and patterning of life events, they argue, contribute to confusion about midlife, to ambivalence toward it, and to our difficulties in preparing for and adapting to the middle years. They draw on empirical data from a study of two Radcliffe College classes to illustrate incongruities between women's expectations and the realities they later encounter.

INTRODUCTION: THE STUDY OF WOMEN IN MIDLIFE 3

Margie Lachman provides a detailed description of how the concepts and methodologies of life-span developmental psychology can be applied to the study of midlife in women. She analyzes the concept of development, arguing that the definition of development is critical to studies of the midlife period. Reviewing principles of research design and measurement, including an analysis of common errors, she provides a framework for approaching a variety of topics relevant to generating a sound data base on women's middle years.

Carolyn Heilbrun draws on both the lives and works of women writers, from George Eliot to May Sarton, in her exploration of new patterns and models for women's middle years. She argues that intensity of experiences in these years—energy and delight, creativity and generativity—arise from one's work and from relationships with other women, rather than from the classic erotic plot centering on marriage that until recently summed up women's adult lives.

ROLES AND RELATIONSHIPS. Chapters in this section both draw on and challenge role theory and the literature on women's psychological well-being. Authors analyze the economic underpinnings of women's life situations and address issues of responsibility and care in a variety of relationships.

Helena Lopata and Debra Barnewolt draw on classic theories of roles and role conflict as background for their empirical study of how women themselves experience their roles. Surveys of Chicago-area women reveal how women in diverse life situations (specifically with regard to parenting and work) rank the relative importance of different roles at present, in the past, and in the future. The authors provide a typology of roles and examine such influences on women's perceptions as age, cohort, and role involvement.

Judith Long and Karen Porter's chapter critically reassesses the existing literature on roles and role conflict, including the concept of dual roles. They point out that prior literature assumes the primacy of family responsibilities for women and views paid employment as a deviant activity. Exploring the reasons for women's economic vulnerability, particularly in old age, the authors show how women's typical marital and occupational "careers" have contributed to their poverty. The public policy implications of traditional views of women are discussed, with special attention given to implications for the Social Security system.

Grace Baruch reviews existing literature about women's psychological well-being, showing how diversity in the definitions of well-being lead to inconsistencies in findings. She critically reviews data bearing on age and stage theories, including current concepts of the midlife crisis. Well-being is then examined in relation to women's roles as paid workers, mothers, wives, and daughters. Using data from a study done with

Rosalind Barnett of women aged 35 to 55, she identifies specific attributes of different roles that may improve or impair well-being.

The extent and permanency of changes important for women's progress toward equal opportunity are questioned by Diane Alington and Lillian Troll. They provide a brief history of women as students to illustrate how the larger society may exploit as well as simultaneously encourage women. Discouraging turnabouts in social attitudes and blatant barriers remain, but on a more optimistic note the authors argue that the family can promote as well as restrict women's opportunities. Woman as "late bloomer" is portrayed as a repeated and heartening phenomenon.

Two chapters focus on the mother – daughter relationship in later life. Ann Stueve and Lydia O'Donnell take the perspective of the daughter, Vivian Wood, Julia Hay, and Jane Traupmann that of the mother. Stueve and O'Donnell ask, how do middle-aged daughters frame their commitments to their elderly parents? Drawing on their study of daughters with at least one parent over 70, they show the diversity of attitudes and of patterns of responsibility, and analyze these in relation to daughters' age, stage of the family life cycle, and employment pattern. Their findings challenge the gloomy picture of the middle-aged woman as inevitably and persistently caught in the middle of onerous duties to parents and children.

In their analysis of the role of mother in later life, Vivian Wood, Julia Hay and Jane Traupmann focus on issues of independence and reciprocity, which are central values in our society. The maintenance of equity, that is, of fairness, in the relationship between parents and children, specifically mother–son and mother–daughter, was the major topic of their study of Wisconsin women aged 50 and older. They report on how feelings of being overbenefited or underbenefited in relationships with parents play themselves out in women's relationships with their children.

Jeanne Spurlock's chapter on black women at midlife emphasizes the diversity of experience in what is too often seen as a homogeneous group. She corrects for prior neglect and stereotyping of black middle-aged women who, despite their greater poverty compared with white women, are characterized by determination and joy as well as struggle. Difficulties in relationships with men are common, but coping capacities are strengthened by the extended family, and the church.

Beatrice Whiting brings the perspective of her studies of other cultures to her analysis of the lives of American women. Seeking universal dimensions that will permit comparisons across disparate societies, she provides a framework of basic psychological needs and shows, for example, how the need for physical contact goes relatively unmet in older women in our society. She also points to ways in which men's needs may be frustrated by changes in women's lives, contributing to the potential for backlash.

ENHANCING WELL-BEING. The enhancement of well being can occur in a variety of institutions such as the educational and health-care systems, and in a variety of relationships, including the therapeutic.

Catherine Delorey explores the major threats to women's health, including those from disease and from deficiencies in the health care system. Data from her own study of midlife women and their physicians indicate the persistence of myths and stereotypes about women's health. Overemphasis on, and distortion of, the experience of menopause exemplifies these problems. Delorey describes the progress of the women's self-help health movement and offers recommendations for improvement in an area critical to women's well-being.

Mary Parlee argues in her chapter that studies of the middle years have not yet adequately addressed the interrelation of psychological and biological aspects of midlife changes. Analyzing the reasons for this neglect, Parlee focuses on assumptions embedded in a biological perspective—for example, labeling a depression as "post-partum" rather than "new-mother depression"—and reviews both barriers to and progress in understanding the psychology of menopause.

Diversity is once again the major theme in Nancy Schlossberg's chapter on women as adult learners; older women are now major figures in the population explosion of adult students. She analyzes three kinds of barriers—situational, dispositional, and institutional. Learning is discussed in the context of women's lives within the family, since the phases and transitions they experience there often are the triggers for the pursuit of additonal education. Describing the experiences of women who return to school, she offers suggestions for improving the person–environment fit between the individual woman and the educational institution.

The difficulties and dilemmas women and their therapists face when new roles and old feelings collide are the subject of two chapters on therapeutic issues of today's midlife women. Rosalind Barnett examines how problems women bring to therapy are related to social changes affecting their lives. Old expectations die hard, the departure from familiar patterns is rarely painless, and being different from one's mother is both inevitable and difficult. Too often, women doubt their own perceptions and capacities, and their femininity. Drawing on current research and on case material, Barnett argues that concepts of choice and risk are valuable to both patient and therapist in understanding and resolving psychological problems.

Malkah Notman's chapter continues the process of examining what is new and what is old about issues women currently present to therapists. Realistic limitations on one's life choices exist, and "classic" psychological issues important in the past have not disappeared—anxiety over competition with one's mother, for example. Case material illustrates such persistent problems as well as those arising from new patterns. For example, a mother may pressure her daughter to be more "liberated" than the daughter might wish to be.

Finally, Zella Luria and Robert Meade present a lively, comprehensive, and tough-minded view of the sexual realities of later life. They review the few empirical studies that bear on the sexuality of women in the middle years, placing Kinsey's research in historical context. The implications of men's earlier mortality for older women's sexual choices are explored; they are diverse, varying with such factors as age, race, marital status, and sexual preference. Luria and Meade suggest that such social changes as the sexual freedom of the baby boom generation, and the increased power women will derive from occupational advancement mean that current patterns may not apply to the next generation of women reaching midlife.

FUTURE DIRECTIONS

We believe that a combination of social and ideological changes are allowing the study of midlife to flourish, providing a more accurate, less stereotypic and less gloomy picture of these years. An overemphasis on negative images, we would argue, arose from two kinds of bias in theory and research. First, the study of midlife has until recently focused on men (e.g., Levinson, 1978). Major themes in this work involve anguish over mortality and over the inadequacy of one's achievements. The relevance of such themes to the understanding of women's lives is being called into question (Baruch, Barnett, and Rivers, 1983). The large differential in life expectancy between males and females—now nearly 8 years—may well influence the intensity of such concerns. A man of 45 stands at a very different "distance from death" from a woman of the same age. Recent studies suggest she is unlikely to share his sense of imminent mortality or his sense of inadequate accomplishment in the world. For those midlife women who were young adults in the 1940s and 1950s, an era when, far from being held to unattainable standards of professional accomplishment, achievement outside the role of wife and mother was unexpected, almost forbidden, the female version of "too short a time left, too much to do" is often "I have almost too many years left, and the chance to fill them with more than I ever thought I could."

A second source of bias affecting our images of midlife women involves the inordinate attention given to supposedly critical and negative experiences with menopause and "the empty nest." As many chapters in this volume emphasize, these are neither central marker events for most women, nor are they main causes of distress. The loss of a youthful appearance also may be little mourned by the healthy middle-aged woman busy with work commitments, and more and more women are in that category. Such predictable changes, especially if they occur "on time," rarely prove burdensome.

These two strands of research and theory have caused middle age to be viewed with, at best, ambivalence. No wonder that the notion of helping women to anticipate, understand, and prepare for their middle years has yet to take hold. This volume, we hope, will offer a more balanced and useful view of midlife. The serious and distressing problems that many women face are not neglected, but neither are the opportunities for growth and change that we now know are characteristic, not just possible, in adulthood.

We recognize that biases in the study of midlife women are in no way ancient history. Nevertheless, recent developments in the social sciences are yielding valuable new approaches to the study of midlife. First, the study of adult development within the framework of life-span psychology has called attention to the potential for growth and change throughout the life course. An important by-product of this view has been the development of new conceptual and methodological approaches to the study of midlife that provide a standard for judging old ideas and testing new ones. Second, the aging of the members of important, well-known longitudinal samples, such as the Berkeley and Oakland growth studies, are providing rich data on the years beyond adolescence in the context of individual life histories (Eichorn, Clausen, Haan, Honzik, and Mussen, 1981). Third, we also are benefiting from the aging of many women researchers who, as younger adults, pioneered new approaches to the study of women, and who are now drawn to the study of the middle and later years. Many are represented in this volume.

Finally, and perhaps least often acknowledged, social scientists are increasingly having to recognize the influence of the Women's Movement, as well as of the social changes it both reflects and catalyzes (Giele, 1982). New ideas and opportunities, we believe, have changed the nature of the realities women face as they grow older, and mostly in a positive direction. The extent to which this is so is debated throughout this volume, but the feeling that one's life is over after 40—that the primary task as mother is done and the best years past—seems less and less widespread among today's midlife women. New educational and occupational opportunities, although far from adequate, are transforming the midlife experience for many women.

REFERENCES

Baruch, G., Barnett, R., & Rivers, C. *Lifeprints: New patterns of love and work for today's women.* New York, McGraw-Hill, 1983.
Eichorn, D. H., Clausen, J. A., Haan, N., Honzik, M. P., & Mussen, P. H. *Present and past in middle life.* New York: Academic Press, 1981.
Giele, J. Z. (Ed.), *Women in the middle years: Current knowledge and directions for research and policy.* New York: Wiley, 1982.
Levinson, D. J. *The seasons of a man's life.* New York: Ballantine, 1978.
Veroff, J., Douvan, E., & Kulka, R. *The inner American: A self-portrait from 1957 to 1976.* New York: Basic Books, 1981.

PART I
Conceptual Approaches to Midlife

Chapter 1

Life Events and the Boundaries of Midlife for Women

JEANNE BROOKS-GUNN AND BARBARA KIRSH

> The shock . . . of middle age is a threshold shock. A door is closing behind us and we turn sorrowfully to watch it close and do not discover, until we are wrenched away, the one opening ahead. (Fromm-Reichmann, F., 1959)

The difficulty of studying midlife in women is illustrated dramatically by the above statement. Midlife typically is characterized as a transitory rather than as a distinct phase of the life cycle. As a phase defined primarily by the end of youth, it is accorded little importance in developmental conceptualizations, in literature, or in the media. Midlife also is defined as the time to prepare for old age and death, the time when one begins to count forward rather than backward (in terms of years to live rather than years lived). This view is reflected in research methodologies that relate behavior in midlife to outcomes in old age. Midlife adjustment, sexuality, satisfaction, and health are considered possible predictors of adjustment to old age but are rarely considered outcomes of earlier behavior (see, as a notable exception, the Berkeley and Oakland growth studies; Eichorn, Clausen, Haan, Honzik, and Mussen, 1981).

An approach that treats midlife both as an antecedent and as an outcome embeds midlife within the life cycle. Life-span developmental psychology stresses that no one life phase may be considered without reference to other phases and that a developmental orientation may be applied to the study of adulthood as well as to childhood and adolescence (Brim and Kagan, 1980).

The metaphor of a door opening as well as closing also alludes to

---

JEANNE BROOKS-GUNN AND BARBARA KIRSH • Educational Testing Service, Rosedale Road, Princeton, New Jersey 08541.

the importance of change and the multidimensional and multidirectional nature of change. As Brim and Kagan (1980) state:

> Growth is more individualistic than was thought, and it is difficult to find general patterns. The life span development view is sharply opposed to the notion of adult stages, arguing that stages cast development as undirectional, hierarchical, sequenced in time, cumulative, and irreversible—ideas not supported by commanding evidence. The facts instead indicate that persons of the same age, particularly beyond adolescence, and the same historical period are undergoing different changes; one person may show an increase in certain attributes while another shows a decline in the same aspects of behavior and personality.

In addition, midlife, if viewed as embedded within the life cycle, rather than as the beginning of the end, may be characterized as more than preparation for death, retirement, loss of relationships, and illness. Instead, it may be portrayed in terms of generativity, satisfaction, and competence, as many of the chapters in this volume suggest.

In this chapter, midlife is discussed in terms of the life events that often occur at this time and are often considered markers of midlife, and of the boundaries of midlife that may or may not be fluid, depending on historical changes and individual perceptions. How individuals and society prepare for midlife—given that some life events associated with midlife are normative while others are not, that boundaries of midlife are fluid, and that midlife is sometimes not accepted as a life phase—will be considered. Finally, why so many individuals are ambivalent about midlife will also be discussed.

BOUNDARIES OF MIDLIFE

The life-span developmental approach, by stressing the multidimensional and multidirectional nature of change, makes clear that the boundaries of any life phase may be more fluid than rigid (Brim and Baltes, in press). It follows that an individual may not be readily classified as to a particular life phase (if, indeed, such categorization were even desirable).

However, the need to classify life stages seems to be universal; throughout history, life phases have been outlined, with chronological age boundaries often given. In current Western society, midlife is often thought to *begin* at age 35. Yet this is the point in which one-half of one's life is *over*, in terms of male life-expectancy norms. If "middle" is the halfway point between two times, then 35 would be men's mid-point, not the beginning of middle age for men, who have a life expectancy of 78, and 39 would be women's midpoint.

While the boundaries seem quite fixed in people's minds, they are in reality quite fluid. With the historical changes that have occurred for women in midlife from the 1920s to the present, it seems that the definition of midlife may have been shifted upward. The boundaries may be constructed by the society and the individual and may be less tied to chronological age. There are several possible reasons for the upward shift. First, young adulthood is more protracted: Education is prolonged, marriage and childbearing are delayed, and career decisions are made more cautiously. Consequently, many individuals in their 30s report that they have not entered midlife yet. When they are queried, the typical response is that they have not bought a house, begun a family, or been married for any length of time, have just separated or divorced, are in the midst of changing jobs, or are embarking on retraining activities. Implicit in these statements is the construction of midlife vis-à-vis its embeddedness in a series of life events, as discussed in the preceding section.

Second, the health of the midlife woman, especially those in the middle class, is relatively good. The belief that midlife ushers in ill health, or at the very least fatigue, aches, and pains, may not be corroborated by experience. Instead of inferring that midlife does not necessarily result in health-related problems, women infer that they have not yet reached midlife. The adage "You're only as old as you feel" is indicative of this view.

Third, midlife may be a time of enhanced sexuality for many women (see Luria and Meade, Chapter 17 of this volume). Greater enjoyment and comfort with one's own sexuality are not expected by many midlife women. Again, the inference is that midlife has not been reached rather than that midlife may mark increased sexual enjoyment for many.

Fourth, midlife typically is believed to coincide with the time at which active parenting ends, when children leave their parents' home. As more women have children later, and as more reblended families are formed, women may have children and adolescents in their home throughout their 40s and 50s. Again, a woman's perception of herself as being in midlife may be postponed.

Fifth, the change in life expectancy alters the boundaries of midlife. When life expectancy was in the 60s, being 50 or 55 had a very different meaning than it does today, when life expectancy is in the 70s and almost in the 80s. Perhaps the upper boundary of midlife remains elastic because the length of old age has remained fixed. In other words, if old age is defined as the last 15 years of life, then the increase in life expectancy would lengthen midlife but not old age.

Finally, being old carries a stigma in the United States. A recent essay in the *New York Times* (1982) begins: "I am old. These hateful words are all but forbidden in these United States. The simple declaration marks the worst kind of deficit. Such a stamp is applied by a nation addicted to the mindless worship of youth."

In order to avoid the appellation of old age, the term *middle age* is expanded upward. While middle age may not be perceived as positively as youth, it is still preferable to old age. The old age stereotype encompasses notions such as senility, incompetence, illness, and debilitation. If these terms define old age, and a 55- or 60-year-old woman does not possess these traits (or perceive herself to possess them), then the term *middle age* would be offered to distinguish one from other similar-aged individuals who possess these undesirable traits. Strangely enough, the majority of 55- and 60-year-olds do not "fit" the stereotype, remaining healthy, competent, independent, and active. The pervasiveness of beliefs about old age may underline the necessity to counteract them by expanding the upward boundary of middle age.

Markers of Midlife

One of the major problems in conducting research on midlife, especially for women, is that many different markers or life events have been used to delineate this period; these multiple life events overlap conceptually, methodologically, and descriptively. Not only do they overlap but they are taken from different disciplines, making cross-discipline comparisons difficult. Within any particular field, this plethora has not been problematic, however, because little interdisciplinary research has been conducted on midlife. Notable exceptions include the attempt to relate the onset of menopause to changes in the parenting role and/or the employment role. For example, the early work on the "empty nest" syndrome demonstrated that for many midlife women hospitalized for depressive symptoms, the primary problem was loss of their major role (in this case that of parent with dependent children) rather than a decline or change in circulating hormones (Bart, 1970). In any case, as researchers from different fields begin to review each other's work and to collaborate, the discrepancies between their markers will become more jarring and the failure to consider life events simultaneously more untenable.

Another problem is that even within a field or subspecialty, while consensus may exist as to the type of marker deemed most appropriate, individual variance in the experience of life events makes generalization difficult and research designs problematic.

At least six different markers of midlife may be found in the literature. While some focus on physical, psychological, or social life events, others combine all three aspects.

The first and simplest marker is chronological age. Age typically represents physical, psychological, and sociocultural indices of changes. For example, even though age is clearly a physical marker, women who remain very active physically may be physiologically similar to women 5 years younger than they are. In addition, cultural differences may make the use of age as a marker problematic. Spurlock (Chapter 10) has argued that midlife begins earlier for black women due to their relatively poorer health and nutrition, limited access to medical care, earlier childbearing, and shortened life expectancy compared to whites. Finally, historical changes in age as a marker may have occurred, partially as a function of changes in health status and longevity.

Second, parenting status is almost always considered a relevant marker. For women, midlife has been characterized as the middle stages of parenting (i.e., being parents of older children, teenagers, or young adults). Research on women's midlife crises focused on the end of active child-rearing. However, the assumption that midlife will coincide with a specific stage of parenting is no longer viable. First, a significant number of parenting careers are either earlier or later than the norm. In the white middle class, a number of women have chosen to begin childbearing in their 30s, so that midlife may coincide with early stages of parenting. At the other extreme are teenage parents, who will have grown adult children before they are 40. Indeed, if teenage pregnancy does perpetuate itself within families (and there is limited evidence that this is the case), teenage mothers will be grandmothers before they are 40. Second, using childbearing as a marker omits those women who remain childless. Childless women, teenage parents, and older parents may constitute one-third of all women in America today.

The more relevant use of child-rearing as a marker encompasses the concept of off-time and on-time life events. Neugarten (1979) has discussed the concept of a life clock in which major events occur in a more or less systematic and time-ordered fashion. Teenage pregnancy typically is defined as an event that is unplanned and/or unanticipated, an event that places the women off time vis-à-vis the norm for child-rearing. However, the perception of being off time or on time regarding one's cohort may be more important than one's actual status vis-à-vis the societal norm. In black urban America today, having a child at 17 to 19 is not perceived as being out of phase, although having one at age 15 is (Furstenberg, 1976). Similarly, in segments of middle-class society, having a firstborn after age 30 is typically not perceived as off time by the mother (although it may be perceived as off time by the grandmother). Perceptions of timeliness may affect life satisfaction, adjustment, and expectations more than actual timeliness, as is suggested by research on pubertal girls. Although the mean age of menarche is about 12½ in

America today, great individual variations occur. Girls who begin to menstruate prior to seventh grade or after eighth grade are defined, by most researchers, as early or late, respectively (Brooks-Gunn and Ruble, 1982, 1983). However, when girls are asked about whether or not they are early, late, or on time, 20% are classified differently than their actual status would suggest; in other words, some girls who are off time believe they are on time and vice versa (Tobin-Richards, Boxer, and Petersen, 1983). In addition, their perceptions of timeliness are more strongly associated with self-esteem than are actual physical indices of pubertal status (Tobin-Richards *et al.*, 1983). Thus, with regard to midlife and parenting, perceiving oneself to be in phase may be more important than being in phase normatively.

The next most important marker, in terms of the research literature, is change in work life events. Since employment and child-rearing often covary, especially in earlier cohorts, it is often difficult to treat employment as an independent variable. At the same time, for certain subgroups of women, employment may be a relevant dimension, especially for those groups who alter their employment situations at midlife—entering the work force for the first time, reestablishing work patterns after children enter school, moving from part time to full time, or moving to a higher position. These four work life events may occur in midlife, with the first three being much more likely to occur in midlife women than men (see Long and Porter, Chapter 5, this volume). As women's employment histories seem to be more fluid and less linear than men's employment histories, employment's usefulness as a marker for midlife may not be as great.

A more profitable approach might be to identify certain clusters of women for whom work-life events were altered during midlife. Lopata and Barnewolt (Chapter 4, this volume) describe groups of women in terms of the importance of family and employment to them. Several subgroups of women are identified, each of which has distinguishing characteristics. Another approach would be to look at those women who change their employment patterns at midlife versus those who do not. One might expect those women who are in flux to show different patterns of physical adjustment, life satisfaction, role negotiations, and power within the family from those of the women whose patterns remain fairly stable over time.

Fourth, the activities that women engage in during midlife as well as the mix of these activities have been considered significant life events in midlife. It has been assumed that during midlife, child-rearing demands decrease while other demands (employment, community, and other family members) increase. At the same time that child-rearing demands decrease, other relational demands may be placed on the woman, particularly those of older parents, grandchildren, and husband. In general, the literature using these markers has placed the responsibility upon the women herself. Demands of parents, grandchildren, and children are assumed to be the responsibility of the midlife woman rather than the midlife man. Midlife men seem to be perceived as having some control over the amount of time these demands place upon them, while the midlife woman is not perceived to have much control, being required to take on additional relational requests. Whether employed women are allowed to be "excused" from these tasks, to provide support through financial remuneration, or to request additional time from husbands, rather than being expected to add these responsibilities, is under study (Brody, 1980). Given that older parents expect their midlife daughters to be more responsive than their sons and that midlife daughters (and daughters-in-law) provide more support than do sons (Wood et al., Chapter 8), one might expect employed women and their older parents to experience some difficulty adjusting to such demands.

Fifth, hormonal changes are occurring at this time and may or may not be a significant life event. Hormonal changes precede the onset of menopause, are gradual, and vary greatly across individual women. One indication of these gradual changes is the greater incidence of infertility in midlife women than in younger women. Such infertility is a significant and often unanticipated life event for midlife women who planned their child-rearing careers for their 30s and 40s.

Since the experience of life events may not be normative during midlife, research needs to focus on (a) the appropriate referent group (or groups), rather than comparing individuals to societal norms that may not be salient to the individual (as in the example of urban teenage mothers); (b) women's perceptions of the timeliness of specific events, which may differ from the actual timeliness vis-à-vis specific referent groups; (c) the importance of others' beliefs about timeliness in determining an individual's reaction to a life event (as in the example of the mother who wishes to have a grandchild earlier than her daughter wishes to have a child); and (d) the relationship of differing measures of timeliness to an individual's life satisfaction and feelings of effectance and self-worth. In addition, discrepancies in the timeliness of life events need to be examined; for example, one may feel on time with regard to child-rearing but off time with regard to employment. Is it more disruptive to the individual to be off time with regard to certain life events than to others, or is the notion of off time more cumulative?

In sum, many of the life events associated with midlife are associated only in a probabilistic sense, in that all individuals do not experience them, or experience them at different times or in a different sequence. The variability of midlife markers and the lack of cohesion among them makes it difficult, if not impossible, to discuss transitions to midlife. How one prepares for a transition that is so fluid as to make the term *transition* possibly untenable will be discussed later.

HISTORICAL CONTEXT OF MIDLIFE EVENTS

The transition to midlife may be more or less fluid, depending on the historical context within which it is embedded. Some of the movable markers that determine the elasticity of boundaries are entrance into and progress through educational institutions, age at marriage, moving away from the nuclear family, age of parenting, and widowhood. While these events are experienced by the individual, societal changes influence the probability that a number of individuals will experience a life event at a particular time (Riley, 1973). Important variables in a cohort's movement through life include mortality, fertility, marital status, nationality (immigration), rural–urban residence, and education.

Rossi (1980) suggests that our models of adult development arose out of a specific historical period, that of perhaps the most stable time (1950s and 1960s) in the past century. Patterns of predictable life events are predicated on this model. Instead of using as the normative group those adults who experienced the Great Depression as children or adolescents, World War II as adolescents or adults, and the return to large families and low labor force participation by women in the 1950s, one needs to compare them to other cohorts. Indeed, some demographers have stopped talking about the rapid and surprising decline in the birth rate through the late 1960s and 1970s and instead have focused on the rapid rise in fertility rates immediately following World War II.

Other sociologists have discussed the importance of historical context in defining life phases and interpreting life events. Hareven (1978) suggests that three aspects of life-course analysis are particularly relevant: (1) the synchronization of individual with family transitions, (2) the interaction between life-course transitions and historical changes, and (3) the cumulative impact of earlier life-course transitions on subsequent ones. Analyzing historical changes in definitions of life phases, Uhlenberg (1978) finds three somewhat universal age strata—childhood (0–15), adulthood (15–60), and old age (60+). Although he believes that social conceptions have changed over the century, the

> context of each age category has persisted over this period: Children are expected to live with parents, attend school, and be socialized into the culture; young adults are expected to establish families and take on adult work responsibilities; middle-aged adults are expected to complete the rearing of their children and maintain stability in their occupations; and the elderly are

expected to progressively relinquish various roles and complete the life course by dying. (p. 67)

It is interesting that although Uhlenberg does not differentiate between young and midlife adult phases in his three strata, he does so in his discussion of the context of the categories. In other conceptions, young and midlife adults are usually separate, as are childhood and adolescence.

Uhlenberg (1978) outlines a typology of five family life courses women typically follow into midlife. These are that (1) women marry, bear children, and are still alive and married at the age of 50 (the normatively expected); (2) women die before they reach 50; (3) women never marry and survive to 50; (4) women are married without children and reach 50; and (5) women bear children and survive to 50, but their marriages are not intact because of death or divorce. Uhlenberg compared these life courses for cohorts born in 1870, 1890, 1910, and 1930. The most dramatic changes over time have been in (1) increasing life expectancy, so that more women in the later cohorts reach midlife and more reach midlife with their spouses; (2) increasing rates of marriage, so that fewer of the 1930 cohort are single compared to the older groups; (3) declining age at marriage; and (4) changes in childlessness and never-married status. Childlessness increased dramatically from the 1870 cohort (9%) to the 1890 cohort (14%) and the 1910 cohort (16%), who were young adults during World War I and the Depression. Women born in 1930 had the lowest childlessness rate (4.5%), bearing their children during the late 1940s to the early 1960s. Declines in early widowhood over the 1870–1930 period have been matched by higher divorce rates, but women tend to remarry after divorce, so that families are more likely to be intact in midlife for the 1930 cohort than they were for the older women. Uhlenberg's conclusion is that the rates of conformity with the norms of women's role performance increased from the 1870 cohort to the 1930 cohort. He predicted in 1974 that women would enter midlife from subsequent birth cohorts with far less conformity to these family roles because of divorce and because of norms allowing voluntary childlessness and nonmarital status.

One of the more fascinating aspects of Uhlenberg's analysis is the obvious omission of employment as a marker of status. By concentrating on the family life course, the notion is reinforced that women follow a limited life script. That women are defined by marriage and children means that most of their script is written by the end of young adulthood. They are going to experience significant life events only in terms of divorce, remarriage, or the death of a spouse. As an example, one of the most popular and often quoted statements from the teenage pregnancy literature suggests that for the young unmarried mother, 90% of her life script is written, most of it dismal. Such a view does not allow for changes, for resilience, or for growth, all of which have been found in studies of teenage parents (Furstenberg, 1976). Given this subtle but farily prevalent belief, it is no wonder that the study of midlife women has languished. The movement from young to middle adulthood is considered a nonevent.

In addition, it is doubtful that a similar analysis would be undertaken for men, even though most men could be classified within the five life-course categories. The cohorts of men born in 1870, 1890, 1910, and 1930 also experienced the changes in age of marriage, childlessness, life expectancy, divorce, and remarriage. However, discussions of men's midlife courses concentrate on work life (Levinson, 1978; Vaillant, 1977).

It is a common experience for the baby boom cohort (born between 1946 and 1964) to seek markers of age status and not find firm enough passage rites to convince them of changed status. For example, when large numbers of baby boomers left home for college, a passage rite occurred, removing them from the nuclear family; but the enormous numbers of the cohort encouraged the formation of a new stage—the youth culture of the 1960s and early 1970s—rather than the expected move into adulthood. The age of 21 had been a legal marker of adult status, but the law shifted downward to 18 with the population explosion, giving full legal rights to vote, join the military, drink (in most states). This fluctuating marker reduced the legal coming-of-age to one celebrated more for the adolescent pleasures of driving and drinking than for the responsibility of being a full citizen.

Other markers continue to shift—protracted education, high rates of premarital sex and cohabitation, divorce and remarriage, and changing values whereby women can delay or decline marriage and still derive high levels of life satisfaction. (Although this was probably always the case for individuals, societal beliefs seem to be more accepting of these alternatives than ever before.) Marriage and the end of education have become less salient markers of attainment of adult status.

Some former midlife markers have changed, and others are new for women and are still being defined. What existed as clear age boundaries for former generations (or at least appear clear in retrospect) often fade or blur as other cohorts approach them, partly because of changing characteristics of those younger cohorts. The upper limit of middle age, as discussed earlier, was probably 55 to 60, with the years beyond that classified as old age. Yet the large number of people beyond 55 who do not feel "old" alter the upper boundary of midlife.

The older members of the baby boom generation currently are witness to some unexpected changes in their parents' life-style and attitude changes, new love relationships after divorce or death of a spouse, further education, new hobbies, career switches, geographic moves—all dependent of course, on financial stability and health. It is difficult for people in their 30s and 40s to feel middle-aged when their parents exhibit "youthful" rather than elderly behavior.

The high divorce rate has had an impact on markers surrounding middle age. Abrupt changes in life-style usually accompany divorce, unsettling women economically, geographically, and emotionally. A divorced 45-year-old woman may well lead a life similar to that of a 35- or even 25-year-old unmarried woman—wear the same clothing styles, attend the same singles events, live in the same apartment complexes (since their incomes could well be comparable). They may both be single parents of children still at home, and be searching for a better job and good love relationships.

Finally, the tremendous recent emphasis on physical fitness occurred as the baby boom generation reaced "middle age." This may be interpreted as a conscious effort to continue young adulthood in appearance, activities, and values (Jones, 1980).

Preparation for Midlife

In general, preparation for life events or transitions occur for those events that are anticipated. Two approaches to the issue of preparation for life events have been suggested, each of which involves the distinction between anticipated and unanticipated life events. Brim and Ryff (1979) have hypothesized that a taxonomy of life events characterized by three properties might be useful for examining anticipatory socialization. The three properties of life events that they believe to be relevant are (1) age-relatedness, or the relationship of an event to chronological age, (2) the social distribution of an event, or if an event occurs, the number of persons who will experience it, and (3) the likelihood of occurrence for an individual, or the probability of an event occurring to any given person. From this three-dimensional classification system, eight types of events may be generated. For some of these events, anticipatory socialization occurs and for some it does not. Events that are studied typically are those for which preparation does take place—those events that are highly age-related, are shared by many, and are likely to occur to any given individual. These are the events studied by sociologists and psychologists, as they are normative, age-graded, and well labeled. At the other extreme are events for which preparation does not take place—events that are not likely to occur to an individual, are not predictable in terms of timing, and are not common enough to allow for shared experiences with many others (Brim & Ryff, 1979). However, many life events are not so clear-cut: They may have some relationship to age or there may be a moderate likelihood of occurrence, as in the case of divorce. Many of the examples of events in the middle given by Brim and Ryff are midlife events—death of a father or husband, children's marriages, becoming a grandparent, "topping out" in one's career. The individual may not prepare for such events, given their weak relationship with the three dimensions discussed earlier. These events contrast with many of those in young adulthood, which are more normative and age-graded. Children and adolescents are overtly taught how to perform familial and occupational roles in preparation for young adulthood. This preparation has predominantly meant becoming a wife and mother for women, and husband, father, and economic provider for men. Once these roles are established in adulthood, however, the expectations and socialization for the next stage (midlife) are generally unfocused, at best.

The value of the anticipation of life events is that the individual is provided information regarding the event (and the appropriate social roles and sanctions surrounding it) and is encouraged to seek out information. The individual may search for role models who have experienced the upcoming event or may be contacted by a potential role model who wishes to "pass on" information to the individual. She may be introduced to or seek out new social referent groups such as professional women's organizations, single parents' organizations, parent–teacher organizations, and so on. The individual may begin to rehearse a new set of behaviors related to the life event. More generally, information gathering may be at a cultural level, where attitudes and beliefs are acquired or at least become more salient, given the anticipated change. With regard to childhood and adolescence, the ways in which sex roles are acquired and changes integrated into one's self-definitions have been studied in great detail (Maccoby and Jacklin, 1974; Brooks-Gunn and Ruble, 1983). During midlife, little research on anticipatory socialization has been conducted. In fact, it is not clear (1) whether or not anticipatory socialization takes place, (2) what form it might take (active seeking, passive reception, active offering), (3) whether or not individuals desire more preparation or are at least aware of the lack of preparation, or (4) whether or not life events would be experienced differently if anticipatory socialization took place.

Another way to look at anticipatory socialization is in terms of the timing of life events. The notion of an event being on time implies that the event is normative and occurs at the time when it is expected to occur. Off-time events, in this framework, are still expected (i.e., early puberty, late menopause, late parenting) but occur at a time when they are not anticipated. Whether or not the lack of anticipatory socialization or the perception of being out of phase affects an individual's experience of a life event is not well understood. The most information comes from the study of maturational status in adolescence, vis-à-vis one's peers. Methodologies comparable to those used for untangling the effects of being early or late, perceiving oneself to be so, and the composition of the referent group with respect to maturational timing in puberty might be developed for midlife events; events with biological links (such as menopause, parenting, and physical changes) might be most amenable to such an approach.

Returning to the concept of unanticipated events, rather than off-time events, it is clear that socialization occurs; it is just that it is often after the fact. In this case, *post hoc* socialization may occur in the observation of role models, seeking new referent groups, asking friends for information, and being offered information, these processes being the same as an anticipatory socialization. Typically, this is studied under the rubric of adaptation to life changes rather than as socialization. The term implies that the process is internal, intrapsychic, and individualistic.

Another problem arises when a cohort anticipates one set of experiences, because of the experience of previous cohorts, and then finds itself in a very different set of conditions. In fact, some have hypothesized that vast changes in major social institutions may be expected when the experiences of a cohort contrast sharply with those of the previous cohort (Ryder, 1965). An example of such contrast is the situation of the generation that grew up with the Depression and World War II, followed by their children of the baby boom. In this case, one's anticipatory socialization may not be adequate. For example, many of our female friends lament, as they juggle the responsibilities of children, spouses, parents, community, and employment, "If mother had only told me it would be like this." Of course, mother could not, as she was much less likely to have been employed during her childbearing years, to be rearing children alone, or to have parents live well into their 80s. Perhaps the interest in research on role models arose out of the unmet need of women researchers themselves for anticipatory socialization experiences.

Another example of inadequate socialization due to the reliance on experiences of the preceding cohort involves more indirect forms of socialization, specifically cultural awareness of maternal employment. In a national survey of families (*General Mills Family Report*, 1977), 80% of all adults felt that women with young children should not work outside the home, except in cases of extreme economic need. Clearly, such a cultural belief could discourage women from seeking information about managing young children while employed, even though many women are available to provide such information.

Even within a cohort, an event may be experienced quite differently. Elder (1974) has presented a fascinating analysis of the life experiences and adjustment of two cohorts who were young during the Great Depression. Those who were young children and those who were entering adolescence during the Depression had different experiences and outcomes. Within the cohort just entering midlife, life courses have been quite divergent, even in women from similar backgrounds (Zadeh, 1975).

Another approach emphasizes personally normative events that may be experienced as crises even though they occur for a number of (or all) individuals. Erikson's conceptualization of life development was instrumental in the acceptance of this view of adult development. Studies on midlife men (Vaillant, 1977; Levinson, 1978) are examples. Development is seen as potentially enhanced by satisfactory coping with such events as divorce, death of parents and spouse, and children leaving home. Although an individual cannot fully prepare for these events, being independent, capable of financial decisions, and open to change, for adaptation to new experiences and acquaintances would be essential for adaptation to these common events.

The Radcliffe Study[1]

In order to examine the question of whether or not women are prepared for midlife and, if so, whether various cohorts perceive their preparation differently, two cohorts of Radcliffe College graduates are being examined. This study involves women who finished Radcliffe in 1947 and in 1962, years noted for striking contrasts in historical and cultural circumstances. Questionnaires completed by these two groups provide rich information on early influences, college experiences, adult attitudes toward self and society, and also on the actual roles and activities chosen for each decade of adult life. Each stage of life for the Radcliffe alumnae was subject to different historical events and cultural values, so early influences such as family structure and class background may interweave in contrasting ways with individual proclivities and personalities in influencing adult life patterns. Eighty-three women from the class of 1947 completed a questionnaire at their 35th reunion; thus, they were in their mid-50s, just finishing midlife. In contrast, the Radcliffe class of 1962 was tested at their 20th reunion, when they were in the early 40s. More than one-half of the 1962 class completed the questionnaire.

---

[1]We wish to thank the Henry A. Murray Center for the Study of Lives, at Radcliffe College, for their support of B. Kirsh and for provision of data from their archives.

Preparation for Careers

Few of the graduating class of 1947 had assumed they would have careers; few prepared for them. They had expectations of idyllic married life, and most of them did marry soon after college (68% by the end of 1950). They had more children at younger ages than the class of 1962. Fifteen percent of the younger women had given birth after the age of 40. In 1982, of the 83 women attending their 35th reunion, 14 had no children, 5 had one child, 17 had two, 20 had three, 16 had four, 7 had five, 1 had six, and 3 had seven. These highly educated women had participated enthusiastically in the baby boom between 1946 and 1964.

Even with relatively large families, this group had 31 master's degrees and 15 doctoral or professional degrees. Only 10 of these 83 women attending the reunion were not working; the rest listed a wide variety of occupations, including professor, therapist, librarian, lawyer, writer, business executive, and clerical worker. Many had started their careers late in life when child-care responsibilities decreased or when they became single again. About half of the women at the reunion were still married to their first husband; 12 had remained single, 6 were widowed, 10 were in their second or third marriages, and 9 had divorced and not remarried.

More of the 1962 graduates had established careers than had the 1947 graduates. The social context had changed in the 15 years between their graduations. The earlier class had grown up through the Depression and World War II and anticipated unlimited domesticity and financial security after college graduation. They hoped for and had large families, spending their 20s and 30s at home with children and chores, or doing some volunteer work. They had given scant thought to their futures beyond these early adult years. Most of them voiced surprise at how unprepared they were for midlife. Substantial effort was essential in order to adapt to new life-styles and gain self-knowledge, as changes affected them both from external, or social, sources and from internal, or personal, sources. Difficulty in coping with drastically changed circumstances was a common theme among the 1947 graduates at the time of their 30th reunion.

Preparation for Changes in Sexuality

When the Radcliffe graduates from the class of 1947 were surveyed 30 years after college about their attitudes toward changing sexual standards, very few of the women accepted the changed attitudes or behaviors for themselves. Many voiced worry and disapproval as to the negative consequences they had seen, in terms of broken marriages and personal unhappiness. A common response was that they had had to learn to accept the changed sexual standards because of conflicts over their children's sexuality, but they said they personally remained "conventional" and "old-fashioned." Several women endorsed the decrease in hypocrisy and sexual double standard but worried about the bewildering choices faced by other women, particularly adolescents, in making choices about sexual behavior.

This cohort of women, now in their 50s, were caught unprepared for social change in the norms regarding sexuality. They grew up in a time when delayed gratification (economically and sexually) was endorsed as a way to get through the Depression and World War II. They married early and produced relatively large families; now, many of them are unexpectedly single because of divorce or widowhood, and those that remain married must reestablish relationships with husbands in new family situations without children's intrusions. They clearly feel the pressure to be more sexual at a time of increasing physical symptoms of aging. One woman complained: "I feel my age. Arthritis spreading from back to knees to ankles. Memory giving me trouble (no one prepared me for this so young!)."

And yet some studies suggest that women's sexuality increases with age in terms of interest and ease of arousability. This is in contrast to a decline of sexuality with age in men. Rubin (1979) found that many of the marriages she studied had been plagued with sexual problems in the early years, but that when sexual norms relaxed and fear of pregnancy faded with age, couples improved their sexual relationships during midlife. Among Rubin's sample, over 60% of the women had been virgins before they were married. Both cultural and life-stage factors have helped improve their sex lives to a point where, according to Rubin, roughly 90% of these midlife women have experienced orgasms.

Preparation for Changes in Relationships

Midlife typically entails a reevaluation and renegotiation of many relationships. Long marriages are altered by children leaving home, allowing more time for companionship between spouses; at the same time, many women return to work, go to school, or change careers as their children enter adolescence and young adulthood. A new world away from the home generally serves to engender feelings of competence and instrumental orientation in women whose daily lives have been oriented around family and home. Frequently, household chores, decision making, and financial matters are areas of negotiation where women feel more independent. There can be strains in a long marriage when the midlife woman moves out into the work world around the same time her husband begins to relax in his occupational role and wants to appreciate more leisure and home-centered activities.

Relationships between the midlife woman and her parents change, also. She often has more responsibilities and worries in caring for aging parents, helping them with decisions and practical matters they had previously felt adequate to attend to themselves. Often relationships between elderly parents and the midlife child improve and they come to appreciate each other in more mature ways. With the death of one parent, the midlife woman generally has a greater role in the physical and emotional well-being of the remaining parent. Also, the midlife individual faces mortality of both parent and self as signs of aging and illness increase (Wood et al., Chapter 9, this volume).

The women in the 1947 Radcliffe class report that they experienced years of turbulence with their adolescent children, but now, in their 50s, they have far better understanding of and relationships with their grown children. The women mention areas of disapproval of their children's life-styles—particularly in the realms of sexuality and values toward money and career—but they have come to accept their children's lives as entities separate from their own. This acceptance of separateness enhanced the parent–child relationship.

Of course, midlife women who are single experience different sorts of relationships with men and other women than their married peers. Women in the 1947 and 1962 Radcliffe classes reported happy surprise at finding romance and fulfilling love relationships in their 30s, 40s, and 50s. These relationships could be characterized as less sex-role-stereotyped and more companionate than earlier marriages or relationships. Reliance on women friends, often from college, was strong, especially among single women. These friends formed a support network rivaling or sbustituting for family relationships, particularly for the 1962 cohort.

THE AMBIVALENCE SURROUNDING MIDLIFE

Not only is midlife an ambiguous phase, as illustrated by the fluidity of its upper boundary, the lack of consensus on the timing of certain life events, the multiplicity of markers used to define the midlife experience, and the lack of any conceptual framework embedding midlife in the life cycle, but individuals feel ambivalent about it as well. To become an adult is often seen as equivalent to the end of exploration and growth. The adolescent perceives the adult world as muted rather than vivid, dead rather than passionate and alive. This is reflected in the following quote:

> To much of the public . . . the mode of authority in America, the mode that deals with real experience, the mode that is neither dead (as the adult mode

seems to be) nor compromised (as the childish world of television seems to be), is the adolescent mode—mode of exploration, becoming, growth, and pain. (Troll, 1982)

The author is suggesting that even adults agree with the unspoken premise that to be adult is to be grown up and "mature" in the sense of having closed all doors to exploration. If popular opinion assigns such attributes as aliveness, excitement, and growth to the young, what remains for the rest of us—stodginess, inertia, absence of feeling? Even though adulthood is perceived this way in literature, the media, and even research, most individual adults would state that they value growth and perceive pain as a measure of progress (Spacks, 1981). However, even if individuals perceive their own lives to be rich and intense, at the same time their general perception of adulthood reflects the notion of "living death." Thus, the private experience of adults may be very different from the public view of adults. This is why the study of the midlife experience as embedded in the life cycle is so important, as it illustrates the possibility of growth and change throughout life. However, popular conceptions of midlife suggest that growth is truncated for women but not for men.

It is not surprising that adults may be ambivalent about the onset of midlife, given that they share the general belief in midlife as a negative event or a nonevent, even in the face of contradictory evidence from their own and their friends' lives. Direct contradiction to this pessimistic view of adulthood is also being put forth by a variety of authors today, as seen in this volume. Midlife may be a time of great growth, expansion, and satisfaction.

A large part of the ambivalence about midlife is probably due to the feelings and experiences related to physiological changes associated with aging. Much of the life-course research on adulthood either ignores or denies these effects, although Rossi (1980) recently has made an eloquent plea for the inclusion of biological change into our models of adult development. Not only do physiological events need to be studied with regard to co-occurrence with social and psychological events, but women's perceptions about such changes need to be explored.

In a study of 68 women aged 33 to 56 and their families, Rossi (1981) asked the women what age they would most like to be. Not surprisingly, none wanted to be older. One-half wished to be under 30. The mean desired age was 32 to 33 years, regardless of the current age of the woman. Rossi found that while chronological age did not predict the desired age, the actual symptoms of aging did (eyesight, shape of body, condition of teeth, energy level). In addition, having a large family, being older when the first child was born, and being less educated contributed to the desire to be younger. Analyses of the individual contributions of factors such as attractiveness, fatigue, and medical problems to negative feelings about one's actual age or to the desire to be younger would provide needed information about the ambivalence surrounding midlife.

Finally, it is commonly believed that by midlife there is no plot line left for women, or that the plot line is completely predicated upon the woman's marital and parental status. (The plot line is as follows: Leave father's home, enter husband's home, rear children; the rest of the plot remains unfinished.). If women are defined only in relationship to others (children and husband), then the end of parenting is the termination of their plot line. However, with the advent of multiple roles for midlife women, especially that of employment, a new plot line may be written that focuses on achievement and creativity. In fact, Heilbrun (Chapter 3) argues that the central theme of midlife for women is achievement, rather than relationships. Men, she claims, have known about the importance of achievement for a long time. She advocates that women take into account the possibility for enlarging the sphere of work during midlife. This view may be a reaction to the tacit assumption that midlife women continue their role as the bearers of responsibilities to the family, with the additional concerns of older parents taking the place of parenting. Instead of arguing that midlife offers the possibility of work satisfaction, one might argue that this possibility exists throughout the life-span. The processes by which women are limited in their achievement of such satisfaction may be similar across the life-span, rather than being specific to each stage.

REFERENCES

Bart, P. B. Mother Portnoy's complaints. *Trans-Action*, 1970, 8(1–2), 69–74.
Brim, O. G., and Baltes, P. (Eds.). *Life span developments and behavior* (Vol. 5). New York: Academic Press, in press.
Brim, O. G., and Kagan, J. *Constancy and change in human development*. Cambridge, Mass.: Harvard University Press, 1980.
Brim, O. G., and Ryff, C. On the properties of life events. Kurt Levin memorial address. Paper presented at the APA Meetings, New York, September 1979.
Brody, E. "Women in the middle" and family help to older people. *Gerontologist*, 1981, 21, 471–485.
Brooks-Gunn, J., and Ruble, D. N. The development of menstrual-related beliefs and behaviors during early adolescence. *Child Development*, 1982, 53, 1567–1577.
Brooks-Gunn, J., and Ruble, D. N. The experience of menarche from a developmental perspective. In J. Brooks-Gunn and A. Petersen (Eds.), *Girls at puberty: Biological and psychosocial perspectives*. New York: Plenum, 1983.
Eichorn, D. H., Clausen, J. A., Haan, N., Honzik, M. P., and Mussen, P. H. (Eds.). *Present and past in middle life*. New York: Academic Press, 1981.
Elder, G. H. *Children of the Great Depression*. Chicago: University of Chicago Press, 1974.

Furstenberg, F. F., Jr. *Unplanned parenthood*. New York: Free Press, 1976. General Mills Company. *General Mills Family Report*, 1977.

Hareven, T. (Ed.). *Transitions: The family and the life course in historical perspective*. New York: Academic Press, 1978.

Jones, L. *Great expectations: America and the baby boom generation*. New York: Coward Press, 1980.

Levinson, D. J. *The seasons of a man's life*. New York: Ballantine Books, 1978.

Maccoby, E. E., and Jacklin, C. N. *The psychology of sex differences*. Stanford: Stanford University Press, 1974.

Neugarten, B. L. Time, age and life cycle. *American Journal of Psychiatry*, 1979, *136*, 887–894.

New York Times. December 18, 1982.

Riley, M. A. Aging and cohort succession: Interpretations and misinterpretations. *Public Opinion Quarterly*, 1973, *37*, 35–49.

Rossi, A. S. Life-span theories in women's lives. *Signs*, 1980, *6*, 4–32.

Rossi, A. S. Aging and parenthood in the middle years. In P. Baltes and O. Brim (Eds.), *Life span development and behavior*. New York: Academic Press, 1981.

Rubin, L. *Women of a certain age*. New York: Harper, 1-79.

Ryder, N. B. The cohort as a concept in the study of social change. *American Sociological Review*, 1965, *30*, 843–861.

Spacks, P. M. *The adolescent idea*. New York: Basic Books, 1981.

Tobin-Richards, M. H., Boxer, A. M., and Petersen, A. The psychological significance of pubertal change: Sex differences in perceptions of self during early adolescence. In J. Brooks-Gunn and A. Petersen (Eds.), *Girls at puberty: Biological and psychosocial perspectives*. New York: Plenum Press, 1983.

Troll, L. *Continuations: Adult development and aging*. Monterey, Calif.: Brooks/Cole, 1982.

Uhlenberg, P. Changing configurations of the life course. In T. Hareven (Ed.), *Transitions: The family and the life course in historical perspective*. New York: Academic Press, 1978.

Vaillant, G. E. *Adaptation to life: How the best and the brightest came of age*. Boston: Little, Brown, 1977.

Zadeh, P. *Radcliffe Alumnae Quarterly*, 1975.

Chapter 2

Methods for a Life-Span Developmental Approach to Women in the Middle Years

MARGIE E. LACHMAN

The central thesis of this chapter[1] is that the study of women in midlife can be enriched if it is placed in a change-oriented, life-span framework. This message is conveyed by the title of this book—*Women in Midlife*—which places middle age in the context of the life span. The book's title also conveys a message about the current state of the field of life-span human development. Until recently, researchers have focused primarily on the young and the old. Thus, there is a gap in our knowledge about the middle of the life-span. This neglect of the middle years is particularly true with regard to the study of women, but the situation is slowly being rectified (see Baruch, Barnett, and Rivers, 1983; Eichorn, Clausen, Haan, Honzik, and Mussen, 1981; Giele, 1982; Lowenthal, Thurnher, and Chiriboga, 1975; Rossi, 1980; Rubin, 1979; Stewart and Platt, 1982; as well as this volume).

This chapter suggests an organizing conceptual framework and compatible methodological procedures for the study of women in midlife. First, conceptual features of a life-span developmental view are presented. Second, two measurement topics are discussed: (a) reliability of change and (b) age-related validities. Third, two research topics are presented: (c) multidimensionality of change and (d) research designs

---

[1] I would like to thank Avron Spiro III and John R. Nesselroade for their helpful comments on an earlier version of this chapter.

MARGIE E. LACHMAN • Psychology Department, Brandeis University, Waltham, Massachusetts 02254.

for the study of development. For each topic, some of the common pitfalls that plague developmental researchers are presented and recommendations for overcoming these problems are proposed. Methodological points are illustrated with examples from research on personality and intellectual functioning in adulthood.

Since only a limited number of issues can be addressed within the confines of a single chapter, this chapter is a selective rather than a comprehensive presentation of developmental research methods. In particular, methodological issues and exemplary topics from life-span developmental psychology are emphasized. For the interested reader, a number of sources provide a broader coverage of developmental methodology (e.g., Achenbach, 1978; Baltes, Reese, and Nesselroade, 1977; Wohlwill, 1973). Although the chapter's content is primarily derived from a psychological perspective, the issues raised should be applicable to those from other disciplines who are interested in the study of women in midlife and in the critical evaluation of research on this subject. One of the advantages of adopting a life-span developmental approach for the study of midlife is that it is a pluralistic and multidisciplinary perspective. Indeed, the life-span perspective, which will be discussed in the next section, has its counterparts in a number of fields other than psychology, including sociology, economics, history, and biology (Baltes, Reese, and Lipsitt, 1980).[2]

LIFE-SPAN DEVELOPMENTAL APPROACH

What features of a life-span developmental approach can be useful for research on women in the middle years? In this section the basic assumptions and characteristics of a life-span developmental approach are presented and applied to the study of women in midlife (Baltes *et al.*, 1980; Brim and Kagan, 1980; Lerner and Ryff, 1978). The goals of life-span research are to examine the nature and course of development and to search for the antecedents and consequences of developmental change. Life-span researchers engage in the description, explanation, and optimization of development. One of the basic assumptions of a life-span view is that development occurs throughout life. This assumption, however, cannot be subjected to empirical scrutiny without specifying a definition of development.

Definition of Development

Within a life-span view, the definition of development is less restrictive than that usually associated with child development perspec-

---

[2]The descriptive term, *life-course,* rather than *life-span,* has been used in sociology, history, and economics (Elder, 1978; Rossi, 1980).

tives (Lerner, 1976; Harris, 1957). In child development models, development typically is characterized by the presence of stages, an end-state orientation, structural reorganization, invariant sequences, and unidirectional and universal changes (Flavell, 1970; Kohlberg, 1969; Wohlwill, 1973). This view has come to be known as the "strong" model of development. In contrast, a "weak" view of development includes any change that is reliable in its definition of development (Baer, 1970). In the most extreme version of the "weak" view, change and development are synonymous.

In a life-span view, development is represented along a continuum of change rather than at either the "strong" or the "weak" extreme (Baltes and Nesselroade, 1979). A life-span view imposes fewer restrictions than many child development models for classifying change as development. According to a life-span conception, developmental changes during adulthood may be characterized by multidirectionality, reversibility, and variability (nonuniversality) across individuals, cultures, and historical time. This broader definition of development may include structural reorganization, invariant sequences, and other features that are characteristic of child-oriented viewpoints, but other forms of change are also included (Reese and Overton, 1970; Looft, 1973). Indeed, some researchers have applied stage models to the study of adult personality development (e.g., Erikson, 1963; Labouvie-Vief, 1982; Levinson, 1978; Vaillant, 1977). Even when stage models are applied to the study of adulthood, however, they may take on forms different from those associated with the structural-cognitive models of child development (e.g., Piaget, Werner). For instance, adult models often include the specification of an invariant sequence, but not of structural reorganization (Levinson, 1978). Others have found that normative stage models are less useful for studying adult development and instead have focused on nonnormative life events as an organizing framework for the study of adult development (Hultsch and Plemons, 1979). The pluralistic conception of a life-span developmental perspective allows for the possibility of multiple influences and diverse outcomes.

Sources of Development

The diverse nature and course of life-span development has its origins in the interaction of biological (heredity) and environmental (experiential) factors. According to the model developed by Baltes and his colleagues (Baltes, Cornelius, and Nesselroade, 1979; Baltes *et al.*, 1980), heredity and experience are the underlying determinants of three major sets of influences that control development: (a) normative age-graded, (b) normative history-graded, and (c) nonnormative.

Normative age-graded influences are those that occur regularly within a culture with respect to timing and duration in the life-span. The menopause is one example of a normative age-graded developmental phenomenon for women in midlife. Normative history-graded events are those that occur in a uniform way for the majority of members of a given cohort.[3] The effects of historical change may be reflected in birth cohort differences. By definition, different cohorts are exposed to different historical/cultural events and they experience the same event at different points in the life-span. The Great Depression, for instance, was found to have long-term (i.e., from childhood to old age) consequences for women (Elder and Liker, 1982) and a differential impact for the 1920 and 1928 birth cohorts (Elder, 1979). Finally, nonnormative events are those that do not follow a regular pattern but rather can occur at any time for any person or group. These events may include rare occurrences, such as diseases (e.g., Parkinson's disease) or an earthquake, as well as more common events when they occur at unexpected or nontraditional times in the life-span (e.g., early widowhood or returning to school in midlife). Baltes et al. (1980) have speculated that age-graded influences are more salient, relative to other influences, in child development and late old age, whereas during midlife, nonnormative events are expected to be the most important set of influences. However, further research is needed to examine the interactive role of the three primary sources of development and their impact at different points in the life-span.

VARIABILITY AND PLASTICITY IN DEVELOPMENT. It has been proposed that age- and history-graded influences and nonnormative life events interact to produce the differential and normative patterns that are characteristic of life-span development (Baltes et al., 1980). In response to their joint effects, life-span development is characterized by both regularity and variability. Thus, within a life-span view, development during the middle years may reflect a great deal of regularity, but also interindividual (between-person) variability and intraindividual (within-person) plasticity (Baltes and Baltes, 1980). Interindividual differences can take on meaning at a number of different levels within a life-span view. One form of interindividual variability can be found at the level of cohort. Between-cohort differences can be a marker of historical-cultural changes. Consider a hypothetical example using the dimension of life satisfaction. In Figure 1A it is shown how two cohorts of women may differ in level of satisfaction and in the direction and course of change. Cohort 2 is always more satisfied with life than Cohort 1; moreover,

---

[3]The term *cohort* is used throughout this chapter to refer to birth cohort, that is, those who are born during the same period of time. In general, cohort can refer to any group of individuals that experiences a given event within the same time period.

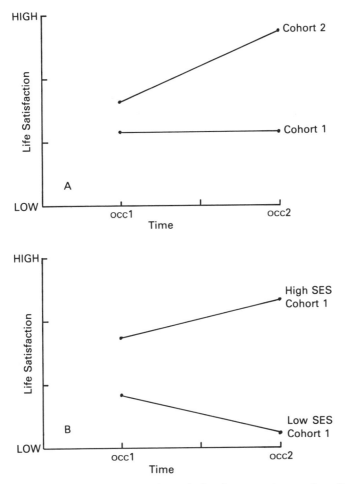

Figure 1. (A) Between-cohort differences in life satisfaction change over two occasions. (B) Within-cohort differences in life satisfaction by socioeconomic status (SES) over two occasions.

Cohort 2 becomes more satisfied over time, whereas Cohort 1 does not change in level of satisfaction over the life-span.

Another form of interindividual variability can be found at the intracohort (within-cohort) level. In Figure 1B we see that for Cohort 1, the middle-class women are always higher in life satisfaction than the lower-class women, and the former group increases in satisfaction as the members get older, whereas the lower-class women become less satisfied as they age. These data illustrate that variability is possible at many levels. Elder (1979) has shown that the personality development of women may vary as a function of their birth cohort, and that within cohorts, patterns of development may be further differentiated according to factors such as social class and educational status.

Although we may be able to obtain an accurate description of age and cohort differences in change, both age and cohort are merely markers or indexes for underlying processes. Identification of age- and cohort-related change does not tell anything about the how and why of development. It is for this reason that several researchers have challenged the role of age and cohort as the primary organizing variables for life-span developmental psychology (Wohlwill, 1970). To go beyond the level of description of cohort differences requires theoretically guided models and explanatory methods. The methods and interpretations will depend on the status that is assigned to the cohort variable (Baltes et al., 1979). In psychology, cohort differences are usually considered in terms of limitations on external validity. Are the results found for one cohort applicable to other cohorts? For sociologists, however, cohort usually is a theoretically meaningful variable that requires explanation. Why do cohorts develop differently? Elder (1979) has suggested that one way to shed light on cohort differences is to examine subgroups within cohorts. Analysis of group differences in exposure to various events or experiences can provide useful information about the processes underlying cohort differences.

In addition to differences in change patterns between persons, a life-span view acknowledges and seeks to chart within-individual variability or plasticity (Baltes and Baltes, 1980). There is an emphasis placed on determining the range of potential behaviors that could be achieved and the conditions under which optimal development can be realized (Denney, 1982). To accomplish this, research efforts should be directed at identifying the antecedents of developmental change. Knowledge about various influences on development can have direct implications for intervention and treatment programs. Within a life-span view, a strong emphasis is placed on preventive and optimization, rather than remedial, forms of intervention (Danish, Smyer, and Nowak, 1980; Turner and Reese, 1980).

Life-Span Development and Women in Midlife

Although the origins of a life-span development view have been traced to the 18th century (see Baltes, 1979; Reinert, 1979), its application to the study of women in midlife is a more recent endeavor (Giele, 1982; Neugarten, 1968; Rossi, 1980). One emphasis of a life-span view is on the dynamic nature of middle age. The key factor is *change,* which can occur on a number of levels (e.g., individual, cultural) and in a variety of forms (e.g., differential, normative, qualitative, quantitative). In nondevelopmental views, middle age often is defined in a static way with fixed chronological age boundaries. The most apparent weakness of these latter views is evident just if one considers that the age range associated with middle age varies widely across persons and cultures (Shannon and Kedar, 1979–80).

A second emphasis suggested by a life-span approach is the complexity of change patterns during midlife. In some nondevelopmental approaches, midlife is approached in terms of a series of events (e.g., menopause, "empty nest," widowhood) without regard to the context in which these events occur. A life-span view focuses on the interrelationships among different events and areas (e.g., family, work) of life (Elder, 1978). The empty nest, for example, cannot be fully understood unless something is known about other aspects of a woman's life. For example, we would want to know information about her relationship with her children when they were at home, the quality of her marital relationship, whether she is working outside of the home, her health status, whether she has a sick parent to care for, and other factors.

A third emphasis of the life-span approach is that each period of life is part of an integrated whole. Thus, middle age cannot be treated as an isolated period. In some cases, early experiences may be transformed by later experiences (discontinuity). In other cases, experiences in midlife may be a direct outgrowth of earlier events (continuity). A fourth emphasis of a life-span view is on the historical and cultural relativity of development; development is embedded within a historical context. What holds true for a cohort of middle-aged persons in one historical–cultural context may not hold for those in other contexts.

Research Issues

To summarize, life-span developmental researchers are concerned with the description, explanation, and optimization of behavior-change processes that occur from birth to death. It is recognized that development may be multidirectional, multidimensional, and variable. Moreover, development occurs at both the individual and societal levels. A number of methodological challenges arise in life-span research because of these features. Four goals for life-span research are considered here. First, it is necessary to adopt techniques that enable the reliable measurement of change. A second task for life-span researchers is to develop and utilize measurement instruments that are valid for the age range to be studied. Third, it is important to employ designs that can capture the complexity and diversity of change. A fourth priority is to identify methods for examining individual and cultural/historical patterns of change. In the remainder of this chapter, research methods that can assist in accomplishing these four objectives will be considered.

Measurement Issues

Researchers have identified two broad classes of measurement: (1) open-ended or unstructured and (2) fixed-choice or structured. Both of these measurement strategies are potentially useful for the study of women in midlife. For exploratory work, open-ended questions are generally desirable because they do not limit the respondents' range of answer choices. Open-ended responses can be usefully applied in developing fixed-choice questions or they can be subjected to an objective coding system in order to quantify the responses. For descriptive and explanatory hypothesis-testing, structured measurement is usually more appropriate. In this format, respondents are given specific choices from which to select answers. In the domain of personality assessment, for example, three types of structured data sources have been identified (Block, 1977; Cattell, 1965). These are life-ratings (e.g., checklists of daily activities or moods, behavioral observations), questionnaires (e.g., self-report personality inventories), and objective tests (e.g., experimental tasks). Regardless of the particular form of inquiry, there are two measurement issues that must be addressed: reliability and validity of measurement. The following discussion will focus on issues of reliability and validity that have particular relevance for developmental research. In order to address these specific issues, however, it will be useful to begin by presenting a general overview of the reliability and validity concepts.

Assessment of Reliable Change

The primary goals of life-span research are the identification and the explication of change processes. A necessary prerequisite to fulfilling these goals is to achieve reliable measurement. Measurement reliability implies accuracy, precision, and consistency in the assignment of numbers to characterize behavior. The assessment of reliability provides an index of the accuracy of measurement. According to classical measurement theory (Lord and Novick, 1968), if a measure is reliable, a response or recorded outcome should be repeatable. There are many factors that can interfere with measurement accuracy, and, in practice, measurements always contain some degree of error. It is unsystematic or random fluctuations that contribute to unreliability of measurement. For instance, random variation in measurement may result from extraneous factors related to the testing conditions, the experimenter, or the subjects (Nunnally, 1978). These random fluctuations or measurement errors must be distinguished from systematic changes across occasions. The latter, so-called true changes, are not troublesome in terms of measurement reliability and, moreover, are at the very heart of developmental analyses. As will become apparent throughout this discussion, one of the notable tasks that faces the developmental researcher is the separation of "true" developmental changes from unsystematic or unreliable fluctuations in scores. Methods for separating systematic and unsystematic changes will be presented after a brief discussion of reliability.

Several methods can be applied to the analysis of measurement reliability. Each of these forms takes into account different information about the sources of random fluctuations (Ghiselli, Campbell, and Zedeck, 1981). The decision to use a given method should be based on one's research goals as well as on the measurement information that is available. The four most common forms of reliability are consistency (test–retest), equivalence (alternate forms), homogeneity (internal consistency), and interrater agreement. Space limitations make it impossible to go into detail on these aspects of reliability. For those readers who are interested in a more in-depth coverage of reliability issues, any of the following are useful sources: American Psychological Association (1974); Anastasi (1968); Ghiselli *et al.* (1981); Lord and Novick (1968); Nunnally (1978).

RELIABILITY VERSUS CHANGE. We will concentrate our discussion on the consistency form of reliability because of the unique problem it raises for the developmental researcher. Consistency reliability is frequently referred to as test-retest reliability, since it is calculated as the correlation between two administrations of the same test. As such, it is an index of the degree to which scores remain constant over time. To the extent that a measure is consistent, individuals should receive the same score on repeated administrations over short time intervals (e.g., 1 week, 1 month).

For the developmental researcher, perhaps the most serious drawback of this form of reliability is that it confounds true change in the measured attribute with error of measurement in the scale. The retest correlation coefficient indicates the degree to which individuals maintain their relative rank ordering over time. In the context of reliability, if the estimate is relatively low, this is taken as evidence that the instrument is unreliable. However, such an outcome also could reflect legitimate rank-order change in a reliably measured dimension; that is, people may actually change their relative status on a given dimension. To minimize the extent of "true" change in reliability assessments, the measurement specialist usually recommends that the retest coefficient be estimated within a relatively short (e.g., 1-month) period. This strategy will be effective in controlling change in many cases since few dimensions would be expected to undergo systematic change over such a short time period. There are, however, some problems that arise with this strategy. First, if the retest interval is too short, the subjects may remember their responses and thereby create an illusion of reliability by recording the same responses from memory. Second, there are instances (such as when assessing moods or other psychological states) when short-term, even daily, changes would be entirely possible and likely. For example, emotional states such as anxiety have been found to undergo short-term changes (Nesselroade and Bartsch, 1977). Under such circumstances, the consistency reliability index makes it difficult to separate "true" change from measurement error. If a state anxiety inventory was administered on two occasions over a 2-day period and a relatively low (e.g., .30) retest correlation was found, this could be a result of unreliability of the anxiety scale that was used, but it also could be indicative of change in the mood of anxiety. In situations where short-term developmental changes or mood fluctuations are anticipated, the use of the test-retest form of reliability assessment is contraindicated. Other forms, such as homogeneity, are usually more appropriate under these circumstances.

Stability

To deal with the confounding of measurement error and change, developmental researchers have made a useful distinction between the reliability of a measure and the stability of a phenomenon (Baltes *et al.*, 1977). Reliability refers to whether an instrument is measuring an attribute in a repeatable or consistent manner. Stability, however, describes the nature and extent of change in the dimension that is being measured. Note that high stability describes the "no change" end of the continuum, and its opposite, lability, implies change or low stability.

The conceptual distinction between reliability and stability is useful since change is viewed as a phenomenon of interest, rather than as a form of error, in developmental research. One operational problem that has been noted in developmental analyses is the difficulty in separating random from true sources of fluctuations in scores. Test–retest reliability is operationally equivalent to the stability coefficient since both are computed as the correlation between performances on the same instrument on two occasions.

As an index of change, the stability coefficient reflects the degree to which the individual rank orders in scores have changed over time. If there are changes in rank order, this is indicative of interindividual differences in change. Consider a case where a scale of life satisfaction is administered on two occasions at a 1-month interval and the stability correlation coefficient is .35. If this is the only reliability information that is available, it would be difficult to determine whether people had changed in their life satisfaction or the assessment of life satisfaction was unreliable. Therefore, we need to obtain a reliability estimate such as the split-half index of homogeneity, which controls for cross-occasion fluctuations. Let us assume in this case that the split-half index was .85. This provides evidence that the assessment is fairly reliable according to homogeneity criteria, and, therefore, there is reason to attribute the differences in scores to reliable interindividual changes in life satisfaction over time.

For some time now, researchers have noted the challenges that face the developmental researcher in separating legitimate change from noise in measurement (Bereiter, 1963). Several sophisticated procedures have been developed to carry out this task (e.g., Carmines and Zeller, 1979; Heise, 1969; Jöreskog, 1979; Wheaton, Múthen, Alwin, and Summers, 1977). While these methods require familiarity with concepts that are beyond the scope of the present chapter, they should be examined by the reader who is interested in learning about techniques for the separation of unreliability and change.

One simple procedure for aiding the diagnosis of change, the correction for attenuation, will be suggested here. The correction for attenuation is based on the assumption that reliability of a measure marks the upper-bound limit for a correlation involving that measure (Ghiselli *et al.*, 1981). The correlation between two measures cannot exceed the product of the square roots of the reliabilities of the two measures. Thus, since a stability coefficient is a correlation between the same measure on two occasions, it is restricted by the measure's reliability. For example, if a life satisfaction scale has an internal consistency of .92 at occasion 1 and .90 at occasion 2, the stability coefficient could not exceed .91 ($\sqrt{.92} \times \sqrt{.90}$). If the stability estimate is .49 in our example, this is indicative of change, since .91 is the upper bound given the reliabilities. An estimate of stability is meaningful only when considered in relation to reliability. For instance, the same stability of .49 could be indicative of no reliable change (high stability) if the internal consistency of the life satisfaction scale at each occasion was .50. Note that the problem with using only the statistical significance for interpreting change is that even if the stability coefficient is different from zero, it may be indicative of change. In the example above, a coefficient of .49, although statistically significant with a sample of 15 or more, should be interpreted as reliable change if the reliability is high. Indeed, with a stability coefficient of .49, only 24% of the variance at occasion 2 can be accounted for by occasion 1 scores.

The correction for attenuation is a procedure that places the stability coefficient within the context of measurement reliability (Nunnally, 1978). It involves making an adjustment to a correlation, in this case the stability, to compensate for measurement error. The correction for attenuation estimates the stability correlation under the assumption that reliability at both occasions is perfect (i.e., 1.0). To continue with the life-satisfaction example in which the reliabilities are .90 and .92, if we had corrected for attenuation, the .49 stability would increase to .54. If the reliability at both occasions had been .50, the stability estimate of .49 when corrected would increase to .98. In general, the lower the reliabilities of the measures, the greater the effects of the correction for attenuation on the correlation coefficient.

Several researchers have pointed out the importance of correcting for attenuation in personality research, where often the reliabilities of measures are relatively low (.30 to .50) (Block, 1977; Epstein, 1979). Without correcting for measurement error, it is possible that the degree of stability will be underestimated, as illustrated in the above example. The goal of such efforts is to get the most accurate measurement possible and at the same time to permit sensitivity to developmental changes. It must be noted that stability is always a relative phenomenon, and in isolation the stability coefficient is not a meaningful index (Wohlwill, 1973). Reliability of measurement provides a useful standard for the evaluation of stability versus change.

Validity of Measurement

In addition to reliability of measurement, a major goal for researchers is to achieve validity of measurement. Validity refers to the degree to which an instrument measures what it is intended to measure. The relationship between reliability and validity is sometimes overlooked by researchers. Reliability is a necessary, but not a sufficient, condition for validity of measurement. If a measure is not accurate or consistent, it cannot be considered valid; however, even if a measure is reliable, this does not assure its validity. Before the validity of an instrument can be assessed, its purpose or goals must be specified. Traditionally, discussions of measurement validity have focused on three classical forms—content, criterion-related, and construct validity (American Psychological Association, 1974; Ghiselli *et al.*, 1981; Nunnally, 1978).

DEVELOPMENTAL ISSUES OF MEASUREMENT VALIDITY. Because life-span developmental research involves the assessment of behaviors across multiple age groups and multiple occasions, a number of special validity concerns arise. These issues are referred to here as age-related validity and structural validity. Like the traditional forms, they focus on whether a measure is measuring what it is supposed to measure. However, since developmental research involves age and time comparisons, additional questions arise as to whether a measure is valid for different age groups or on different occasions. Although these aspects of validity are singled out here as of particular concern for developmental research on women in midlife, they may be considered special cases of the classical validity forms. Thus, to understand fully the nature of age-related and structural validities, the reader should be familiar with the traditional validity forms mentioned above.

Age-Related Validity. One of the challenges facing the researcher of life-span development is how to measure the same construct in multiple age groups. If one is interested in how a given phenomenon such as attachment (see Lerner and Ryff, 1978) develops from birth to death, it becomes important to determine how to measure the construct in a meaningful way for the entire range of age groups that will be examined. The problem is particularly salient in the study of middle age and aging because the majority of measures have been developed and standardized on children and young adult samples; thus, the validities for middle and older age groups are unknown.

The age-validity problem has been clearly illustrated with the case of psychometric intelligence (Baltes and Willis, 1979). Intelligence tests generally have been carefully developed and standardized for the purpose of predicting school performance in children and adolescents. Nevertheless, researchers have employed these same instruments to study changes in intelligence in middle and old age, without first determining their meaning for these age groups (Labouvie-Vief, 1977). Results based on the inappropriate use of intelligence tests or other measures may be misleading. If middle-aged adults score lower on a test than college students, does this mean that they have less intelligence or is it an inference based on improper measurement? Rather than continue to apply youth-centered criteria and standards for evaluating intellectual performance in middle and old age, researchers have begun to ask: What are the proper criterion measures for middle age (Labouvie-Vief and Chandler, 1978)? For example, Schaie (1977–1978) has suggested that in middle age, the function of intelligence is to integrate long-range goals and to solve real-life problems. Thus, measurement instruments should include content that is related to these aspects of functioning.

Two general strategies can be used to deal with the age-validity problem. The first is to conduct studies that are aimed at validation of existing measures for age ranges that were not included in initial scale development procedures. For example, Costa and McCrae (1980) have examined the usefulness for middle- and old-aged adults of the 16 Personality Factors inventory originally validated by Cattell, Eber, and Tatsuoka (1970) for young adult samples. In their investigations of the factor structure of the 16 PF, they found the same personality factors at all age levels and concluded that the inventory is valid for middle- and older-aged adults. This procedure, whereby the validity of an extant measure is determined for multiple age groups, has some drawbacks. First, this strategy does not allow for unique, age-specific dimensions. Second, test items are not always appropriate or predictive for a wide age range.

An alternative to validating existing scales is to develop new age-specific measures for the constructs of interest (e.g., Lachman, Baltes, Nesselroade, and Willis, 1982). This allows for consideration of constructs that may be relevant only for a specific age group. Research by Clayton and Birren (1980), for instance, has indicated that wisdom is a characteristic that is unique to later life. In the field of intellectual aging, Demming and Pressey (1957) recognized the need for age-specific measurement more than two decades ago. More recently, this need has been addressed by several researchers in the field of intellectual aging who have revived the search for meaningful measurement procedures and more adequate criteria for evaluating performance in middle and old age (Quayhagen, Gonda, and Schaie, 1979; Popkin, Schaie, and Krauss, 1980; Schaie, 1978). These researchers have directed their efforts to the development of age-relevant assessment devices in order to construct measures that are ecologically valid for adults in middle and old age.

In addition to not allowing for unique age-specific constructs, another problem with trying to validate existing scales is that the items may not be appropriate for all age groups. For example, when questions about behavior and habits in school are included in achievement motivation questionnaires, they are not likely to be meaningful for middle-aged adults. Achievement motivation can have a different meaning and may be manifested in different contexts (e.g., career) for middle-aged groups. This argues for developing age-specific measures for life-span research. A concern related to age validity is whether measures are valid across sexes. Are questions that have been validated on males appropriate for females? As has been pointed out with regard to age, there may be constructs that are unique for one sex group, or the same variable may take on different meanings for men and women. Many of the theoretical constructs and measurement instruments for adult development have been standardized on samples of males. One challenge that faces researchers of women in the middle years is to determine the validities of these existing theories and concepts for women. Another is to develop new conceptions of development that may or may not be applicable to men (e.g., Gilligan, 1982).

Two solutions to the age- and sex-related validity problems have been suggested. The researcher is encouraged both to examine the validities of extant measures for middle- and old-aged and male and female samples and to develop new age- or sex-specific measures for the unique aspects of women's adult development. Even if these two strategies are followed, there still is a major validity issue that cannot easily be solved by either. The problem arises because in many studies researchers are interested in comparing multiple age groups simultaneously. Therefore, one must consider whether the same construct is being measured at all age levels. This question of whether the same psychological measure is valid for multiple age groups is analogous to the pharmacological case, where the same drug may have different benefits or side effects when administered to different age groups. In the realm of personality research, this issue arises, for example, when a self-report item means something different to members of different cohort groups. Consider an item from the Extraversion scale of the Eysenck Personality Inventory (Eysenck and Eysenck, 1963), which asks whether the respondent can let go and enjoy gay parties. In my own experience with administering this scale, I have found a striking difference in the responses of college students and older adults to this item: The majority of college respondents have asked for clarification as to the meaning intended by "gay parties," whereas only one of all the older adult subjects did so. The college students were unclear whether the item referred to jolly parties or homosexual parties. The older respondents seemed to take the former interpretation for granted (or else they were more timid about asking for clarification). As this example illustrates, the validation process must take into account that the meaning of an item, or the construct that it represents, may vary with the age or cohort of the respondents.

Cross-age validation requires careful construction and pilot-testing of measures. One useful method for testing the age equivalence of measures is factor analysis. This procedure permits the assessment of whether measures have the same underlying structure or pattern for all ages (Labouvie, 1980; Nesselroade, 1977). The confirmatory factor-analysis method developed by Jöreskog (1979) is particularly applicable since it enables the testing of the equivalence of a factor solution simultaneously for multiple groups (Jöreskog and Sörbom, 1978). The same techniques can be adopted for examining whether a measurement structure is equivalent for males and females. The multioccasion extension of the age-validity problem is referred to here as structural validity and is discussed in the next section.

Structural Validity. Structural validity or measurement equivalence over time is another validity problem that commonly arises in life-span developmental research. When an instrument is administered on multiple occasions in the context of a longitudinal study, the measurement validity may be subject to change. For example, if the development of creativity is studied by asking subjects to think of novel uses of common objects on several occasions, does this task measure creativity in the same way on each occasion? The definition of creativity in this context involves novel applications of familiar objects. If subjects are given the same task on repeated occasions, however, the task no longer involves novelty. Thus, the nature of the creativity assessment changes, and the task may become more a measure of memory than of creativity. Even if different items (i.e., alternate forms) are used on each occasion, the validity of the task still may change due to the fact that the subjects are asked to "be creative" on more than one occasion.

Structural validity is related to age validity because, with longitudinal designs, people will necessarily be of different ages on each measurement occasion. The major difference is that the structural equivalence problem involves repeated assessment of the same persons and is aimed at determining whether retesting changes the validity of a test. This phenomenon of the changing structural or measurement validity of tests is similar to the internal validity problem of retesting, which will be discussed later.

In addition to changes in test structure over time, in longitudinal research there is also the problem of the "aging of tests" (Gribbin and Schaie, 1977). In Schaie's longitudinal study of intelligence, the original version of the Primary Mental Abilities (PMA) test (Thurstone and Thurstone, 1948) had been adopted at the first occasion of measurement in 1959. By the second occasion of a measurement, the PMA had been revised (Thurstone, 1962). Schaie (1979) noted that the original edition was better suited for the older cohorts but that the new version was more appropriate for the younger cohorts. This was particularly true for the verbal meaning subtest, because there are cohort differences in the popular word meanings and frequency of word usage. In order to preserve the longitudinal continuity of measures, Schaie decided to retain the 1948 edition for all subsequent measurement occasions. This decision was supported by the results of a study in which both the 1948 and 1962 versions of the PMA were given to the youngest cohorts in the longitudinal study (Gribbin and Schaie, 1977). By examining factor structures of the various subtests, the validity of the 1948 edition was found to be acceptable for the youngest cohorts. As mentioned for age validity, factor analysis is one useful method for checking the structural validity of a test. Factor-analysis procedures can be used to determine whether the internal structure of a measure and/or the correlations among factors remain stable over time (Labouvie, 1980).

Summary

In this section we have discussed several key measurement issues that may confront researchers studying development during middle age. Reliability and validity are crucial in order to ensure accuracy and meaningfulness of one's measurements. Both reliability and validity, however, are sensitive to sampling, testing conditions, and other variable factors. Therefore, it is recommended that the reliability and validity of a measure to be investigated for every intended purpose (Nunnally, 1978). In developmental research, when multiple age groups and testing occasions are investigated, it is particularly important to investigate the reliability and validity of measurement for all groups. For example, it is unreasonable to assume that if a measure of achievement motivation is reliable or valid for college-aged males in 1960, it will be appropriate for middle-aged women in 1980. For this reason, examination of the measurement properties of instruments is critical in life-span developmental research. In the next sections we will focus on research design issues for the study of development in midlife.

RESEARCH DESIGN ISSUES

Multidimensionality of Change

As mentioned earlier, the study of adult development from a life-span perspective involves the description and explanation of intraindividual change and interindividual differences in change (Baltes *et al.*, 1980). In order to gain a full and complete picture of development, it is useful to examine multiple aspects of change. In the following sections, several components of change are considered. Particular attention is devoted to two major categories: quantitative and qualitative changes (Baltes and Nesselroade, 1973). Quantitative change refers to differences in the magnitude or level of change, whereas qualitative change is represented by shifts in pattern or by reorganization of structure.

QUANTITATIVE CHANGE. Developmental studies, traditionally, have been focused on changes in the group average or the mean. There are, however, at least two other indices that are informative with regard to the quantitative description of change. These are the correlational stability index and the variance. Each of these components of change offers unique information, and when considered in concert, they can capture and illustrate the multidimensional nature of change.

In many accounts of adult development, researchers focus only on mean level changes. Although this kind of analysis provides relevant information, it refers to only one aspect of change. It can indicate whether a group shows more or less of a given trait at different times. Examining change at the group level, however, may mask individual changes. As can be seen in Figure 2A, it is possible for individuals to change over time yet to have the mean level remain constant. Examination of only group level changes in this case would obscure change at the individual level. One way to obtain a more complete picture of individual change is to compute individual change scores (i.e., Occasion 2 score minus Occasion 1 score).

The stability (test-retest) coefficient provides another meaningful index of individual changes (see earlier discussion of stability). Specifically, it indicates the extent to which individuals maintain their relative rank orders over time. The stability coefficient is sensitive to individual changes in rank orders; thus, a low stability coefficient is indicative of interindividual differences in change. In Figure 2A, individuals' positions have fluctuated from the first to the second occasion. This pattern is an example of high negative stability since those with high scores at Occasion 1 have lower scores at Occasion 2 and those with low scores at Occasion 1 have higher scores at Occasion 2. The outcome in Figure 2A presents a powerful case for considering multiple aspects of change. If only the mean were examined, it would appear as if no change had occurred, whereas, in fact, at the individual level there was change.

Another picture of change is illustrated in Figure 2B. Here there is perfect stability—i.e., rank orders are maintained—but the overall group mean has increased. Again, a focus on only one dimension would present a limited view of change versus stability. In Figures 2C and 2D, two other combinations are presented: respectively, mean change and low stability (rank-order change) and no change in either mean or rank order. These examples illustrate how consideration of multiple aspects of change can enrich the study of development and provide a more complete picture.

A third component of change is represented by the variance of a measure. The variance is a marker of the extent of individual differences. As such, it allows for comparison of variability across age groups and occasions. Several researchers have considered whether interindividual variability increases with aging (Baltes et al., 1980; Fries and Crapo, 1981). The focus of this inquiry has been on comparing estimates of the variance of a measure for young and old age groups. To date, the variance has been given very little attention as an index of change. Moreover, few studies even contain information about the variance (Bornstein and Smircina, 1982).

QUALITATIVE CHANGE. Although most research questions are formulated in terms of quantitative aspects of change, there is another class

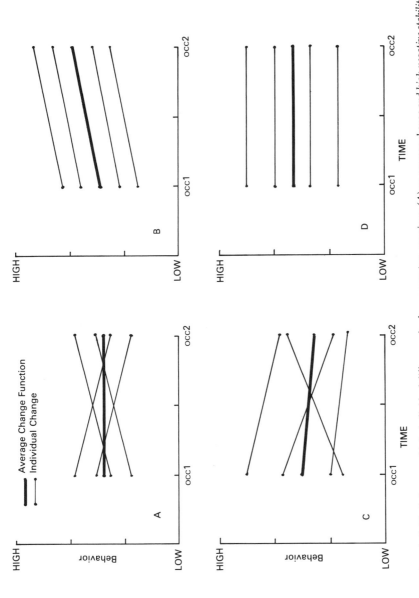

Figure 2. Intraindividual change and interindividual differences in change over two occasions: (A) no average change and high negative stability; (B) average change and high correlational stability; (C) average change and low correlational stability; (D) no average change and high correlational stability. Based on Baltes, Reese, and Nesselroade (1977).

of questions that have as their focus changes in structure or pattern. This approach to change requires a multivariate approach since it involves consideration of changing relationships among several variables.

The factor-analytic model is one approach that easily lends itself to the examination of qualitative change. In a factor-analysis framework, structural changes can be manifested in terms of changes in factor patterns (e.g., number of factors, patterns of factor loadings) or the factor correlation matrix. For further discussion of qualitative changes within the factor model framework, see Baltes and Nesselroade (1973) or Nesselroade (1977).

Research on the integration-differentiation-reintegration hypothesis of intellectual development (Reinert, 1970) illustrates the application of factor analysis to examine structural change components. This hypothesis states that during the life-span the organization of intellectual abilities changes from a general, undifferentiated, or global intelligence to a more specialized, multidimensional intelligence, and later to a new form where abilities are again more integrated. Baltes, Cornelius, Spiro, Nesselroade, and Willis (1980) found that the structure of intelligence in old age is represented by fewer factors and by higher intercorrelations between factors than have been found in young adults. The data, then, support the hypothesis that, with aging, there are structural changes that are reflective of a reintegration in intellectual functioning.

Structural changes in intelligence and in other domains are an interesting substantive research focus in their own right. In the "strong" conceptions of development, as discussed earlier, development involves structural reorganization of behavior over time (Kohlberg, 1969). The investigation of structural change, however, is also desirable from a methodological standpoint. It is recommended that structural invariance of a construct be demonstrated prior to examining quantitative aspects of change (Baltes and Nesselroade, 1973). It is necessary to establish that the same construct is being measured at different occasions and/or in different groups before examining increments or decrements in that dimension. Empirically, of course, it is possible to have both structural and quantitative changes. However, if there is both structural reorganization and quantitative change, it is difficult to know how to interpret quantitative increases and decreases in scores (Baltes and Nesselroade, 1973). For example, reports of intellectual declines in adulthood must be interpreted with caution if these dimensions are also undergoing structural changes. Under these circumstances, the entire nature or structure of intelligence has changed.

In summary, consideration of both quantitative and qualitative aspects of change should enable the researcher to capture the multidimensionality, multidirectionality, and complexity of life-span development.

Although changes in level are the most commonly studied, examination of correlational stability as well as structural aspects may shed additional light on midlife development. It is interesting to consider that at different points in the life span certain forms of change may be more prevalent. Schaie (1977–78) has proposed a model for the life-span development of cognitive functioning in which qualitative changes occur from the late 30s to the early 60s and quantitative intellectual changes occur in early and late adulthood. He suggests that the structural changes in cognitive functioning during the middle years yield a new pattern, which facilitates integrating long-range goals as well as solving real-life problems with greater flexibility. Some researchers have proposed that there is structural reorganization in cognitive functioning throughout the adult years (e.g., Labouvie-Vief, 1977, 1982), while others have suggested that there are few or no structural changes in adulthood (Flavell, 1970). Use of the methods described here would enable the researcher to test empirically these various positions on the nature of midlife development.

In this section, several forms and indices of change have been discussed. Since each component adds a unique piece of information about the nature of change and development, it is useful to examine as many forms of quantitative and qualitative change as is possible. However, there are specific design requirements that are necessary in order to consider certain change components. For example, the stability coefficient can be examined only in longitudinal studies since multiple occasions of measurement are required to compute the stability coefficient. Intraindividual changes in level, variance, or structure also can be studied only within a longitudinal framework. In cross-sectional studies, it is possible to look only at interindividual (age) differences in means, variances, or structure. Differences across age groups, as will be pointed out in the next section, can provide only an approximation and sometimes an inaccurate account of developmental change. Quantitative changes such as those described here can be considered in either the univariate or the multivariate case, whereas qualitative changes, specifically, require multivariate analysis (see Harris, 1975; Morrison, 1976; or Nesselroade, 1977, for coverage of multivariate techniques). In the next section, specific designs for the study of change will be considered.

Classical Developmental Research Designs

Given the major focus of life-span developmental research on intraindividual changes and interindividual differences in change over time, it is crucial to employ research designs that permit a direct assessment of change. Traditionally, the cross-sectional and longitudinal methods have been used in developmental research. There are, however, some major flaws and widespread misunderstandings associated with these designs (Baltes *et al.*, 1979). First, the cross-sectional and longitudinal designs will be described and particular attention will be devoted to their strengths and weaknesses. Then, some alternative designs for developmental research will be specified.

CROSS-SECTIONAL DESIGNS. As mentioned earlier, one goal for life-span developmental research is to identify age-related changes in behavior. The cross-sectional design involves the assessment of multiple samples from different age levels at one time. As such, the cross-sectional method provides information about age group differences, but not necessarily about age-related changes. As illustrated in Table 1, the cross-sectional method involves a comparison of samples of different age groups who also are from different birth cohorts. For instance, the 20-year-olds in 1980 were born in 1960 and the 40-year-olds were born in 1940. Thus, any outcome that indicates differences between the 20- and 40-year-olds in 1980 will, by design, reflect birth cohort (1960 vs. 1940) differences as well.

One major weakness associated with the cross-sectional method is that it provides no direct information about intraindividual changes; it can approximate change only through the observation of group (age-cohort) differences. For example, questions as to whether the 1960 cohort when 40 (in the year 2000) will show characteristics similar to those of the 40-year-olds from the 1940 cohort cannot be addressed with the cross-sectional design. Nor can it be determined whether the 1940 cohort at 20 in 1960 was like their 20-year-old counterparts in 1980. In the cross-sectional design, age and cohort effects are confounded; groups differ not only with respect to age but also with respect to cohort. Because cohorts may differ in the way they were reared and in the set of historical events that they experienced as they were growing up, we can expect to find differences in their patterns of life-span development.

Table 1. Cross-Sectional and Longitudinal Methods[a]

Time of measurement	Cohort			
	1960	1940	1920	1900
1980	20	40	60	80
1960				60
1940				40
1920				20

[a]Entries are age levels. Horizonal rectangle is cross-sectional method. Vertical rectangle is longitudinal method.

Other problems associated with the cross-sectional method become apparent when considered within a quasi-experimental design framework (Campbell and Stanley, 1963; Labouvie, Bartsch, Nesselroade, and Baltes, 1974; Schaie, 1977). The classical cross-sectional design does not have experimental design status because (a) the independent variable, age, cannot be directly manipulated, and (b) respondents cannot be randomly assigned to age groups. As such, there are several threats to the internal validity of the cross-sectional design, and, as a consequence, we cannot be certain that age is the factor responsible for any differences between groups. Campbell and Stanley (1963) have discussed eight factors that threaten the internal validity of preexperimental and quasi-experimental research designs: maturation, history, selection, experimental mortality, testing, instrumentation, statistical regression, and selection by maturation interaction. These factors will be addressed here as potential sources of invalidity for the cross-sectional and longitudinal designs. Note, however, that not all of these factors pose threats for developmental research designs. In fact, maturation, rather than being a source of invalidity, is the major variable of interest for developmental research (Baltes *et al.*, 1977). Other factors such as history and selection can also provide a meaningful focus for developmental study and thus need not always be considered design threats.

One threat to the internal validity of cross-sectional designs is selection bias. Those middle-aged and older adults who are available for research tend to be positively selected relative to others from their cohorts. Cross-sectional comparisons, then, can underestimate age differences because the older groups are likely to be positively biased with regard to such factors as intelligence and health. Moreover, it is difficult to find different age-cohort groups who are equivalent on all variables. Cohorts often differ on variables (e.g., education and socioeconomic status) that are known to be related to psychological outcomes (Krauss, 1980). Such differences between cohorts should be taken into consideration when selecting research samples. When these differences between cohorts cannot be controlled, it may be more appropriate to conduct within-cohort analyses (Krauss, 1980). Examination of differences in developmental outcomes within a cohort may reveal something about the processes associated with between-cohort differences.

Another problem of selection in the cross-sectional design is that each cohort has a unique life history and there are no controls for the conditions that existed prior to the research. Baltes (1968) has referred to this as a problem of generation effects. In his research on the Great Depression, Elder (1979) has illustrated that the timing of historical events has had a differential impact on the development of cohorts. Thus, any differences found between age groups could also reflect differences in cohort-related histories. Indeed, cohort differences have been found in a number of domains, including intelligence (Baltes *et al.*, 1979; Schaie, 1979) and personality (Elder, 1979; Nesselroade and Baltes, 1974). These cohort differences in performance could be due to differential patterns in the timing of major events (e.g., the Great Depression) or the regular course of cultural change (e.g., exposure to television, computers, or lifelong education).

Another problem that threatens the internal validity of cross-sectional designs is instrumentation. The interview conditions, test format, or test administrator may vary across age groups and be responsible for differences in behavioral responses. For example, 20-year-olds are likely to be interviewed in the context of a school setting, such as an introductory psychology course for academic credit, whereas older persons may be tested in a senior center or in the home. Any differences between age groups could reflect these conditions, rather than true age differences.

As already discussed, there are several problems with the cross-sectional design that place limitations on its usefulness for life-span developmental research. However, the cross-sectional design is widely used because of its economy with regard to time. Researchers cannot always wait for their subjects to grow older in order to study adult development. Thus, the cross-sectional method is more practical than long-term longitudinal designs because multiple age groups can be examined with only one occasion of measurement. Despite this advantage, it is rarely the case that cross-sectional results can be unquestionably interpreted as age changes. Only if all age cohorts have been selected from the same parent population and have experienced the same life histories, and, therefore, differ only with respect to age, are cross-sectional age differences interpretable as average intraindividual age changes (Baltes and Nesselroade, 1979). This assumption, however, is difficult to test and is unlikely to occur due to rapid changes in historical–cultural conditions and the selective sampling issue already mentioned. Thus, in most cases the cross-sectional method can only provide an approximation to intraindividual (age) change. Nevertheless, cross-sectional findings can be suggestive of developmental trends. The results can then be followed up to determine whether the same patterns can be replicated over time.

LONGITUDINAL DESIGNS. The longitudinal method is often considered the *sine qua non* of developmental research (McCall, 1977). The term *longitudinal* implies there are multiple assessments of the same persons over time (Baltes and Nesselroade, 1979).[4] This design is illustrated in

---

[4]Procedures that involve the sampling and measurement of independent groups or panels from the population at different times also have been included in the definition of longitudinal studies (Schaie and Hertzog, 1982).

Table 1. Notice that the 1900 birth cohort is followed from 1920 to 1980, during which time they age from 20 to 80 years. Because of its direct focus on intraindividual change, the longitudinal method is usually considered more appropriate than the cross-sectional method for the study of development. Although in a longitudinal study the same people are followed over time and behavior changes can be charted across different ages, this method does not always offer a clear-cut assessment of age-related change. Since there are a number of threats to the internal validity of longitudinal designs, it is not always possible to isolate age as the ("causal") factor responsible for differences. The major sources of invalidity for the longitudinal design are history, instrumentation, testing, mortality, and statistical regression.

In the single-cohort longitudinal design, history rather than age may be the factor that is responsible for the results. A given outcome may be due to environmental events that occurred over the period of investigation. This would imply that the same results would have occurred for other age-cohort groups had they been included in the design. As an example, consider a hypothetical 5-year longitudinal study of depression in a cohort of women during the transition to midlife. If depression was found to increase in these women over this 5-year period, it would not be clear whether the change could be attributed to the midlife transition or to environmental events. For example, it could be that changes in the economy and unemployment conditions led to the changes in depression. If several age cohorts had been followed over the same period, all, regardless of age, might have shown similar increases in depression.

Instrumentation effects, similar to those mentioned for cross-sectional research, also can jeopardize the internal validity of longitudinal designs. For example, the conditions of test administration can vary greatly across occasions and thereby distort the results. In addition, there is the problem of retesting. The same questions are usually asked repeatedly, so that responses may change due to familiarity with the questions or to participation in the study, rather than to aging. Posttest-only control groups can be added to determine the extent of retest effects (Nesselroade and Baltes, in preparation).

Another design threat involves the mortality or selective attrition of subjects from one occasion to the next. Anyone who has done longitudinal research, even over a short period of time, knows how rare it is to maintain all the members of one's sample over time. For many reasons (e.g., illness, lack of interest, death), people may drop out of the sample. The internal validity problem arises when there is an interaction between maturation and attrition, that is, if those who remain in the study develop in a way that is different from those who drop out. For instance, if we are interested in whether introversion increases over the adult life-span, we must determine whether those who drop out are more introverted. If so, we could get a false picture of decreasing introversion (i.e., increasing extraversion) with aging.

A final threat to the internal validity of longitudinal designs is statistical regression. Because of measurement unreliability, extreme scores tend to regress toward the mean over time (Cronbach and Furby, 1970; Furby, 1973). Since it is rare to achieve error-free measurements (see earlier discussion of measurement reliability), regression to the mean is a common threat in longitudinal research. The problem of statistical regression is that extreme scores (either high or low) are often the result of unique patterns of random error that will not occur in the same way twice. Therefore, scores will change in a predictable way; that is, they will approach the mean. This phenomenon of regression is manifested when high scores decrease and low scores increase from the first to the second occasion (Baltes, Nesselroade, Schaie, and Labouvie, 1972; Furby, 1973). Rather than abandon the study of change altogether, as some researchers have suggested (Cronbach and Furby, 1970), it seems more reasonable to search for ways to control or compensate for the effects of regression to the mean. One way to protect against regression to the mean is to use highly reliable measures. It is very rare, however, to obtain perfectly reliable assessments. The problem of statistical regression can be alleviated, in many cases, by including more than two measurement occasions in one's design (see Nesselroade, Stigler, and Baltes, 1980).

The various factors mentioned above interfere with the interpretation of the results of cross-sectional and longitudinal studies. In some cases the problems can be addressed through the use of control groups, but in other circumstances the results may be hopelessly confounded. In such cases design decisions ultimately become a matter of priorities and trade-offs.

EXTERNAL VALIDITY OF DEVELOPMENTAL DESIGNS. Thus far we have considered threats to the internal validity of developmental research designs. In addition to these weaknesses, the conventional developmental designs also suffer from limitations in external validity. External validity is concerned with the generalizability of research findings across persons, measurement variables, treatments, settings, and time. Can the results found be applied to other people in other places at other times? In longitudinal studies, the findings for one cohort may not be applicable to other cohorts who have grown up under a different set of historical conditions. Thus, under conditions of rapid cultural change, there are restrictions placed on the generalizability of findings from single-cohort research. Another external validity problem involves selective attrition. If those who drop out of a study differ from those who remain, then the results will be limited in generalizability. For example, if those who remain in a longitudinal study are better educated, the results may not be applicable to those with less education. It is recommended, therefore, that statistical tests of differences between the dropouts and the longitudinal sample be performed in order to determine the extent of selective attrition (for examples of methods of testing for differential dropout, see Nesselroade and Baltes, in preparation; Siegler and Botwinick, 1979).

There is, unfortunately, a trade-off between internal and external validity. If one conducts a highly controlled, internally valid study in the laboratory, this is usually done at the expense of external validity concerns. On the other hand, if one tries to maximize external validity by conducting research in real-life settings, the amount of rigor and control over internal validity invariably will suffer. Traditionally, psychologists have given primary attention to internal validity at the expense of external validity. However, some life-span developmental psychologists have suggested that at least equal concern should be given to external validity (Baltes *et al.*, 1977; Bronfenbrenner, 1979; Hultsch and Hickey, 1978; Schaie, 1978). The underlying value is that researchers have an obligation to design research that has application and relevance beyond the specific observations made in one study in an artificially contrived situation.

Sequential Research Designs

As discussed in the previous section, there are a number of serious weaknesses associated with the conventional cross-sectional and longitudinal designs. In the cross-sectional design, age and cohort effects are confounded, and in the longitudinal design, age and time of measurement are confounded. Moreover, major discrepancies have been found between the results of cross-sectional and longitudinal studies. In the domains of personality and intelligence, for instance, cross-sectional results have been indicative of decrements in functioning beginning in midlife. On the other hand, longitudinal findings have revealed few changes and little evidence of declines in functioning throughout adulthood (Baltes *et al.*, 1977). It was the widespread occurrence of these contradictory findings in cross-sectional and longitudinal studies that stimulated the development of more sophisticated models and data-gathering strategies. These new strategies are referred to as sequential designs. The major advantage of these designs is that they provide replication of age effects and controls for various sources of invalidity.

Sequential designs have been approached from a variety of different perspectives (e.g., Baltes, 1968; Glenn, 1977; Ryder, 1965; Schaie, 1965).

The approach recommended by Schaie and Baltes (1975) will be presented here for illustrative purposes. They have identified two types of sequential strategies: cross-sectional and longitudinal sequences. The major distinction is that in the former, independent samples are tested over time, and in the latter, the same sample is repeatedly tested over time. Cross-sectional sequences involve the replication of a cross-sectional study over the same age range for at least two times of measurement. Longitudinal sequences require repeated measures of at least two cohorts over the age range of interest on at least two occasions. Thus, sequential designs are straightforward extensions of the conventional cross-sectional and longitudinal designs. Through the replication across either cohorts or time, it becomes possible to separate age from cohort or time effects. Thus, it is possible to disentangle the effects that are confounded in cross-sectional and longitudinal designs.

In Table 2 the horizontal segments represent cross-sectional sequences. On three occasions (1940, 1960, 1980) samples ranging in age from 20 to 80 are assessed. With this design, it is possible to examine whether the same developmental pattern holds true for more than one cohort. Since the groups at each occasion are independent (i.e., new representatives of each cohort are selected on each occasion), there can be no retesting effects.

The vertical sections in Table 2 depict longitudinal sequences. Three cohorts (1920, 1940, 1960) are followed over a 60-year period as they age from 20 to 80. Since the same age range is observed across multiple cohorts, it is possible to determine whether age changes are generalizable across cohorts that are developing during different historical periods.

It must be recognized that sequential designs are not the developmental researcher's panacea. In fact, because of their status as quasi-

Table 2. Cross-Sectional and Longitudinal Sequences[a]

Time of measurement	Cohort					
	1960	1940	1920	1900	1880	1860
2040	80					
2020	60	80				
2000	40	60	80			
1980	20	40	60	80		
1960		20	40	60	80	
1940			20	40	60	80

[a] Entries are age levels. Vertical rectangles are longitudinal sequences. Horizontal rectangles are cross-sectional sequences.

experimental designs, there are still potential threats to the validity of these designs. For example, the problems of testing and selective attrition, which plagued single-cohort longitudinal designs, still can be troublesome in sequential longitudinal designs. Through the use of control groups, however, it becomes possible to address some of these concerns (Schaie and Hertzog, 1982). For example, the use of cross-sectional sequences in combination with longitudinal sequences is one effective way to control for effects of retesting. The cross-sectional sequences, which are independent assessments, can serve as a posttest-only control group for the longitudinal sequences. Differences between cross-sectional and longitudinal sequences could be attributed to effects of retesting.

As mentioned earlier, there are several approaches to sequential designs. The methods presented here represent the position agreed upon by Schaie and Baltes (1975). Initially, Schaie (1965) and Baltes (1968) disagreed on several points, which have since been resolved. In their discussion, three major issues were raised: (a) the need for two-factor versus three-factor models, (b) the use of sequential designs for descriptive versus explanatory purposes, and (c) the use of sequential designs as data-analytic versus data-collection strategies. Their resolution of these issues is briefly summarized below. (For more extensive coverage, see Baltes et al., 1979; Schaie and Hertzog, 1982; Schaie and Baltes, 1975.) First, it was concluded that only two factors are necessary for the sequential methods, since the third factor is always inextricably linked to the other two, and, therefore, it is represented in the interaction of the other two factors. Second, sequential designs can only provide descriptive information about development. Age and cohort variables may be indicators of change, but they do not reveal anything about the underlying sources of development. Third, sequential strategies are data-collection strategies. With cross-sectional or longitudinal sequences, it is possible to collect all data necessary to separate the variables that are confounded in the conventional designs. The recommended data collection arrangement for developmental psychologists interested in intraindividual change and interindividual (cohort) differences in change is the age-by-cohort matrix. However, there are other possible arrangements (time by cohort or age by time) that are more appropriate when designs include only a few occasions of measurement or a few cohort groups. As for data analysis, there are several appropriate techniques that can be applied to the sequential designs. The most commonly applied techniques for data analysis are analysis of variance (Nesselroade and Baltes, in preparation) and multiple regression (Buss, 1979–1980; Mason, Mason, Winsborough, and Poole, 1973). Structural equation models represent an alternative analytic method (Rogosa, 1979). With newly developed computer programs for structural equation analysis, it is possible to consider quantitative and qualitative aspects of change simultaneously for multiple cohorts (Jöreskog and Sörbom, in preparation).

In summary, sequential designs may be effective in eliminating the major confounds in the single-occasion cross-sectional and the single-cohort longitudinal designs. This is accomplished by replicating age effects across time and cohorts. One major drawback of the sequential designs is that they are time-consuming and costly since they require multiple assessments on multiple groups. To complete the longitudinal sequences depicted in Table 2 would take 100 years! Fortunately, there are some reasonable variations of the sequential designs, such as the "convergence" method (Bell, 1953), which make it possible under certain conditions to approximate long-term age functions with short-term longitudinal data (Wohlwill, 1973).

Alternative Research Designs

Often it is not possible or feasible to employ longitudinal (repeated-measurement) methods even though one is interested in how a phenomenon or characteristic has changed over time. One alternative means for studying change is the retrospective method. This usually entails asking subjects to recall what they felt, thought, or did on previous occasions. Of course, such retrospective reports are subject to distortion because of the role of intervening events and problems of memory, and methods for checking accuracy should be adopted (Finney, 1981; Gutek, 1978; Powers, Goudy, and Keith, 1978). The retrospective procedure is often used in studies of adjustment to critical life events. With unexpected events such as widowhood, it is difficult to anticipate the event. In these cases the subjects are usually identified after the event has occurred; therefore, retrospective methods may be the most feasible.

For the study of anticipated events such as the birth of a child, it may be possible to follow subjects longitudinally or to use prospective methods. In prospective accounts, subjects may be asked to make predictions about what they think things will be like in the future.

Another procedure for studying adjustment to events was adopted in the Normative Aging Studies at Duke University, where they selected a sample that was "at risk" for one or more life events such as retirement (Siegler, 1977). Thus, they were able to obtain assessments before and after the occurrence of events, and did not have to rely on retrospective accounts. Moreover, they could make comparisons with those in their sample who did not experience the events.

Prospective and retrospective methods provide subjective rather than objective accounts of development. Within a phenomenological framework, subjective expectations and interpretations take on central meaning. These perceptions of change, from past to present and present to future, are more salient than objective indicators of change within a phenomenological framework (Ryff and Heincke, 1981; Thomae, 1970).

Explanatory Research

The developmental designs that have been discussed thus far are useful for descriptive research. They can be applied to chart the course of intraindividual change and interindividual differences in change. The cross-sectional, longitudinal, and sequential designs do not, however, permit the study of the sources or causes of change. In order to go beyond description to the level of explanation, it is necessary to employ other techniques.

AGE SIMULATION. Traditionally, psychologists have applied the experimental paradigm for explanatory research. However, as mentioned earlier, experimental techniques often are difficult to apply in developmental studies because many of the independent variables of major interest (e.g., age, history) cannot be subjected to direct manipulation or random assignment. Some of the desirable features of the experimental designs may be captured with age-simulation strategies (Baltes and Goulet, 1971). Age simulation involves the manipulation of variables hypothesized to be associated with age. Through the examination of age by treatment interactions, the key developmental parameters that lead to existing age differences can be identified.

There are several methods available for age simulation. The most common form involves the application of treatment manipulations of variables such as practice, speed, or sensory deprivation, which are expected to be related to age differences. Other types of simulation involve age-hypnotic regression (Baltes *et al.*, 1977) or computer-generated models (Baltes, Nesselroade, and Cornelius, 1978). The major value of age simulation strategies is that it permits the analysis of sources of development in a shortened period of time. However, because age simulation does not involve the monitoring of developmental changes in their naturalistic form, their major weakness is one of external validity. Questions typically arise as to whether the simulated developmental processes would occur in the same way *in vivo*.

CAUSAL METHODS. Another methodological option for explanatory research is causal modeling (Rogosa, 1979). Causal modeling does not involve the manipulation and isolation of a causal variable, as is true for experimental research. Rather, it involves considering whether a given causal hypothesis is consistent with a particular set of correlational data. Causal modeling involves making explicit statements about the relationships among a set of variables. It is possible to set up competing theoretically based models and to test the adequacy of these models for representing observed data. Earlier versions of causal models such as path analysis and cross-lagged panel models have been greatly improved through the development of computer programs that allow for multiple indicators of latent factors (Jöreskog and Sörbom, 1978). Several techniques are available for the analysis and estimation of causal models. The interested reader should refer to the following sources for an introduction to this area (Jöreskog, 1979; Kenny, 1979; Rogosa, 1979). Although causal models are commonly used in sociology and economics, it is only recently that psychologists have begun to apply them to the study of adult development and aging (e.g., Lachman, 1983). Causal models enable researchers to examine the antecedents of development through the use of naturalistic–correlational data. This combination of explanatory power and emphasis on external validity makes causal models particularly desirable for life-span developmental research.

Conclusions

The goal of the present chapter has been to apply the conceptual and methodological features of a life-span developmental perspective to the study of women in the middle years. For those readers who already have formulated research questions, this chapter has been intended as a source of methodological suggestions and answers. For those who do not yet have specific questions, it also has been the aim of this chapter to facilitate the formulation of research questions on development during midlife. Although one ideally expects to choose an appropriate method or design for study after determining the questions to be researched, there is in reality a two-way interaction between questions and methods. The questions generated are dependent, in large part, on one's knowledge of research methods. For example, those who do know how to measure change properly will be forced to take a nondevelopmental approach to research. Or, those who are not aware of multivariate techniques will be likely to formulate univariate questions. In alerting the reader to some of the critical issues and pitfalls of developmental methodology and by suggesting some solutions, the present chapter has as part of its overall agenda the stimulation of new types of research questions as part of an effort to enrich and advance the study of women in midlife.

References

Achenbach, T. M. *Research in developmental psychology: Concepts, strategies, methods.* New York: Free Press, 1978.
American Psychological Association. *Standards for educational and psychological tests.* Washington, D.C.: American Psychological Association, 1974.
Anastasi, A. *Psychological testing* (3rd ed.). London: Macmillan, 1968.
Baer, D. M. An age-irrelevant concept of development. *Merrill-Palmer Quarterly,* 1970, *16,* 238–246.
Baltes, P. B. Longitudinal and cross-sectional sequences in the study of age and generation effects. *Human Development,* 1968, *11,* 145–171.
Baltes, P. B. Life-span developmental psychology: Some converging observations on history and theory. In P. B. Baltes and O. G. Brim, Jr. (Eds.), *Life-span development and behavior* (Vol. 2). New York: Academic Press, 1979.
Baltes, P. B., and Baltes, M. M. Plasticity and variability in psychological aging: Methodological and theoretical issues. In G. Gurski (Ed.), *Determining the effects of aging on the central nervous system.* Berlin: Schering, 1980.
Baltes, P. B., Cornelius, S. W., and Nesselroade, J. R. Cohort effects in developmental psychology. In J. R. Nesselroade and P. B. Baltes (Eds.), *Longitudinal research in the study of behavior and development.* New York: Academic Press, 1979.
Baltes, P. B., Cornelius, S. W., Spiro, A., III, Nesselroade, J. R., and Willis, S. L. Integration vs. differentiation of fluid-crystallized intelligence in old age. *Developmental Psychology,* 1980, *16,* 625–635.
Baltes, P. B., and Goulet, L. R. Exploration of developmental variables by set manipulation and simulation of age differences in behavior. *Human Development,* 1971, *14,* 149–170.
Baltes, P. B., and Nesselroade, J. R. The developmental analysis of individual differences on multiple measures. In J. R. Nesselroade and H. W. Reese (Eds.), *Life-span developmental psychology: Methodological issues.* New York: Academic Press, 1973.
Baltes, P. B., and Nesselroade, J. R. History and rationale of longitudinal research. In J. R. Nesselroade and P. B. Baltes (Eds.), *Longitudinal research in the study of behavior and development.* New York: Academic Press, 1979.
Baltes, P. B., Nesselroade, J. R., and Cornelius, S. W. Multivariate antecedents of structural change in development: A simulation of cumulative environmental patterns. *Multivariate Behavioral Research,* 1978, *13,* 127–152.
Baltes, P. B., Nesselroade, J. R., Schaie, K. W., and Labouvie, E. W. On the dilemma of regression effects in examining ability-level related differentials in ontogenetic patterns of intelligence. *Developmental Psychology,* 1972, *6,* 78–84.
Baltes, P. B., Reese, H. W., and Lipsitt, L. P. Life-span developmental psychology. *Annual Review of Psychology,* 1980, *31,* 65–110.
Baltes, P. B., Reese, H. W., and Nesselroade, J. R. *Life-span developmental psychology: Introduction to research methods.* Monterey, Calif.: Brooks/Cole, 1977.
Baltes, P. B., and Willis, S. L. The critical importance of appropriate methodology in the study of aging: The sample case of pyschometric intelligence. In F. Hoffmeister and C. Muller (Eds.), *Brain functions in old age.* Heidelberg: Springer, 1979.
Baruch, G., Barnett, R., and Rivers, C. *Lifeprints: New patterns of love and work for today's women.* New York: McGraw-Hill, 1983.
Bell, R. Q. Convergence: An accelerated longitudinal approach. *Child Development,* 1953, *24,* 145–152.
Bereiter, C. Some persisting dilemmas in the measurement of change: In C. W. Harris (Ed.), *Problems in measuring change.* Madison: University of Wisconsin Press, 1963.
Block, J. Advancing the psychology of personality: Paradigmatic shift or improving the

quality of research. In D. Magnusson and N. S. Endler (Eds.), *Personality at the crossroads: Current issues in interactional psychology*. Hillsdale, N.J.: Erlbaum, 1977.

Bornstein, R., and Smircina, M. T. The status of the empirical support for the hypothesis of increased variability in aging populations. *Gerontologist*, 1982, 22, 258–260.

Brim, O. G., Jr., and Kagan, J. (Eds.). *Constancy and change in human development*. Cambridge, Mass.: Harvard University Press, 1980.

Bronfenbrenner, U. *The ecology of human development: Experiments by nature and design*. Cambridge, Mass.: Harvard University Press, 1979.

Buss, A. R. Methodological issues in life-span developmental psychology from a dialectic perspective. *International Journal of Aging and Human Development*, 1979–1980, 10, 121–163.

Campbell, D. T., and Stanley, J. C. *Experimental and quasi-experimental designs for research*. Chicago: Rand McNally, 1963.

Carmines, E. G., and Zeller, R. A. *Reliability and validity assessment*. Beverly Hills: Sage, 1979.

Cattell, R. B. *The scientific analysis of personality*. Baltimore: Penguin, 1965.

Cattell, R. B., Eber, H. W., and Tatsuoka, M. M. *Handbook for the Sixteen Personality Factor Questionnaire*. Champaign, Ill.: Institute for Personality and Ability Testing, 1970.

Clayton, V. P., and Birren, J. E. The development of wisdom across the life span: A reexamination of an ancient topic. In P. B. Baltes and O. G. Brim, Jr. (Eds.), *Life-span development and behavior* (Vol. 3). New York: Academic Press, 1980.

Costa, P. T., Jr., and McCrae, R. R. Still stable after all these years: Personality as a key to some issues in adulthood and old age. In P. B. Baltes and O. G. Brim, Jr. (Eds.), *Life-span development and behavior* (Vol. 3). New York: Academic Press, 1980.

Cronbach, L. J., and Furby, L. How should we measure "change" — Or should we? *Psychological Bulletin*, 1970, 74, 68–80.

Danish, S. J., Smyer, M. A., and Nowak, C. A. Developmental intervention: Enhancing life-event processes. In P. B. Baltes and O. G. Brim, Jr. (Eds.), *Life-span development and behavior* (Vol. 3). New York: Academic Press, 1980.

Demming, J. A., and Pressey, S. L. Tests "indigenous" to the adult and older years. *Journal of Counseling Psychology*, 1957, 4, 144–148.

Denney, N. W. Aging and cognitive changes. In B. B. Wolman (Ed.), *Handbook of developmental psychology*. Englewood Cliffs, N.J.: Prentice-Hall, 1982.

Eichorn, D. H., Clausen, J. A., Haan, N., Honzik, M. P., and Mussen, P. H. *Present and past in middle life*. New York: Academic Press, 1981.

Elder, G. H., Jr. Family history and life course. In T. K. Hareven (Ed.), *Transitions: The family and the life course in historical perspective*. New York: Academic Press, 1978.

Elder, G. H., Jr. Historical change in life patterns and personality. In P. B. Baltes and O. G. Brim, Jr. (Eds.), *Life-span development and behavior* (Vol. 2). New York: Academic Press, 1979.

Elder, G. H., and Liker, J. K. Hard times in women's lives: Historical influences across 40 years. *American Journal of Sociology*, 1982, 88, 241–269.

Epstein, S. The stability of behavior: I. On predicting most of the people much of the time. *Journal of Personality and Social Psychology*, 1979, 37, 1097–1126.

Erikson, E. *Childhood and society* (2nd ed.). New York: Norton, 1963.

Eysenck, H. J., and Eysenck, S. B. G. *Eysenck personality inventory*. San Diego: Educational and Industrial Testing Services, 1963.

Finney, H. C. Improving the reliability of retrospective survey measures: Results of a longitudinal field survey. *Evaluation Review*, 1981, 5, 207–229.

Flavell, J. H. Cognitive changes in adulthood. In L. R. Goulet and P. B. Baltes (Eds.), *Life-span developmental psychology: Research and theory*. New York: Academic Press, 1970.

Fries, J. F., and Crapo, L. M. *Vitality and aging.* San Francisco: Freeman, 1981.
Furby, L. Interpreting regression toward the mean in developmental research. *Developmental Psychology,* 1973, *8,* 172–179.
Ghiselli, E. E., Campbell, J. P., and Zedeck, S. *Measurement theory for the behavioral sciences.* San Francisco: Freeman, 1981.
Giele, J. Z. (Ed.). *Women in the middle years: Current knowledge and directions for research and policy.* New York: Wiley, 1982.
Gilligan, C. *In a different voice: Psychological theory and women's development.* Cambridge, Mass.: Harvard University Press, 1982.
Glenn, N. D. *Cohort analysis.* Beverly Hills: Sage, 1977.
Gribbin, K., and Schaie, K. W. The aging of tests: A methodological problem of longitudinal studies. Paper presented at the 30th Annual Meeting of the Gerontological Society, San Francisco, November 1977.
Gutek, B. A. On the accuracy of retrospective attitudinal data. *Public Opinion Quarterly,* 1978, *42,* 390–401.
Harris, D. P. (Ed.). *The concept of development.* Minneapolis: University of Minnesota Press, 1957.
Harris, R. J. *A primer of multivariate statistics.* New York: Academic Press, 1975.
Heise, D. R. Separating reliability and stability in test-retest correlation. *American Sociological Review,* 1969, *34,* 93–101.
Hultsch, D. F., and Hickey, T. External validity in the study of human development: Theoretical and methodological issues. *Human Development,* 1978, *21,* 76–91.
Hultsch, D. F., and Plemons, J. K. Life events and life span development. In P. B. Baltes and O. G. Brim, Jr. (Eds.), *Life-span development and behavior* (Vol. 2). New York: Academic Press, 1979.
Jöreskog, K. G. Statistical estimation of structural models in longitudinal-developmental investigations. In J. R. Nesselroade and P. B. Baltes (Eds.), *Longitudinal research in the study of behavior and development.* New York: Academic Press, 1979.
Jöreskog, K. G., and Sörbom, D. *LISREL IV: Estimation of linear structural equation systems by maximum likelihood methods.* Chicago: International Educational Services, 1978.
Jöreskog, K., and Sörbom, D. Simultaneous analysis of longitudinal data from several cohorts. In H. Winsborough and O. D. Duncan (Eds.), *Analyzing data for age, period, and cohort effects,* in preparation.
Kenny, D. A. *Correlation and causality.* New York: Wiley, 1979.
Kohlberg, L. Stage and sequence: The cognitive-developmental approach to socialization. In D. A. Goslin (Ed.), *Handbook of socialization theory and research.* Chicago: Rand McNally, 1969.
Krauss, I. K. Between- and within-group comparisons in aging research. In L. W. Poon (Ed.), *Aging in the 1980s: Psychological issues.* Washington D.C.: American Psychological Association, 1980.
Labouvie, E. W. Identity versus equivalence of psychological measures and constructs. In L. W. Poon (Ed.), *Aging in the 1980s: Psychological issues.* Washington, D.C.: American Psychological Association, 1980.
Labouvie, E. W., Bartsch, T. W., Nesselroade, J. R., and Baltes, P. B. On the internal and external validity of simple longitudinal designs. *Child Development,* 1974, *45,* 282–290.
Labouvie-Vief, G. Adult cognitive development: In search of alternative interpretations. *Merrill-Palmer Quarterly,* 1977, *23,* 227–263.
Labouvie-Vief, G. Dynamic development and mature autonomy: A theoretical prologue. *Human Development,* 1982, *25,* 161–191.
Labouvie-Vief, G., and Chandler, M. J. Cognitive development and life-span developmen-

tal theory: Idealistic versus contextual perspectives. In P. B. Baltes (Ed.), *Life-span development and behavior* (Vol. 1). New York: Academic Press, 1978.

Lachman, M. E. Perceptions of intellectual aging: Antecedent or consequence of intellectual functioning? *Developmental Psychology*, 1983, *19*, 482–498.

Lachman, M. E., Baltes, P. B., Nesselroade, J. R., and Willis, S. L. Examination of personality-ability relationships in the elderly: The role of the contextual (interface) assessment mode. *Journal of Research in Personality*, 1982, *16*, 485–501.

Lerner, R. M. *Concepts and theories of human development*. Reading, Mass.: Addison-Wesley, 1976.

Lerner, R. M., and Ryff, C. D. Implementation of the life-span view of human development: The sample case of attachment. In P. B. Baltes (Ed.), *Life-span development and behavior* (Vol. 1). New York: Academic Press, 1978.

Levinson, D. J. *The seasons of a man's life*. New York: Knopf, 1978.

Looft, W. R. Socialization and personality throughout the life span: An examination of contemporary psychological approaches. In P. B. Baltes and K. W. Schaei (Eds.), *Life-span developmental psychology: Personality and socialization*. New York: Academic Press, 1973.

Lord, F. M., and Novick, M. R. *Statistical theories of mental test scores*. Reading, Mass.: Addison-Wesley, 1968.

Lowenthal, M. F., Thurnher, M., and Chiriboga, D. *Four stages of life*. San Francisco: Jossey-Bass, 1975.

Mason, K. O., Mason, W. M., Winsborough, H. H., and Poole, W. K. Some methodological issues in cohort analyses of archival data. *American Sociological Review*, 1973, *38*, 242–258.

McCall, R. B. Challenges to a science of developmental psychology. *Child Development*, 1977, *48*, 333–344.

Morrison, D. F. *Multivariate statistical methods* (2nd ed.). New York: McGraw-Hill, 1976.

Nesselroade, J. R. Issues in studying developmental change in adults from a multivariate perspective. In J. E. Birren and K. W. Schaie (Eds.), *Handbook of the psychology of aging*. New York: Van Nostrand Reinhold, 1977.

Nesselroade, J. R., and Baltes, P. B. Adolescent personality development and historical change: 1970–1972. *Monographs of the Society for Research in Child Development*, 1974, *39*(1, Serial No. 154).

Nesselroade, J. R., and Baltes, P. B. Sequential strategies and the role of cohort effects in behavioral development: Adolescent personality (1970–1972) as a sample case. In S. Mednick and M. Harway (Eds.), *Longitudinal research in the United States*, in preparation.

Nesselroade, J. R., and Bartsch, T. W. Multivariate perspectives on the construct validity of the trait-state distinction. In R. B. Cattell and R. M. Dreger (Eds.), *Handbook of modern personality theory*. Washington, D.C.: Hemisphere, 1977.

Nesselroade, J. R., Stigler, S. M., and Baltes, P. B. Regression toward the mean and the study of change. *Psychological Bulletin*, 1980, *88*, 622–637.

Neugarten, B. L. (Ed.). *Middle age and aging*. Chicago: University of Chicago Press, 1968.

Nunnally, J. C. *Psychometric theory* (2nd ed.). New York: McGraw-Hill, 1978.

Popkin, S. J., Schaie, K. W., and Krauss, I. K. *Age-fair assessment of psychometric intelligence*. Paper presented at the 33rd Annual Scientific Meeting of the Gerontological Society of America, San Diego, November 1980.

Powers, E. A., Goudy, W. J., and Keith, P. M. Congruence between panel and recall data in longitudinal research. *Public Opinion Quarterly*, 1978, *42*, 380–389.

Quayhagen, M., Gonda, J., and Schaie, K. W. *Are familiar tasks always meaningful?* Paper

presented at the 32nd Annual Meeting of the Gerontological Society. Washington, D.C., November 1979.
Reese, H. W., and Overton, W. F. Models of development and theories of development. In L. R. Goulet and P. B. Baltes (Eds.), *Life-span developmental psychology: Research and theory*. New York: Academic Press, 1970.
Reinert, G. Comparative factor analytic studies of intelligence throughout the human life-span. In L. R. Goulet and P. B. Baltes (Eds.), *Life-span developmental psychology: Research and theory*. New York: Academic Press, 1970.
Reinert, G. Prolegomena to a history of life-span developmental psychology. In P. B. Baltes and O. G. Brim, Jr. (Eds.), *Life-span development and behavior* (Vol. 2). New York: Academic Press, 1979.
Rogosa, D. Causal models in longitudinal research: Rationale, formulation, and interpretation. In J. R. Nesselroade and P. B. Baltes (Eds.), *Longitudinal research in the study of behavior and development*. New York: Academic Press, 1979.
Rossi, A. S. Life-span theories and women's lives. *Signs: Journal of Women in Culture and Society*, 1980, 6, 4–32.
Rubin, L. B. *Women of a certain age: The midlife search for self*. New York: Harper & Row, 1979.
Ryder, N. B. The cohort as a concept in the study of social change. *American Sociological Review*, 1965, 30, 843–861.
Ryff, C. D., and Heincke, S. G. *The subjective organization of personality in adulthood and aging*. Paper presented at the Biennial Meeting of the Society for Research in Child Development, Boston, April 1981.
Schaie, K. W. A general model for the study of developmental problems. *Psychological Bulletin*, 1965, 64, 92–107.
Schaie, K. W. Quasi-experimental research designs in the psychology of aging. In J. E. Birren and K. W. Schaie (Eds.), *Handbook of the psychology of aging*. New York: Van Nostrand Reinhold, 1977.
Schaie, K. W. Toward a stage theory of adult cognitive development. *International Journal of Aging and Human Development*, 1977–78, 8, 129–138.
Schaie, K. W. External validity in the assessment of intellectual development in adulthood. *Journal of Gerontology*, 1978, 33, 695–701.
Schaie, K. W. The primary mental abilities in adulthood: An exploration in the development of psychometric intelligence. In P. B. Baltes and O. G. Brim, Jr. (Eds.), *Life-span development and behavior* (Vol. 2). New York: Academic Press, 1979.
Schaie, K. W., and Baltes, P. B. On sequential strategies in developmental research: Description or explanation. *Human Development*, 1975, 18, 384–390.
Schaie, K. W., and Hertzog, C. Longitudinal methods. In B. B. Wohlman (Ed.), *Handbook of developmental psychology*. Englewood Cliffs, N.J.: Prentice-Hall, 1982.
Shannon, J., and Kedar, H. S. Phenomenological structuring of the adult lifespan as a function of age and sex. *International Journal of Aging and Human Development*, 1979–80, 10, 343–357.
Siegler, I. *Stress and adaptation in later life: Description of study population sample, major life events, and resources*. Paper presented at the 30th Annual Scientific Meeting of the Gerontological Society, San Francisco, November 1977.
Siegler, I. C., and Botwinick, J. A long-term longitudinal study of intellectual ability of older adults: The matter of selective subject attrition. *Journal of Gerontology*, 1979, 34, 242–245.
Stewart, A. J., and Platt, M. B. Studying women in a changing world: An introduction. *Journal of Social Issues*, 1982, 38, 1–16.
Thomae, H. Theory of aging and cognitive theory of personality. *Human Development*, 1970, 13, 1–16.

Thurstone, L. L., and Thurstone, T. G. *SRA primary mental abilities: Intermediate ages 11–17.* Chicago: Science Research Associates, 1948.

Thurstone, T. G. *Primary mental abilities for grades 9–12.* Chicago: Science Research Associates, 1962.

Turner, R. R., and Reese, H. W. *Life-span developmental psychology: Intervention.* New York: Academic Press, 1980.

Vaillant, G. E. *Adaptation to life.* Waltham, Mass.: Little, Brown, 1977.

Wheaton, B., Múthen, B., Alwin, D. F., and Summers, G. F. Assessing reliability and stability in panel models. In D. R. Heise (Ed.), *Sociological methodology, 1977.* San Francisco: Jossey-Bass, 1977.

Wohlwill, J. F. The age variable in psychological research. *Psychological Review,* 1970, 77, 49–64.

Wohlwill, J. F. *The study of behavioral development.* New York: Academic Press, 1973.

Chapter 3

Middle-Aged Women in Literature

CAROLYN G. HEILBRUN

> The upshot of all such reflections is that I have only to let myself *go!* So I have said to myself all my life—so I said to myself in the far-off days of my fermenting and passionate youth. Yet I have never fully done it. The sense of it—of the need of it—rolls over me at times with commanding force: it seems the formula of my salvation, of what remains to me of a future. I am in full possession of accumulated resources—I have only to use them, to insist, to persist, to do something more—to do much more—than I *have* done. The way to do it—to affirm one's self *sur la fin*—is to strike as many notes, deep, full and rapid, as one can. All life is—at my age, with all one's artistic soul the record of it—in one's pocket, as it were. Go on, my boy, and strike hard; have a rich and long St. Martin's summer. Try everything, do everything, render everything—be an artist, be distinguished, to the last. (James, 1947, p. 106)

Henry James was nearly 50 when he wrote those words in his notebook; 10 years later he would begin *The Ambassadors*, the first of his last three great novels. Its hero is a man of 55, a man who has failed to live his life until now—even, perhaps, to recognize that he has not lived it. Henry James and his generation of American men provide all of us with a model for late achievement. Two friends from his youth, Henry Adams and Oliver Wendell Holmes, were, like James, to flower late: Adams did not write *Mont-Saint-Michel and Chartres* until he was 65 and his *Education of Henry Adams* until he was almost 70. Holmes reached his full powers when he was appointed to the Supreme Court at 61 (Matthiessen, 1944, p. 30). Henry's brother, William James, whose youth was a long exercise in indecision, did not produce his first book, the important *Principles of Psychology*, until he was 47.

    I speak of men because it is possible, even likely, that the pattern of male lives in the 19th century suggests the pattern of female lives in the

---

CAROLYN G. HEILBRUN • Department of English, Columbia University; home address: 151 Central Park West, New York, New York 10023.

20th. More than a hundred years ago, for example, young men were troubled by the whole question of "vocation," by the hard task of choosing the path of life that promised the most passion and the most joy. Vocation was new for men at that time, and not allowed for women. Maggie Tulliver in George Eliot's *The Mill on the Floss* wishes she might have a steady purpose in life, and says to her brother: "You are a man, Tom, and have power, and can do something in the world," and Tom replies, "Then if you can do nothing, submit to those who can" (Mintz, 1978, pp. 45, 62). Today, young women need no longer submit and, like the men of the 19th century, long to be called to something but are uncertain what that something may be. Similarly, a middle-aged man like Strether in James's *The Ambassadors*, who has always failed to "live," who has swerved from the direct assault of experience, fearing it, "always considering something else; something else, I mean, than the thing of the moment," (1964, p. 26) not only adumbrates the condition of middle-aged women today but, indeed, reflects that condition.

When we move from middle-aged men to women, seeking an image of middle-aged women in literature, we must look not only at characters in novels but also at the women who created those characters. So ignored has the middle-aged woman been, so rare a bird is she as a protagonist in literature that we must watch first how the idea of middle age struck the women artists themselves, and then explore how she has been represented in literature.

Inevitably, happily, one begins with Colette. More and more does she appear to present, in her life, the paradigm of female autonomy, and in her writings the way toward treasured solitude and the vitality of the open life. Colette was born into one destiny and lived, in later years, to achieve another. From an idyllic childhood (though no childhood is idyllic in the sense of being without conflict, without repressed resentment against even the most loving mother) Colette, dowry-less, was married off to a man very much older than she, a profligate and pimp of other people's talents. She had never dreamed of being a writer, had never consciously thought of it: Her recent biographer has been struck by "the exceptional process by which [Colette] was brought to write," and "the time required before she achieved recognition as a writer" (Sarde, 1981, p. 16). The exceptional process, of course, was that of being forced by her husband to write books about her girlhood experiences (the Claudine books), which—incredible though it seems—were published under *his* name. Colette was just 50 when she first published a novel under her own name, the single name she had chosen for herself: Colette. Meanwhile, she had married twice, appeared in music halls and on the stage, been a journalist and a lover of men and women. When she died, she was the first woman ever accorded a state funeral in France.

With the early process we need not concern ourselves here. It is sufficient to record that Colette needed to be forced into her profession, into the practice of what now strikes us as the natural flowering of an inborn talent. Indeed, she wrote that she had no early desire to write. "what a blessing that I could experience such an absence of literary vocation!" (Mallet-Joris, 1981, p. 7). The blessing, of course, is mentioned in the knowledge of achievement. Yet this, as Mallet-Joris says, tells us much about the question of "creativity" in women (Mallet-Joris, 1981, p. 8). So entrenched is the long cultural constraint against women having ambitions as opposed to erotic daydreams that some pressure appears necessary to overcome the dire effects of confining women, as Freud does, to what literary critics now call the erotic plot (Freud, 1957, pp. 176–177). In the past decade and more, expectations of and encouragement for some commitment to a life not confined to the need for love and children have been provided women by the culture as a whole. It is clear, however, that few women, not even a Colette, can be expected without great external support or coercion to overcome societal sanctions against nonerotic ambitions.

But it is the middle-aged Colette who must interest us here. Her fame came late, as has the fame of many notable women writers in our own time. May Sarton's fame has steadily increased as she grows older, and Doris Grumbach became a successful novelist very late. Stevie Smith, the English writer, was to declare: "I am becoming quite famous in my old age, isn't it funny how things come 'round?" (1981, p. 313). It is those who achieve great stature long after youth who offer us, like Donne's lovers, a pattern for our lives.

As Colette's biographer said of her at 50: "Man had finally been shorn of his magical and commanding force; he no longer either barred doors or opened them. For Colette, the days of compromise and sharing were over." She entered on a period that Valery has named *Le Bel Aujourd'hui*, the "lovely present" (Sarde, 1980, p. 360). The ambition for middle-aged women must be to render the present "lovely," which means not that it is calm and without pain—such contentment may be found in a front porch rocker—but that it offers its own intensity, and is experienced in non-nostalgic relation to the past. Renunciation must be part of it, as with Colette's Lea in *The Last of Cheri*, who, Sarde tells us, resembles Colette in her "penchant for renunciation for the sake of freedom, in the abstention Colette praised so highly" (1980, p. 351). And what is renounced, abstained from? Love. Not, of course, love of friends, colleagues, companions, even family if they are capable of becoming friends. What is renounced is the erotic dream that can take, in its most acceptable middle-aged form, the wish for an "escort," for that acknowledgment of personhood that, in the restricted world of femininity, only a man can bestow. Colette herself saw the opportunities of middle age as a project "when you set out across the undulating barrier" (Sarde, 1980, p. 379). At this time also, Sarde tells us, Colette rejoiced no longer to feel a rival for men, but rather to discover that as a woman she could now enjoy "the highest type of female relationship, without boasting or braggadocio, void of any desire to save face, full of jokes and mutual understanding" (p. 383). This friendship with women is one of the rare prizes of middle age, ironically offered not to those who are refugees from married life but to those who share new experiences in the public sphere. For the ultimate joy of middle age is work.

Many women artists have agreed. Käthe Kollwitz wrote in her diary that she found familial ties growing slacker; "for the last third of life there remains only work. It alone is always stimulating, rejuvenating, exciting and satisfying" (Kearns, 1976, p. 125). Women, an Isak Dinesen character says, "when they are old enough to have done with the business of being women, and can let loose their strength, must be the most powerful creatures in the world" (1972, p. 119). The feminists among us hope for a time when "the business of being woman" shall not be distinguished from the business of being human, and Dinesen's middle-age change into power will not be so noteworthy. Meanwhile, her phrase is apt.

The messages from and to middle-aged women are all alike in this: that life for such women can indeed be an undiscovered country, but to enter it requires not only amazing courage but the secret knowledge that men have not kept the joys of accomplishment to themselves because these joys are negligible. They claimed them because, among other reasons, they alone can make life, once youth is past, compelling. The hard part is for women to see youth go, and believe something lies beyond. Fromm-Reichmann has put it well: "The shock . . . of middle age is a threshold shock. A door is closing behind us and we turn sorrowfully to watch it close and do not discover, until we are wrenched away, the one opening ahead."

Middle-aged women, until very recently, found more encouragement in life than in art. Indeed, middle age itself has had such a bad press that it is startling to find it praised at all, even by men. Samuel Butler, here, as elsewhere, set out to shock, and did: "To me it seems that youth is like spring, an overpraised season. . . . Autumn is the mellower season, and what we lose in flowers we more than gain in fruits. Fontenelle at the age of 90, being asked what was the happiest time of his life, said he did not know that he had ever been much happier than he then was, but that perhaps his best years had been those when he was between fifty-five and seventy-five" (Butler, n.d., p. 38). Women of middle age seldom appeared in novels of the 18th and 19th centuries, unless as someone's mother or surrogate mother, and then only to affect the younger women's erotic plot, her finding a husband and thus a "destiny." The significant fact about women, in fiction as in life, is that, after youth and childbearing are past, they have no plot, there is no story to be told about them. In 1908 Arnold Bennett found it easy enough to startle the world in this regard: "I had always revolted against the absurd youthfulness, the unfading youthfulness of the average heroine. And as a protest against this fashion, I was already, in 1903, planning a novel (*Lenora*) of which the heroine was aged forty, and had daughters old enough to be in love. The reviewers, by the way, were staggered by my hardihood in offering a woman of forty as a subject of serious interest to the public" (Bennett, 1928, vi–viii).

Young women and girls do not have individual stories, only variations upon the same story, the waiting for sexual maturity, the selection by an acceptable man, or not, and the children who will follow. Simone de Beauvoir put it concisely: "She is twelve years old and already her story is written in the heavens. She will discover it day after day without ever making it; she is curious but frightened when she contemplates this life, every stage of which is foreseen and toward which every day moves irresistibly" (1957, p. 298). For women in literature who avoid, or are deprived of, this erotic-marriage plot, no story remains to be told. Such women cannot write their own stories; no narrative will ever be told about them. So in George Gissing's *The Odd Women*, two of the three sisters do not marry and are thus wholly unworthy of narrative: They have no story. Their youngest sister, Monica, lives out the erotic plot, which ends in marriage and death. Gissing's novel, indeed, explores the question of whether any other narrative *is* possible for women.

The question is answered in certain 20th-century novels, where it appears that the middle-aged woman may, at her rebirth, hold the secret of a new plot. Virginia Woolf's (1925) Clarissa Dalloway, who has just broken into her 52nd year, will undergo a profound transformation in *Mrs. Dalloway*. Clarissa Dalloway is to be contrasted with Woolf's more typical, and more conventionally appealing, middle-aged woman, also over 50, Mrs. Ramsay, of *To the Lighthouse*. Mrs. Ramsay has all the seductive, overwhelming charm of the beautiful mother but has no story of her own, and is eventually drained of life by the unremitting demands and needs of others. Her urging of all women to marriage marks her inability to reconsider the pattern of her own life, or to question the promise of the marriages she has encouraged. Lily Briscoe, 44, must resist the attractions and advice of Mrs. Ramsay, must release herself from that feminine source of power if she is to paint her own picture at the end of the novel, and have her own vision.

But Mrs. Dalloway, unlike Mrs. Ramsay, will become Clarissa by the end of the novel, that is to say, will become herself. The first sentence of the novel is: "Mrs. Dalloway said she would buy the flowers herself." The last two lines are: " 'It is Clarissa,' he said. For there she was." *Mrs. Dalloway*, almost infinitely reverberative, most not be simplified by description as the story of how a middle-aged woman reinvents her self (the novel is careful to separate these two words), but that transformation is at the heart of the novel. Clarissa glances in the mirror, seeing herself (one word):

> How many million times she has seen her face, and always with the same imperceptible contraction! She pursed her lips when she looked in the glass. It was to give her face point. That was her self—pointed; dartlike; definite. That was her self when some effort, some call on her to be her self, drew the parts together, she alone knew how different, how incompatible and composed so for the world only into one centre, one diamond, one woman who sat in her drawing-room and made a meeting point, a radiancy. . . . (p. 55)

Many elements figure in the transformation—her past, the return of an old lover and present friend, her husband's being invited to lunch without her, "how it is certain we must die" (p. 267). Central to the story is also the passage into madness and death of a young man, his sanity destroyed by the war. Clarissa and he are, in a sense, doubles, and this identification of a young man, condemned to a monstrous "manly" death, and an older woman, restricted to a properly "ladylike" life, is one of the revolutionary themes of the work. It was with this novel that Virginia Woolf, as she said, found her own voice at last. She was 44 at the publication of *Mrs. Dalloway*, the same age as Lily Briscoe when Lily became certain of what she wished her destiny to be, and painted her picture.

Doris Lessing has been, in our own time, the outstanding portrayer of middle-aged women in the crisis of discovering that they exist only in their relationships to others; they are only ancillary. In "To Room 19," Lessing wrote the terrible and terrifying story of a woman who deserts her profession, marries, has the "ideal" life, and eventually goes in search of her lost self in a lonely London room in a sleazy hotel; she seeks nothing but solitude. Her husband believes she has a lover; he sets detectives to spy on her. Realizing that she is soon to lose the room, she kills herself. The story is shattering and, in its honesty, incomprehensible to those women who fear to consider themselves entitled to a destiny separate from a family's, or who do not wish to face the anxiety and dubious rewards of singularity. The rewards are dubious, not because they are unimportant, or not life-enhancing, but because all birth, but especially birth at middle age, is painful and does not lead (as women have been taught their lives must lead if they are good and loving) to peace, acceptance, and appreciation. Perhaps the hardest task of middle age is to enter upon a new experience that must be, as all adventure is, painful and risky.

Lessing's bridge from "To Room 19" to *The Summer Before the Dark* is, as Roberta Rubinstein has pointed out, a novella about a 50-year-old man entitled *The Temptation of Jack Orkney* (Rubinstein, 1979, p. 200). The imminent death of Orkney's father shocks him into awareness of his spiritual drift toward inertia, the temptation of doing nothing. Kate Brown of *The Summer Before the Dark* also will discover that she is, in Rubinstein's words, "on the verge of a shift in her life's preoccupations and identity" (p. 200). Kate will experiment with sexuality, new assurances of her attractiveness, but above all she will dream repeatedly of carrying a dying seal toward water, necessary to its survival. The seal is Kate's identity, her selfhood, her hope of rejuvenation that will not be easy at her age. Rejuvenation for women is not a replay of youthful success—charm, male attentions, serving the needs of children. Rather, Kate must enact all the rejections of age—*not* to be found alluring, enticing—that her society has taught her are the rejections of womanhood and personhood. Even if she can, by dressing a certain way, evoke whistles from construction workers, is this reassuring? She must instead discover a strength, or the chance for strength, that does not end with marriage and "they lived happily ever after" but rather begins with the knowledge of old age and death as they come to all, but not with especial harshness to women. Bearing the great weight of her own self, she struggles toward life.

Women who are artists in life rather than in literature have taught us that work is the great redeemer. But women often deny this because they have been trained to dream, not of opening doors, but of closure, the safe house whose threshold, symbolically speaking, they have needed to cross only once. Women's romances, like television commercials, provide easy resolutions, and a cast of characters who speak as expected. Do the right thing and they will love you. Those who have written of middle age in literature speak less of work, more of the need to eschew closure, to choose risk, to know that, as with those feared paralyzed, pain is the sign of life, the hope for recovery.

In 19th-century novels, the most middle-aged women were allowed was another marriage, another manly chest to subside upon. Perhaps the closest we come in a 19th-century novel to a middle-aged woman's awareness of these modern questions is Daniel Deronda's mother. She is unique, perhaps, in all literature. She is a woman who did not wish to live out the erotic plot, who particlarly detested the role of women in Jewish tradition. The patriarchal tradition has long seen daughters, particularly when they are only children, as the means of acquiring a grandson, a continuation of the paternal line (think of Shakespeare's Juliet). As Daniel Deronda's mother says of her father, "I was to be what he called 'the Jewish woman' under pain of his curse. I was to feel everything I did not feel, and believe everything I did not believe" (Eliot, 1967, p. 692). She tells her son, "Every woman is supposed to have the same set of motives, or else to be a monster. I am not a monster, I have not felt exactly what other women feel—or say they feel, for fear of being thought unlike others" (p. 691). Her father, Daniel's mother says, "cared more about a grandson to come than he did about me: I counted as nothing" (p. 698). "You are not a woman," she tries to explain to him: "You may try—but you can never imagine what it is to have a man's force of genius in you, and yet to suffer the slavery of being a girl. To have a pattern cut out—'this is the Jewish woman; this is what you must be; this is what you are wanted for'; a woman's heart must be of such a size and no larger, else it must be pressed small, like Chinese feet" (p. 694). Daniel's mother was a great artist, a great singer, and in middle age, what can she do but lament? In the modern novel, she may dare more, if not as a girl, then as an older woman. While George Eliot seems almost to have determined to doom this woman, how differently the voice sounds from that of Miss Havisham in Dickens's *Great Expectations*, who, deserted on her wedding day by her bridegroom, froze into permanent dejection and the unending repetition of that terrible moment. Nor might one answer that, had she married elsewhere, she might have lived. As I have suggested, Katherine Anne Porter shows us in "The Jilting of Granny Weatherall" that finding another man and having your life "like any other woman" does not mean that you have found your destiny, that you have been the author of your own story. Granny Weatherall might have said, with a character in Djuna Barnes's *Nightwood*, "I've not only lived my life for nothing, but I've told it for nothing" (1937, p. 165).

Male writers in the 20th century began also to portray middle-aged women characters in new and provocative ways. We might remember Kate of D. H. Lawrence's *The Plumed Serpent*, who is 40 at the book's opening, and profoundly dissatisfied with her life. While many readers and critics have found much that is troubling in this novel, Lawrence's presentation of a middle-aged woman's sense of meaninglessness in life is perceptive, even though her destiny does, in the end, revolve around a charismatic male leader, male violence, and a regrettable (though prophetic) religion. It is the beginning of the book that arrests us.

Closer to the central problems of middle age is Angus Wilson's *The Middle Age of Mrs. Eliot*, a study of the sudden awakening of a self-satisfied woman after the accidental shooting of her husband. She discovers that all her committees, good works, social acceptance have arisen from her position as "Mrs." Eliot, and not from herself as a person. "She thought, if Bill gave everything to me, what was my life for? It had no meaning except in him. They had set out together to climb somewhere; but she had been only a rope, not a guide, for she had never known their destination or asked it, only judged its approach by his look of certainty, reading his face for portents of success or failure. There was not a single way that she could live for him now; or die for him" (1960, p. 103). Wilson, unlike Lawrence, sees her through to a new acceptance of selfhood; he has said that Mrs. Eliot is, of all his characters, the one closest to himself. The need of men to find an identity beyond that of their business or corporation or government agency is one that renders the female character human for them, rather than merely female.

In the years following Betty Friedan's *The Feminine Mystique*, many women authors have given us heroines who strike out in early middle age for themselves, leaving stifling marriages and seeking some degree of autonomy. Many of these might profitably be discussed here, but I shall conclude with a current author who, now just 70, has long written of the middle-aged woman, and did so before the subject became fashionable or even respectable. May Sarton wrote a poem on her 50th birthday, which she celebrated in Greece, praising Athene:

> Not she of the olive,
> But she of the owl eyes,
> A spear in her hand. (1965a, p. 47)

She had first met this Athene in youth, and now, 50, knows this is not a place for the young: It is right, rather, to meet Athene on one's 50th birthday:

> It was the right year
> To confront
> The smile beyond suffering. (p. 49)

Sarton has written of married women, lonely within "happy" marriages, but she has also written of middle-aged women loving other women, finding in these loves the sources of poetry, of art. In *Mrs. Stevens Hears the Mermaids Singing*, she portrays women lovers lost in the happiness of discovering each other, while appearing to those who pass them like two dull middle-aged women: "There was a secret joy when they walked down the street together (for at this time they often set out on long walks) to know that from the outside what people saw was two middle-aged women, but inside they were wild children, wild with joy, feeling each of them that this (surely last and best) love affair was a great present from life, a source of renewed energy" (1965b, p. 165). Sarton is writing of women who find renewed energy and passion in the love of other women late in life. But even for those who will not move into another and different passionate love, intimacy with women is an unexpected reward of their new freedom to move outside of a constrained destiny. Although Sarton has only touched upon this, many women today have noticed how marriages have been preserved because of the wife's discovery of intimacy with other women, the release of honest conversation, the wonder of deep personal trust in friendship. Many marriages have escaped dissolution because of the safety valve provided by these new friendships.

For women as for men, middle age must avoid the feverish and fruitless search for fading youthful passions and reassurances; rather it must seek a new country, new accomplishment, adventure, and the pain that is the price of adventure. Women have often to find these adventures in a new world—of work, institutional struggle, ambition, the agony of competition and compromise. (Men, already living in that world, may find their middle-aged adventure in personal tasks, and the private acts of nurturance.) Erik Erikson has written of generativity as the mature choice—the working for something beyond oneself, for future generations. In late middle age, furthermore, one can afford to take risks the young cannot afford: to speak out, to affront conventional opinion and demands. Women, having been private people, perhaps, may now reach out and work in organized numbers, within existing institutions or in their own new groups. E. M. Forster, writing in the bad times between the world wars, regretted the need for the middle-aged, if they were not to retire from life altogether, to join a movement. He saw the time through which he had lived as a tragedy in three acts. "In the first act the individualist hopes to improve society, in the second, he tries to improve himself, in the third act he finds he's not wanted, and has either to merge himself in a movement or to retire" (Colmer, 1975, pp. 210–211).

Most of us now in late middle age were taught to be, as Forster was, wary of movements. But in the world of today, concerted action is required, and required particularly of those, like women, who have lived their lives devoted to personal and familial pursuits. Generativity today may be possible only in a movement, or at least a communal effort, whether political, artistic, or ideological. If one might end with a prophecy, it is that, even for individualistic artists, generativity for women in middle age will be found in bonding with other women, for mutual support, in an ambience of productive work and accomplishment.

REFERENCES

Barnes, D. *Nightwood*. New York: New Directions, 1937.
Bennett, A. *The old wives' tale* (New ed. with preface). New York: Doubleday, Doran, 1928.
Butler, S. *The way of all flesh*. New York: Modern Library, n.d.
Colmer, J. *E. M. Forster: The personal voice*. London: Routledge and Kegan Paul, 1975.
de Beauvoir, S. [*The second sex*] (H. M. Parshley, Ed. and trans.). New York: Knopf, 1957.

Dinesen, I. The monkey. In *Seven gothic tales*. New York: Vintage Books, 1972.
Eliot, G. *Daniel Deronda*. New York: Penguin, 1967.
Freud, S. The relation of the poet to daydreaming. In *Collected Papers* (Vol. 4). London: Hogarth Press, 1957.
Heilbrun, C. G. On Katherine Anne Porter . . . . In C. Skaggs (Eds.), *The American short story* (Vol. 2). New York: Dell, 1980.
James, H. *The notebooks of Henry James* (F. O. Matthiessen and K. B. Murdock, Eds.). New York: Oxford University Press, 1947.
James, H. *The ambassadors*. New York: Norton, 1964.
Kearns, M. *Käthe Kollwitz: Woman and artist*. Old Westbury, N.Y.: Feminist Press, 1976.
Mallet-Joris, F. A womanly vocation. In E. M. Eisenger and M. McCarty (Eds.), *Colette: The woman, the writer*. University Park: Pennsylvania State University Press, 1981.
Matthiessen, F. O. *Henry James: The major phase*. New York: Oxford University Press, 1944.
Mintz, A. *George Eliot and the novel of vocation*. Cambridge, Mass.: Harvard University Press, 1978.
Rubinstein, R. *The novelistic vision of Doris Lessing: Breaking the forms of consciousness*. Urbana: University of Illinois Press, 1979.
Sarde, M. *Colette: Free and fettered* (Richard Millder, Trans.). New York: William Morrow, 1980.
Sarde, M. The first steps in a writer's career. In E. M. Eisenger and M. McCarty (Eds.), *Colette: The woman, the writer*. University Park: Pennsylvania State University Press, 1981.
Sarton, M. Birthday on the Acropolis. In *A private mythology*. New York: Norton, 1965. (a)
Sarton, M. *Mrs. Stevens hears the mermaids singing*. New York: Norton, 1965. (b)
Smith, S. *Me again: Uncollected writings of Stevie Smith* (J. Barbera and W. McBrien, Eds.). London: Virago, 1981.
Wilson, A. *The middle age of Mrs. Eliot*. New York: Meridian, 1960.
Woolf, V. *Mrs. Dalloway*. New York: Harcourt Brace, 1925.
Woolf, V. *To the lighthouse*. New York: Harcourt Brace Jovanovich, 1949.

PART II
Roles and Relationships

Chapter 4

The Middle Years
Changes and Variations in Social Role Commitments

HELENA Z. LOPATA AND DEBRA BARNEWOLT

Human beings are involved in many social roles in a lifetime, consecutively and within time-bound clusters. One can be a student, worker, wife, and mother either simultaneously or at different times. At any one stage of life, however, a person is involved in a cluster of roles, each with its own cycle of involvement. Each role consists of a set of mutually interdependent relations with members of a social circle for whom duties are performed and from whom rights are received (Lopata, 1971, 1973; Lopata, Barnewolt, and Norr, 1980; Znaniecki, 1940, 1965).

The fact that several social roles are carried forth during the same time or stage of life and that each role involves many different people can lead to problems, as sociologists and social psychologists have long recognized (Biddle and Thomas, 1966; Newcomb, Turner, and Converse, 1965; Ritzer, 1977). These problems have been labeled *role conflict* and *role strain*. *Role conflict* arises when the demands of one role conflict with those of another, as when two or more roles must be engaged in within too short a time period, or when they require psychologically incompatible sentiments or self-concepts. Even the same role can induce occasions of *role strain*, since it involves relations with several circle segments (Gouldner, 1957; Merton, 1968; Merton *et al.*, 1957). Mothers may be faced with conflicting demands from children and their fathers, or may have each child demand attention at the same time. Role strain comes from *role overload*, when circle members make too many demands;

HELENA Z. LOPATA AND DEBRA BARNEWOLT • Department of Sociology, Loyola University, 6525 N. Sheridan Road, Chicago, Illinois 60626.

intersender strain, when two or more members of the social circle make conflicting demands; *intrasender strain*, when the same role partner gives inconsistent messages; and *role–person strain* when the demanded behavior goes against the person's set of values or self-images (this is a slight modification of Kahn *et al.*, 1964; see also Biddle and Thomas, 1966; Goode, 1960; Gross, Mason, and McEadern, 1958; Ritzer, 1977). We can also look at conflict between roles or strain within a role over the life-course. This enables us, for example, to examine the problems of people caught in a social role that they feel interferes with their future plans. Many a young man felt such conflict when faced with induction into the armed services, which would disrupt preparation for his chosen occupation. Strain over the life-span of a role can occur when a mother learns one way of relating with her children, only to find that this style becomes more and more dysfunctional as the children grow. Finally, problems in role performance may come from the ambiguity with which all participants, including the social person, view the role. Mack (1956) analyzed the consequences of occupational indeterminateness and found this to be one of the main problems of the role of housewife. The composition of the social circle of that role and the exchange of duties and rights within it are open to great variation and misunderstanding. On the other hand, as Coser (1975) points out, the complexity of social roles contributes to the complexity and autonomy of personality, and to the feelings of accomplishment and competence.

The complexity of social circles of just four social roles of a woman's role-cluster at the peak stage of involvement can be partially understood from Figure 1. The possibilities of role conflict and role strain, as well as for feelings of satisfaction, are limitless, not only in terms of duties but also in the receipt of rights.

Dealing with Role Strain and Role Conflict

Goode (1960) outlines some ways in which a person or an organization can deal with the inevitable role strain experienced at some time or another within their lives. The person can compartmentalize relations with the various circle segments, postponing and sequencing demands from each. Negotiations can reduce demands or change their timing. Some duties can be ignored or carried out with passive resistance in such ineffectual ways as to push the sender into the job herself or himself or into turning to someone else. There are numerous methods by which workers learn to deal with role overload, intersender or intrasender strain, or role conflict. Roles can be dropped, assisting segments of circles brought in, intermediaries found, and so forth.

Both role strain and role conflict are difficult to avoid and to deal

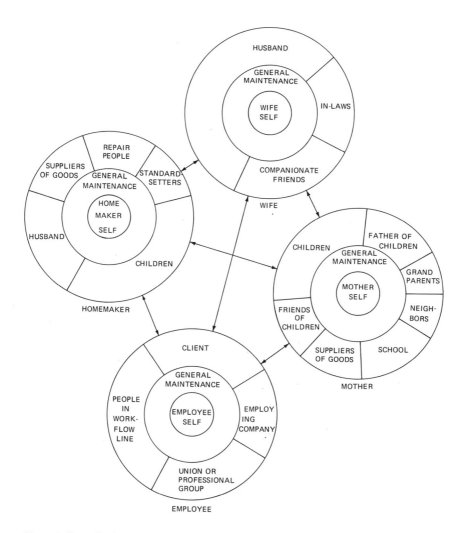

Figure 1. Generalized composition of the social circles of four major social roles of American women.

when there is commitment by the social person to each role and to many segments of each social circle. Women committed to the role cluster of wife/mother/employee/homemaker and the related roles of daughter, daughter-in-law, neighbor, friend, union member, etc., often report role conflict (Bernard, 1971, 1973, 1974, 1975a, 1975b, 1981; Chapman and Gates, 1977; Komarovsky, 1946). Not only do husband and children demand attention at the same time but they require different kinds of behavior and sentiments. Being a perfect housekeeper is often perceived in terms of the product—a spotless and neat home—a difficult accomplishment in the presence of offspring and a not-very- "housebroken" husband (Lopata, 1971). The role of employee requires absence from the home even at times when the roles of wife and mother require presence.

One way in which people deal with role strain is by arranging duties in the different segments of the circle hierarchically, both in terms of the importance assigned to the segment and in terms of the importance assigned to specific duties toward each segment. A woman may feel, for example, that the duties to her children are more important than duties toward the grandparents concerning these children. She may further evaluate time spent companionately with the children as more important than focusing on their physical appearance (even when the grandparents want them "looking pretty"). Role conflict can be partially decreased through a hierarchical arrangement of the roles in the cluster, giving priority to the duties and rights of the roles by order of their assigned importance (Lopata, 1971). Such ranking of roles can be situational, time-bound, or considered as permanent. Problems arise, of course, if members of the different segments of one circle or of different social circles do not agree with the rank order an individual assigns to their segment or role—which is apt to happen if they are more involved in one of the circles than in another. A man may resent having a woman assign the role of wife, when he is the husband, to a second place of importance to the role of mother, even if he is the father of the children (Dyer, 1963; Hobbs, 1965; LeMasters, 1957; Rossi, 1968).

Each society and the smaller social units within it appear to recognize the problems of role conflict and role strain and encourage, or even enforce, hierarchies among different kinds of roles or for different kinds of members. American society has developed strong expectations that men emphasize their occupational role and that circle members of their other roles adjust their demands to those made by that role (Fowlkes, 1980; Pleck, 1975; Whyte, 1956) Wives and children, parents and friends are expected, according to the American success ethic, to reduce their demands upon the male worker, especially the career-minded professional and business executive, if they interfere with the demands of the job (Mortimer, Hall, and Hill, 1978). Although Pleck (1983) claims, on the basis of much research, that the American male has decreased his prior emphasis on his occupational role, others find it still dominant and spreading to other societies. Evans and Bartolome (1980) studied European middle managers who have adopted the American values of success, and concluded that the man's strong commitment to his occupation resulted in a great deal of spillover and strain to family life, with which wives must deal.

The American woman, on the other hand, has experienced several changes in the expected composition and hierarchical arrangement of her social roles over the past century or so. Numerous historians and social scientists have documented the shift in the role structure of married women from kin, community, and occupational involvement to almost exclusive focus upon home roles between the early 1800s and the 1950s (Bernard, 1974, 1981; Easton, 1976; Lerner, 1971; Rothman, 1978; Sicherman, 1975). As the society turned from agricultural to industrial and business life, with its focus on growth and technological change, work became organized into jobs within large complex organizations away from homes, to be performed mainly by full-time, continuously employed men. These men, in turn, were expected to economically support their wives, whose basic roles were homemaker, wife, and mother.

The duties of these roles included the physical and emotional care of the husband and children, home maintenance, and the conversion of objects for home use as one of the stages of production. Women's involvement in economic life away from home was encouraged only prior to marriage, or in cases of dire necessity, and women accepted this definition of the world, or had little power to change it. In any event, by the turn into the 20th century and for many years after, only about one-fifth of the American women worked outside of the home in paid jobs. The figures vary by race and ethnicity, or at least immigrant status, mainly because of necessity, but the ideal remained for married women to stay home and not be involved in paid employment.

Role conflict within the family institution has resulted from the competition between two focal roles of women and the shift in the importance assigned to them at different times in American history. The loosening of authority and power of the patrilineal line accompanying migration, democratization, mass education, and the creation of jobs pushed obligations to in-laws and kin into a position of secondary importance. "Family duties," generalized without specifying the main beneficiary in traditional families, usually consisted of housekeeping tasks, whether performed by the woman directly or through the work of others (Lopata, 1966, 1971). Gradually, however, the romanticization of the role of wife separated it from the general family maintenance and added numerous personal duties. At the same time, the role of mother gained in complexity, with the addition of health maintenance duties accompanying the "germ theory" of illness and child developmental duties thanks to new theories of psychology (Ehrenreich and English, 1979; Rothman, 1978). Thus, the roles of both wife and mother increased in specialized importance, separating from the role of homemaker.

Although the "two-person career"—as sociologists have renamed the situation in which the man takes on the public aspects of a professional or business career while the wife forms the backup support, providing him with needed resources—continues to be idealized in managerial, medical, religious, and even academic worlds, wives are seeking out careers of their own in increasing numbers (Fowlkes, 1980; Mortimer *et al.*, 1978; Vandervelde, 1979). Social scientists have studied ways in which professional and managerial men have been affected by the career demands of their wives, the effects on family life and power distribution of dual-career marriages, and the consequences of career decisions of husbands on the careers of wives (Nadelson and Nadelson, 1980; Poloma, 1972; Poloma and Garland, 1971; Rapoport and Rapoport, 1971, 1976). These studies have been accompanied by research on the role conflict expected to be facing women as they leave the traditional, and supposedly compatibly combined, cluster of housewife/wife/mother and add the role of worker (see Bird, 1979; Lopata and Pleck (1983). A few authors, such as Pleck (1975, 1979, 1983) point to the role conflicts experienced by men because of demands in the roles of worker, husband, father, and home-maintainer. Concern over the alleged role conflict of women arises out of the historically dominant emphasis that they carry the main, even total, responsibility for the maintenance and development—physical, social, and emotional—of the child. Although most American women have small children at home for only a limited number of years of their nearly 80-year-life span, and although only very small children are home during the whole day, the women are expected to keep themselves in a holding pattern in their preparation for adult roles and throughout life in order to be able to stay home during these few years. The emphasis on the ideology defining women as primarily mothers who should be home constantly during the years when their children are young is evident in three ways: first, the failure of the society to provide alternate child care resources; second, the tendency of women to drop out of paid employment after childbirth; and third, the constriction of most discussion about women's employment to those years (Lopata, Barnewolt, and Miller, in press; Lopata, *et al.*, 1980; Lopata and Norr, 1979, 1980).

Awareness of the possibility of role conflict in the lives of American women and of the culturally prescribed, though not consistent, hierarchical arrangement allegedly decreasing this conflict leads to many sociologically interesting questions. Which of the currently discussed roles of women—wife, mother, employee, or homemaker—are chosen as the most important by different types of women? What factors, such as involvement in a role, the composition of the core role-cluster, background, age of children, family income, or own earnings, most contribute to the probability that a woman will select one of these roles as the most important to her at the present time? What are the cohort differences in the role selected as the most important? How do women expect their role focus to change over time? What changes in life circumstances, experienced or projected, influence the hierarchical consistency or flexibility during the middle years of life? We now turn to an examination of the roles women in the middle years of life consider the most important, emphasizing both the similarities and the differences among them.

Methods and Samples

The first study of women's role hierarchies conducted by the senior author utilized questions from several waves of interviews. A 1956 sample consisted of 300 suburban homeowners who were married and had at least one pre-high school child in the home (Lopata, 1966, 1971). Most were white but they varied in social class, with lower-class women showing a definite variation in role orientation from their middle-class counterparts in that they were less oriented to roles outside of the home and to the role of wife. Second- and third-wave interviews used the same schedule, or a more formalized variation, and reached full-time homemakers and employees in older suburbs and in the central city. A total of 571 interviews, including the 300 original ones, were selected out of a total of over 1000 for analysis (Lopata, 1971). Although a subset of the sample responded to a structured question by ranking 12 roles from a set list, most of the respondents were asked an open-ended question: "What are the most important roles of a women (in order of importance)?" The research yielded a sevenfold classification of women:

1. The husband-oriented woman sees her basic role as that of wife, grouping other sets of relations around it; husband-oriented wives have successful husbands.
2. The child-oriented woman believes that the basic unit of the family consists of herself and her children.
3. The house-oriented woman establishes her major area of interest in her home and its maintenance. She often feels that people impinge upon this relation, upsetting her equilibrium by disarranging the house.
4. The life cycle woman decreases her concentration on the role of wife after the children are born but returns to it in later years, either as her children mature or when the retirement, work disengagement, or "phasing-out" stages are reached by her husband.
5. The family-oriented woman blends all roles related to the home,

those of wife, mother, and housewife, into a single "family care" package.
6. The self-directed woman refuses to focus upon any of these roles as basic to her. She is more concerned with herself as a total individual and with satisfying what she defines as her needs than with any role.
7. The woman oriented toward roles outside of her home tends toward such activities as that of worker, community member, volunteer, friend, neighbor, member of a religious organization (Lopata, 1971, pp. 64–66).

The most recent study of American urban women, with interviews in 1978, focused on their construction of reality and included a probability sample of 966 metropolitan Chicago respondents aged 25 to 54. Oversampling of currently nonmarried women resulted in a weighted total of 1,877.[1] The construction of reality theoretical framework aims at the interpretation people have of the world around them and of their place in it. It is concerned with the definition of the situation with which people approach all of the aspects of their lives and their self-images.[2] The role-order question came first in the interview in order to prevent bias arising from the focus of the interview itself and read as follows:

> Please tell me which of these roles is the most important one to you now?
> Which role is second in importance.
> Which role is third in importance?
> Which role is fourth in importance to you now?
> Here is a list of social roles which women can perform at different stages in their lives:
>
> daughter
> student
> worker
> friend
> active/involved citizen
> mother

[1] Research on the changing commitments of women to work and family roles is the basis of this study and was funded by the Social Security Administration (Contract No. SSA600-75-0190, 1975–1979). Dr. Henry P. Brehm was the SSA project officer, Dr. Helena Lopata was principal investigator, and Dr. Kathleen Norr was deputy director. Interviews were conducted in 1977–1978 by the staff of the Survey Research Laboratory of the University of Illinois, Circle Campus. Our thanks go to Kathy Norr, Cheryl Miller, Suzanne Meyering, Marlene Simon, and Jennifer Ettling of the Center for the Comparative Study of Social Roles, Loyola University of Chicago, for their contributions to various stages of the research.

[2] The interview, whose theoretical foundation aimed at the construction of reality of the respondents, contained 31 areas of "competence" and "characteristics" items, which factored into six clusters. These are summarized into leadership, competence, successfulness/intelligence, emotionality, social interaction, and creativity factors.

career woman
homemaker
volunteer worker
wife
member of a church, synagogue, or other religious group
grandmother

The same set of questions was asked for "thinking about when you were 24" and "looking ahead, which of these roles do you think will be the most important one when you are 55?" In the course of this chapter, we will look at the roles the women chose as the most important ones at the present time and through their adult years.

The recent study (1978; see Lopata and Norr, 1979, 1980) involved women who are representative of those who live in the Chicago area, except for the fact that they are more highly educated, due to their relative youth. Thirty-nine percent are Catholic, 48% are Protestant, 4% are Jewish, and the remainder are either without religious identity or scattered among other groups; 73% are white and the majority of the nonwhites are black. The ethnic background of this part of America is reflected in the fact that 46% of the women grew up in families that are closely identified with a national or ethnic group. The women are diversified educationally; 58% have no more than a high school degree, while 20% graduated from college, some of them obtaining more advanced schooling. Most of the women (74%) are married and have children in the home (77%); only 8% live alone. Although almost a third of the youngest women aged 25 to 34 have no children, the percentage drops to 6 for the oldest age cohort. Ten percent of the respondents have never married. As for employment characteristics of the sample, 58% of the women are currently holding a job outside of the home in addition to homemaking activities. The employees are mainly in occupations traditionally held by women. The professional women are mainly in the semiprofessions such as teaching or nursing. The other white-collar workers are concentrated in clerical jobs, and the blue-collar workers are predominantly operatives or service employees.

THE MOST IMPORTANT ROLE OF WOMEN

Table 1 summarizes the role the women consider most important in their lives at the present time. Few women consider a role in which they are currently not involved as the most important, so we have organized the respondents by such involvement in the major roles of American women: employee, wife, mother, homemaker, member of society and its groups, and kin member. Such a small number of the respondents are involved in the role of wife alone, without combining it with em-

Table 1. The Most Important Role by Role Involvement of Chicago Area Women (Percentage Distribution)

Role involvement	Role preference						
	Employee	Wife	Mother	Homemaker	Societal member	Kin member	Total (N)
Employee only	78	0	1	1	14	6	(168)
Employee and wife	17	63	8	7	5	0	(119)
Employee and mother	24	1	63	2	7	4	(174)
Employee, wife, and mother	7	33	48	7	4	0	(617)
Wife and mother	1	34	52	10	2	1	(651)
Mother only	6	0	70	9	11	5	(104)
Total	14	27	45	7	5	2	(1833)

ployment or the role of mother, that they have been removed from this analysis. There are 168 women in the sample who are employees but not wives or mothers, 104 who are mothers but not wives or employees, 119 who combine the role of wife and employee, and 174 involved in both mothering and working outside of the home. By far the largest number of women (651) are wives and mothers but not employees, or combine the home involvements of wife and mother with employment (617). Interestingly enough, there are more women who have not ever entered marriage than who have never been employed for at least 6 months.

Employees who are not also wives and mothers are much more apt to rank the role of worker or career woman as the top role than are women involved in family roles. They are also the most frequent listers of societal roles such as church member, friend, student, citizen, or volunteer, in that order of frequency. Only two women list volunteer as their most important role at the present time, and the number increases to only 24 for the future time period of when they are age 55. The addition of the role of wife immediately moves a woman's role emphasis away from employment, making her husband-oriented, and the addition of the role of mother also dramatically alters the importance assigned the role of worker. The combination of the roles of wife and mother decreases the importance of the employee role, so that only 7% of the respondents involved in all three roles assign first place in order of importance to a role external to the family. Married workers without children are most heavily concentrated on the role of wife, largely due to the fact that the addition of motherhood splits commitment between these two roles. Whether or not a woman is employed does not noticeably influence her tendency to select wife or mother as the most important role, since few choose employee over the role of wife or mother. Women lacking either the role of wife or the combination of wife and employee are the most committed to motherhood. Concentration on the role of mother by nonmarried homemakers is only slightly relieved by the importance of the role of homemaker or member of a set of relations outside of the home. The role of homemaker does not receive "most important" ranking for the most part, but full-time homemakers who are also mothers, whether married or not, are the most likely to rank homemaker as the most important role. The downplaying of this role differentiates the 1978 women from those studied in the 1950s and 1960s, since women in that era were twice as likely as women in 1978 to give it first place in the order of importance. All in all, the role of mother far outweighs any other role, including that of wife, as most important for Chicago area women. We shall now examine the characteristics of women who stress the different roles as important to them now, focusing only on the roles of employee, wife, and mother.

The Work- or Career-Oriented Woman

Although only 14% of the Chicago area women list worker or career woman as the most important role at the present time, distributions vary, depending on several factors. As mentioned before, the work-oriented women do not face competition from the other two roles deemed important for their sex in American society because they are less likely to be married and to have children. Interestingly enough, and contrary to expectations, it is the blue-collar woman, rather than her white-collar counterpart, who is most apt to list the role of employee first in the absence of the roles of wife and mother (see Table 2).

In addition, the blue-collar worker who is married continues to select the role of worker, while the other workers drop their emphasis on the job when marriage is added, with a sizable exception in the case of professional and managerial women. Duncan socioeconomic scores of the respondents' jobs are not, however, significantly related to their role orientation, as far as the employee role is concerned. Educational achievement is not as important an influence on role choice as was anticipated, although it has more impact on women who went to college than on those who ended their education before reaching that level. Family background is also not significantly connected with the placement of the employee role in first order of importance, whether it be indexed by the father's education or occupation, the mother's education

Table 2. The Most Important Role by Role Involvement and Last or Current Occupational Category of Chicago Area Women

Role involvement	Employee role			Wife role			Mother role		
	Professional	White-collar	Blue-collar	Professional	White-collar	Blue-collar	Professional	White-collar	Blue-collar
	(%)	(%)	(%)	(%)	(%)	(%)	(%)	(%)	(%)
Employee only	82	67	88	0	0	0	1	0	0
Employee and wife	26	6	67	62	70	0	0	12	33
Employee and mother	26	28	18	0	0	1	53	61	68
Employee, wife, and mother	9	6	8	44	40	17	37	42	61
Wife and mother	2	1	1	36	34	28	53	51	50
Mother only	0	4	8	0	0	0	100	77	67

or experience in paid employment when the daughter was growing up, or the general socioeconomic status of the home. Also insignificant in influencing the woman's tendency to list the role of worker first are the husband's characteristics, such as his education, occupational category, or Duncan score. The work-oriented women tend to see themselves as leaders and successful people, and they are less likely to see themselves as emotional than are women who give first importance to other roles. It is the age of the children, rather than the age of the respondent, that is the crucial variable. The presence of small children, at least one of whom is under age six, dramatically decreases the choice of employee as the most important role. The work-oriented women tend to live alone, or with someone other than a husband and children. The only other important factors, out of many hypothesized about the women's past or present situation, are the respondent's earnings and her dependence upon these in the absence of other sources of income. This circumstance is usually due to the absence of a husband and thus competition from the role of wife.

THE HUSBAND-ORIENTED WOMAN

Twenty-eight percent of the women in our sample list the role of wife as the most important one at the present time. These respondents tend to be wives who are currently employed but without children. They tend to have entered that role between the ages of 22 and 24 and to have been married a high proportion of time since age 18. The woman's background characteristics appear not to influence her willingness to list the role of wife first. The "strongest" relation exists between the frequency with which the wives list that role and the characteristics of the husband's job and earnings. The more education the husband has, the higher the Duncan score of his occupation, the more often he is in professional or managerial positions, and the more he earns, the more apt is the woman to place the role of wife first in order of importance. Women whose husbands earn little in low-status jobs are definitely not husband-oriented; instead, the focus of their attention is on the mother role. For example, only 25% of the women whose husbands did not finish high school list the role of wife first, but 45% of those with college-educated husbands do so. The distribution is practically duplicated when Duncan socioeconomic status scores are considered (these figures are in the "Now" column of the role of wife in Table 4). If the family income without the respondent's earnings is under $10,000, the wife is not apt to list that role first, with only 4% doing so. However, 39% of the wives living on incomes of over $25,000 (in addition to their own earnings, if any) are husband-oriented. These are similar to findings of the

1956–1965 studies of women living in the same metropolitan area (Lopata, 1971).

THE CHILD-ORIENTED WOMAN

Women oriented toward the role of mother are most often characterized by having a child under the age of 3 at home. Interestingly enough, increase in the number of children tends to decrease orientation toward the role of mother. Women who had their first child at age 27 or later are more apt to list the role of mother first than are women who entered the role at the early age of 19 or less (61 to 43%). The most apt to be oriented toward this role are women who either live alone with their children or share the household with someone else, but not a husband. Child-oriented women tend to be of a lower socioeconomic background and current standing than are the others, mainly because they experience less competition from the role of wife. When compared to women of other role orientations, child-oriented women are not as apt to be employed, thus decreasing the likelihood of role conflict. Both they and their husbands, if any, reached minimal educational levels. Finally, these women are not apt to see themselves as successful leaders, although the factor of emotionality is not related to the frequency of listing the role of mother first. Of course, the self-images are related to socioeconomic background and status, as is the tendency to list the role of mother first, rather than being directly related to that variable.

MULTIPLE CLASSIFICATION ANALYSIS OF ROLE IMPORTANCE

The use of multiple classification analysis enables us to assess the individual and collective impact of nominal and ordinal variables on a woman's likelihood of describing a role as "most important" at the time of the interview. In addition, multiple classification analysis is especially useful because it calculates the impact of each variable controlling for the other variables in the equation. Because not all of the relationships analyzed here are strictly linear in character, the amount of explained variance remains low, but observing the deviation from the mean gives us added insight into the role hierarchies of the women in our study. This enables us to construct a profile of women who are very likely to select a role as important and a correspondent profile of women who are most unlikely to choose that role.

Involvement in the employee role, combined with the exclusion of familial roles, is the most important factor in the choice of worker or career woman as a woman's most important role. In addition, women who have been employed in professional occupations more than 60% of the time since they were 18 years old and who have a high family income are most likely to choose employee as their most important role. Surprisingly, when controlling for the above variables, women with relatively low educational levels of less than high school are also most apt to choose employee as their most important role. Respondents with high levels of education (college completion) are least likely to choose the role of worker or career woman as important when factors of involvement are controlled. Contrary to initial assumptions, older women choose employee as the most important role more often than do young women, probably because of the lesser significance assigned to the role of mother. Deviations from the mean in the opposite direction are not as strong, possibly because the mean proportion of women who choose employee as the most important role is relatively low. The least likely to choose employee are women who are wives and mothers but are not in paid work, who have worked less than 30% of the time since they were 18 years of age, and who did so in blue-collar occupations. Thus, commitment to the employee role is largely dependent on the lack of involvement in competing familial roles, coupled with long duration of involvement in employment, particularly in professional occupations.

Involvement in the role of wife is the single most important factor in determining whether or not a woman will choose that role as most important, but other characteristics of her involvement in that role have additional impact. The woman most likely to choose the role of wife is married and working outside of the home, but is not a mother. In addition, women aged 45 to 54 who were married at age 18 or younger, whose marriage did not end in divorce or death of the spouse, and whose husbands have graduated from college and have high status and high income jobs are most apt to list the role of wife as of greatest importance to them. Those least likely to so rank the role of wife are employees and mothers now aged 25 to 34 who are not currently married and who were between the ages of 22 and 24 when married the first time. From this information we can see that women highly committed to the role of wife have been in that role continuously and with the same man. In addition, their husbands are likely to be occupationally successful men, a finding that shows little change in the last 20 years.

Actual involvement in the role of mother is the main variable when assessing influences on the importance of that role to women. In addition, the other roles in which a woman is involved in tandem with that of mother strongly affect her choice of that role as the most important. Women who are mothers only—that is, who are not wives or employees at the same time—are the most likely to choose mother as the most important role. Those who are both mothers and wives but not employees are the least likely of the women with children to list the role of mother as most important. A variety of factors that reflect the extent of involvement in the role of mother have added impact on the likelihood of choosing that role. Women currently aged 25 to 34, those who entered the role of mother at a relatively late age of 27 or older, those currently with a child less than 3 years old in the home, and those with either an only child or with five or more children were most likely to choose mother as their most important role at the time of the interview. Older women (aged 45–54) who became mothers while still teenagers and had two children who are already grown are least likely to choose mother as the most important role in their lives at this time. It becomes apparent that *active* involvement in mothering young children is statistically the *most significant* indicator of the likelihood of choosing mother as one's most important role.

CHANGES IN COMMITMENTS TO BASIC ROLES IN THE MIDDLE YEARS

The Chicago area women aged 25 to 54 report some very interesting beliefs as to shifts in their focal role within their middle years of life (see Table 3). Of course, the role hierarchies are affected not only by age and stage in the life-course of the woman but also by historical cohort effects. Women in their early 50s in 1978, when they were interviewed, were born between 1923 and 1928. They experienced the depression when very young but were entering marriage and motherhood during the post-World War II baby boom years in which the roles of mother and wife were accentuated in the extreme in American society (Elder, 1974; Friedan, 1963; Lopata, 1971). Women now in their 20s are apt to have been influenced, on the other hand, by feminism and the push of women to paid employment. The differences are somewhat visible in Table 3 in that more of the youngest cohort of women than of the oldest place the role of worker or career woman in first place in order of importance now, when they were age 24, and when they will be age 55. Still, the differences are not large and could be accounted for by the absence of children, indicating the possibility that this much-publicized shift to the world of work might be exaggerated as far as commitment rather than simple involvement is concerned.

Commitment to the role of wife shows interesting variation, by age and in the life-course overview. The youngest women think that they will be much more oriented toward this role when they reach age 55 than are women now approaching age 55. The older women do not see themselves as having gone through a dramatic swing in their commitment to the role of wife, while all the other women see themselves as having major life or family-cycle shifts. The differences between what the young women think will be important to them at age 55 and what

Table 3. Perceived Life-Course Changes in Focal Role by Current Age of Chicago Area Women

Most important role at age	Current age						
	24–29	30–34	35–39	40–44	45–49	50–54	All
	(%)	(%)	(%)	(%)	(%)	(%)	(%)
Employee							
24	25	20	19	14	13	16	19
Now	21	12	9	11	6	15	14
55	18	16	16	15	9	10	15
Wife							
24	35	31	38	36	33	37	34
Now	26	20	28	29	35	31	28
55	47	49	51	49	48	38	47
Mother							
24	24	34	34	31	36	32	31
Now	39	58	51	46	33	31	44
55	14	7	7	13	10	22	12
Homemaker							
24	5	4	2	4	7	1	4
Now	4	6	6	7	12	12	7
55	3	5	4	2	5	5	4
Other							
24	11	11	7	15	11	14	12
Now	10	4	6	7	14	11	7
55	18	23	22	21	28	25	22
Total (N)[a]	500	346	320	251	237	222	1876

[a]100% is obtained by adding percentages in cells of roles at each time period.

women who are now approaching that age think is also evident, though in less extreme, when we look at the role of mother. Women in their 30s, who are the most likely of any cohort to list the role of mother as very important now, expect it to fade into lesser importance when they get older, while women now in the 50-to-54 age range still consider it important much more frequently. The difference in the percentage of women aged 25 to 29 and those 50 to 54 listing the role of mother as important to them at age 24 is probably due to the fact that the youngest women have delayed motherhood until a later age than the older women.

Whether it is a matter of historical cohort differences or stages in the life-course, the older women in our sample are much more apt than are the youngest respondents to list the role of homemaker as the most important to them now, although it is difficult to explain their anticipated drop in importance of this role within the next few years. It is quite possible that they anticipate a reduction in the size of the household as a source of decreasing the complexity of that role (Lopata, 1966). Finally, we find that all women expect an increase in the importance they will assign to social roles outside of the basic four of wife, mother, homemaker, and employee when they reach age 55. Women in the middle years of life are especially apt to ignore roles outside of this cluster, such as friend, member of a religious group, or citizen. They, as well as women who are now aged 45 to 54, expect to turn to these roles in the future. Only 10% of this increase in the number of respondents expecting such a shift is accounted for by an expansion of the role of grandmother; other roles each contribute a few women. There is surprisingly little variation among the different age cohorts in their view of life-course changes in commitments, except for the women in their 30s who are so heavily involved in the role of mother at the present time.

Looking now at the three roles most apt to be listed as of importance at the top level—those of employee, wife, and mother—by actual involvement we find further corroboration of some of the previous statements. The role of employee is considered the most important "now" by many more employed women who are not also wives or mothers than at "age 24" or "age 55." This is very interesting and supports theories of midlife phasing out of interest in one's occupation first developed by Brim and Wheeler (1966) and Neugarten (1973); see also Ritzer (1977). An alternative explanation is that the younger women expect to enter the roles wife and mother and thus to decrease the importance of the role of career woman or worker in the future. This appears to be true of respondents who are now combining the role of employee and wife and who report that they gave the first of these roles greater importance when they were age 24 than they do now.

Life-course variation in commitment is very evident when we look at the roles of wife and mother (see Table 4). Many of the women who are combining marriage and employment, but not motherhood, at the present time may be anticipating having children, since they drop off the commitment to the role of wife at age 55. Full-time homemakers who are wives and mothers anticipate a definite drop of orientation toward the children when they reach age 55. The same is true of women who combine wife, mother, and employee roles. Interestingly enough, few expect to increase the importance assigned the role of worker and few obviously expect to become widowed.

Although most of the associations are not statistically significant,

Table 4. *Perceived Life-Course Changes in the Focal Social Role by Role Involvement of Chicago Area Women (Mean Proportion Selecting Role as Most Important)*

Role involvement	Employee role			Wife role			Mother role		
	24[a]	Now[b]	55[c]	24	Now	55	24	Now	55
Employee only	.56	.78	.45	07	.00	.27	.01	.01	.03
Employee and wife	.24	.17	.17	.54	.63	.56	.02	.08	.20
Employee and mother	.14	.24	.26	.31	.01	.05	.42	.63	.24
Employee, wife, and mother	.12	.07	.10	.35	.33	.54	.39	.47	.08
Wife and mother	.18	.01	.07	.40	.33	.64	.32	.51	.10
Mother only	.10	.06	.15	.21	.00	.04	.49	.70	.29
All	.19	.14	.15	.34	.28	.47	.31	.44	.12

[a] At age 24 (respondents were all between age 25 and 54 at time of interview).
[b] At the time of the interview.
[c] Anticipated at age 55.

some of the variations within the "most important role" assignment related to such variables as the respondent's education, her earnings, family income, and the family income minus her earnings are worth examining (see Table 5). Although education increases interest in the role of employee, it does not influence life-course attachments. The woman most apt to focus on the role of employee, with a peak at the present time, is one who is totally financially dependent upon her earnings and who does very well in bringing home the money. The drop she expects in focusing on the role of employee is probably due to anticipated marriage, or remarriage, since more women give the role of wife as the most important role of age 55 than do so now, if they are currently single breadwinners. The respondents whose family income is produced mainly by someone other than themselves and is high tend to be husband-oriented, as mentioned before, and a dramatic 71% of all women living on a high income not earned directly by themselves expect to be husband-oriented at age 55. Thus, the pattern is clear: The husband's earnings influence the emphasis by the wife on her relation with him, in the past, present, and future, more than any other variable.

Looking at the life-course commitment to the role of wife by the characteristics of the husband, which proved so important in the "now" period, we find an especially strong trend by wives of highly educated men in prestigious jobs to anticipate a strong orientation toward those

Table 5. Perceived Life-Course Changes in the Importance of the Roles of Employee, Wife, and Mother by the Respondent's Education and Earnings, Combined Family Income, and Family Income without Respondent's Earnings of Chicago Area Women (Mean Proportion Selecting Role as Most Important)

Education, Earnings, Income	Employee role			Wife role			Mother role		
	24[a]	Now[b]	55[c]	24	Now	55	24	Now	55
Respondent's education									
Less than high school	.13	.10	.11	.23	.16	.23	.46	.53	.21
High school graduate	.15	.09	.11	.36	.31	.52	.36	.46	.09
Some college	.21	.18	.16	.40	.30	.56	.30	.41	.08
College graduate	.30	.21	.23	.37	.29	.51	.10	.35	.11
Respondent's earnings									
$1,000–$5,999	.17	.06	.10	.38	.34	.52	.26	.43	.08
$6,000–$9,999	.16	.16	.11	.34	.26	.46	.38	.43	.13
$10,000–$14,999	.24	.33	.23	.31	.23	.40	.25	.32	.10
$15,000+	.35	.46	.40	.25	.21	.30	.21	.26	.09
Family income									
Less than $10,000	.18	.16	.17	.20	.06	.15	.40	.53	.23
$10,000–$14,999	.23	.28	.19	.26	.11	.28	.27	.37	.11
$15,000–$19,999	.20	.05	.10	.38	.32	.60	.34	.52	.09
$20,000–$24,999	.16	.10	.13	.47	.41	.64	.25	.36	.07
Income without respondent's earnings									
0	.35	.54	.35	.16	.04	.18	.21	.29	.15
Low	.17	.11	.14	.26	.19	.29	.39	.48	.18
Medium	.16	.07	.12	.39	.35	.56	.33	.47	.10
High	.17	.04	.09	.47	.39	.71	.25	.43	.06

[a] At age 24 (respondents were all between age 25 and 54 at time of interview).
[b] At the time of the interview.
[c] Anticipated at age 55.

Table 6. Perceived Life-Course Changes in the Importance of the Role of Wife by Husband's Education, Occupational Category, and Duncan Socioeconomic Score for Chicago Area Women (Mean Proportion Selecting Wife as Most Important Role)

	Wife role		
Husband's characteristics	24	Now	55
Husband's education			
Less than high school	.27	.25	.33
High school graduate	.36	.35	.55
Some college	.35	.31	.67
College graduate	.52	.45	.69
Husband's occupation			
Blue-collar	.30	.30	.46
White-collar	.33	.42	.67
Professional	.48	.40	.67
Husband's Duncan score			
0–19	.25	.21	.36
20–39	.36	.35	.47
40–59	.31	.37	.60
60–69	.43	.41	.66
70+	.56	.42	.70

men in the anticipated future (see Table 6). The overall pattern is strong, although the measures of significance are lowered by the lack of consistency. Women whose husbands are in low-prestige jobs certainly never anticipate becoming oriented toward them above all other sets of relations.

The lower the education of the woman, on the other hand, the more apt she is to list the role of mother as the most important role to her now and at the age of 24. And although this emphasis is expected to decrease at age 55 for such women, the stress on motherhood continues more frequently than is true of the women at other educational levels. The higher the earnings of the respondent, the less apt she is to list the role of mother as the most important; such women stress the employee role and are apt not to have children. Total family income has an uneven association with emphasis on the role of mother, except that the women with the least amount of funds tend to be more child-oriented in memories of age 24, at the present time, and in the future.

Finally, a look at Table 7 shows interesting trends in the importance assigned to the role of mother. Respondents for whom the role of moth-

Table 7. Perceived Life-Course Changes in the Importance of the Role of Mother by Age of Respondent at the Birth of the First Child, Age of Youngest Child, and the Number of Children for Chicago Area Women (Mean Proportion Selecting Mother as Most Important Role)

Mothering characteristics	Mother role		
	24	Now	55
Age at birth of first child			
19 or younger	.56	.43	.12
20–22	.58	.52	.10
23–26	.30	.49	.10
27 or older	.15	.61	.16
Age of youngest child			
Less than 3 years old	.25	.75	.09
3 to 5 years old	.45	.64	.15
6 to 17 years old	.38	.51	.14
No child less than 18 years old	.18	.12	.09
Number of children			
0	.01	.03	.10
1	.24	.64	.17
2	.33	.51	.08
3–4	.39	.50	.11
5 or more	.55	.49	.18

er was of primary importance in the remembered age of 24 became mothers at age 22 or younger, but even those who were not yet mothers at that time were oriented toward children in 15% of the cases. On the other hand, mothers who entered that role at a later date, as stated before, really focus on it now and even tend to anticipate a similar focus at age 55 more often than do the other women. The age of the youngest child is an important variable; respondents listing the role of mother as the most important to them now typically have small children. The association is very strong, compared to other associations. On the other hand, the connection between the number of children and the perceived importance of the role of mother is uneven. As mentioned before, it is the mother of one child, rather than the one with multiple offspring, who most often concentrates on this role for now. As the number of children goes up, however, the probability of the mother finding this role important at age 24 and carrying over this importance into older years increases, only the mother of one child expects continued concentration on the role of mother as often as does the parent of five or more children. The one-child mother is likely to have that offspring a bit later in life and to have it by choice. She is also more educated than are the mothers of two or three children, and thus more conscious of the importance of the mother for developing the child.

SUMMARY AND CONCLUSIONS

The series of studies of metropolitan women just described indicates how they organize their roles within the role-cluster and over time, assigning hierarchical rank to those in which they are actually involved. The role of employee takes primary focus mainly when the roles of wife and mother are absent from a woman's current life, and only 14% of women aged 25 to 54 in the most recent study assign it first place. Thus, the mass media image of the "new American woman," committed to occupation above family, is simply not reflected in reality, at least among Chicago area women, a finding consistent with those reported in *The Inner American* (Veroff, Douvan, and Kulka, 1981). Even the professionals do not rank it first if they are wives or mothers, and especially if they are both. Husband-oriented women tend not to have children and/or are married to men with a high educational background who are in high-paying and high-prestige jobs. One assumes that such marriages are more demanding of the role of wife and that the woman is more conscious of the contribution made to the home by the husband than are women whose spouse brings home relatively little money from a low-prestige job. Child-oriented women tend to have only one child or to have very young children and to have entered this role relatively late in life. They often lack the role of wife and even employee. The home-oriented woman is almost absent from this sample, although twice the proportion of such Chicagoans existed in the 1956–1965 data (14 to 7%; see Lopata, 1971). Societal and kin roles outside of the family of procreation did not fare well in this study, except among employees who are not married or mothers.

The women in the recent study tend to see their involvement in social roles in life-course terms, expecting a shift from the role of mother to that of wife if they are involved now in child-rearing. Women close to the age of 55, which was used for projections of role importance in the future, tend to see themselves as having shifted emphasis much less often than do the younger women. Those nearing age 55 do not anticipate major changes in the near future, except for an increase of involvement in roles outside of the basic complex of wife and mother. There is no strong projected shift by any women toward the role of employee in the future, in spite of the probability of divorce or widowhood by the time they reach age 55. Roles outside of the home, such as those of friend, member of a religious group, citizen, or neighbor, are expected to increase in importance in their future on the part of women of all ages in 1978, although the respondents now between age 50 and 54 are not as yet so involved. Over twice as many expect roles outside of the family to be of primary importance at age 55 than are so involved at ages 50 to 54.

The strong emphasis on the role of mother, especially by women who have young children and who themselves tend to be in their 30s, as well as the anticipated shift to the role of wife as children become less dependent, reflects American culture and the reality of life. Women's projections into the future show strong differences between what younger women think they will value most when they become age 55 and what women close to that age regard as important at the present time. The younger women think the role of mother will recede in importance much more often than is true of the older women. The younger women are also much more apt to expect the wife role to become very important in the future than older women find it to be. Of course, we do not know if this is a historical or an age phenomenon.

The Chicago area women whom we have studied over the years tend to be relatively traditional. Their stress on the role of mother reflects the value system of American culture. A major difference between the 1956 and the 1978 respondents is the devaluation of the role of housewife, which is not surprising in view of the modern trends in the society. Role conflict is alleviated through the process of assigning hierarchical placement to roles in which the women are actually involved and that demand most from them according to the value system: motherhood when the children are small, wifehood if the husband is in a demanding and rewarding occupation, and employment if those two roles are absent from the role-cluster.

REFERENCES

Bernard, J. *Women and the public interest.* Chicago: Aldine, 1971.
Bernard, J. *The future of marriage.* New York: Bantam, 1973.
Bernard, J. The housewife: Between two worlds. In P. L. Stewart and M. G. Cantor (Eds.), *Varieties of work experience.* New York: Wiley, 1974.
Bernard, J. *Women, wives, mothers: Values and options.* Chicago: Aldine, 1975. (a)
Bernard, J. *The future of motherhood.* New York: Penguin, 1975. (b)
Bernard, J. *The female world.* New York: Free Press, 1981.
Biddle, B. J., and Thomas, E. J. (Eds.). *Role theory.* New York: Wiley, 1966.
Bird, C. *The two-paycheck marriage.* New York: Rawson Wade, 1979.
Brim, O., and Wheeler, S. *Socialization after childhood.* New York: Wiley, 1966.
Chapman, J. R., and Gates, M. (Eds.). *Women into wives: The legal and economic impact of marriage.* Beverly Hills: Sage, 1977.
Coser, R. L. The complexity of roles as a seedbed of individual autonomy. In L. A. Coser

(Ed.), *The idea of social structure: Papers in honor of Robert K. Merton.* New York: Harcourt Brace Jovanovich, 1975, Pp. 237–263.

Dyer, E. D. Parenthood as crisis: A restudy. *Marriage and Family Living,* 1963, 25, 196–201.

Easton, B. L. Industrialization and femininity: A case study of 19th century New England. *Social Problems,* 1976, 23, 389–401.

Ehrenreich, B., and English, D. *For her own good: 150 years of the experts' advice to women.* Garden City, N.Y.: Anchor Books, 1979.

Elder, G. H. *Children of the Great Depression: Social change in life experience.* Chicago: University of Chicago Press, 1974.

Evans, P. A. L., and Bartolome, F. The relationship between professional life and private life. In C. B. Derr (Ed.), *Work, family and the career.* New York: Praeger, 1980. Pp. 281–317.

Fowlkes, M. *Behind every successful man: Wives of medicine and academe.* New York: Columbia University Press, 1980.

Friedan, B. *The feminine mystique.* New York: Norton, 1963.

Goode, W. A theory of role strain. *American Sociological Review,* 1960, 25, 483–496.

Gouldner, A. W. Cosmopolitan and locals. *Administrative Science Quarterly,* 1957, December, 281–306.

Gross, N., Mason, W., and McEadern, A. *Explorations in role analysis: Studies of school superintendency role:* New York: Wiley, 1958.

Hobbs, D. F., Jr. Parenthood as crisis: A third study. *Journal of Marriage and the Family,* 1965, 17, 367–372.

Kahn, R. L., Wolf, D. M., Quinn, R. P., Snoeck, J. D. and Rosenthal, R. A. *Organizational stress: Studies in role conflict and ambiguity.* New York: Wiley, 1964.

Komarovsky, M. Cultural contradictions and sex roles. *American Journal of Sociology,* 1946, 52, 182–189.

Laws, J. L. *The second X: Sex role and social role.* New York: Elsevier, 1979.

LeMasters, E. E. Parenthood as crisis: *Marriage and Family Living,* 1957, 19, 252–355.

Lerner, G. *The woman in American history.* Menlo Park, Calif.: Addison-Wesley. 1971.

Lopata, H. Z. The life cycle of the social role of housewife. *Sociology and Social Research,* 1966, 41, 5–22.

Lopata, H. Z. *Occupation: Housewife.* New York: Oxford University Press, 1971.

Lopata, H. Z. *Widowhood in an American city.* Cambridge, Mass.: Schenkman, General Learning Press, 1973.

Lopata, H. Z. *Women as widows: Support systems.* New York: Elsevier/North Holland, 1975.

Lopata, H. Z., Barnewolt, D., and Miller, C. A. *City women: Work, jobs, occupations, careers.* New York: Praeger, in press.

Lopata, H. Z., Barnewolt, D., and Norr, K. Spouses' contribution to each other's roles. In F. Pepitone-Rockwell (Ed.), *Dual career couples.* Beverly Hills: Sage, 1980. Pp. 111–142.

Lopata, H. Z., and Norr, K. *Changing commitments of American women to work and family roles and their future consequences for social security.* Final report to the Social Security Administration, 1979.

Lopata, H. Z., and Norr, K. Changing commitments of American women to work and family roles. *Social Security Bulletin,* 1980, 43, 3–14.

Lopata, H. Z., and Pleck, J. H. (Eds.). *Research in the interweave of social roles: Jobs and families.* Greenwich, Conn.: JAI Press, 1983.

Mack, R. W. Occupational determinateness: A problem and hypothesis in role theory. *Social Forces,* 1956, 35, 20–25.

Merton, R. The role set. *British Journal of Sociology,* 1957, 8, 106–120.

Merton, R. *Social theory and social structure.* Glencoe, Ill.: Free Press, 1968.

Merton, R. K., Reader, G. G., and Kendall, P. L., eds. *The student-physician.* Cambridge, Mass.: Harvard University Press, 1957.

Mortimer, J., Hall, R., and Hill, R. Husbands' occupational attributes as constraints on wives' employment. *Sociology of Work and Occupations,* 1978, 5, 285–314.

Nadelson, C. C., and Nadelson, T. Dual-career marriages: Benefits and costs. In F. Pepitone-Rockwell (Ed.), *Dual career couples.* Beverly Hills: Sage, 1980. Pp. 91–110.

Neugarten, B. L. *Middle age and aging.* Chicago: University of Chicago Press, 1973.

Newcomb, T. M., Turner, R. H., and Converse, P. E. *Sociol psychology: The study of human interaction.* New York: Holt, Rinehart & Winston, 1965.

Pleck, J. H. *Work and family roles: From sex-patterned segregation to integration.* Paper presented at the annual meeting of the American Sociological Association, 1975.

Pleck, J. H. Men's family work: Three perspectives and some new data. *Family Coordinator,* 1979, October, 481–488.

Pleck, J. H. Husband's paid work and family roles: Current research issues. In H. Z. Lopata and J. H. Pleck (Eds.), *Research in the interweave of social roles: Jobs and families.* Greenwich, Conn.: JAI Press, 1983: 251–333.

Poloma, M. M. Role conflict and the married professional woman: In C. Safilios-Rothschild (Ed.), *Toward a sociology of women.* Lexington, Mass.: Xerox College Publishing, 1972. Pp. 187–198.

Poloma, M. M., and Garland, T. The married professional woman: A study of tolerance of domestication. *Journal of Marriage and the Family,* 1971, 33, 531–540.

Rapoport, R., and Rapoport, R. N. *Dual career families.* Harmondsworth, England: Penguin, 1971.

Rapoport, R., and Rapoport, R. N. *Dual career families re-examined.* New York: Harper Colophon, 1976.

Ritzer, G. *Working: Conflict and change.* Englewood Cliffs, N.J.: Prentice-Hall, 1977.

Rossi, A. Transition to parenthood, *Journal of Marriage and the Family,* 1968, 30, 26–37.

Rothman, S. M. *Women's proper place: A history of changing ideals and practices.* New York: Basic Books, 1978.

Sicherman, B. Review essay: American history. *Signs,* 1975, 1(Winter), 461–485.

Vandervelde, M. *The changing Life of the corporate wife.* New York: Mecox, 1979.

Veroff, J., Douvan, E., and Kulka, R. *The inner American.* New York: Basic Books, 1981.

Whyte, W. H., Jr. *The organization man.* New York: Simon & Schuster, 1956.

Znaniecki, F. W. *The social role of the man of knowledge.* New York: Columbia University Press, 1940.

Znaniecki, F. W. *Social relations and social roles.* San Francisco: Chandler. 1965.

Chapter 5

Multiple Roles of Midlife Women
A Case for New Directions in Theory, Research, and Policy

JUDY LONG AND KAREN L. PORTER

INTRODUCTION

The flexible boundaries of the midlife period are sometimes said to include persons from ages 35 to 64. Midlife is a heterogeneous category, subsuming decisively different life courses. What "midlife" entails is a function, at least in part, of experiences and transitions in earlier periods. Women who currently fall into this category include the first of the baby boom, the veterans of the Feminine Mystique and the Great Depression eras and more than a few flappers. Different birth cohorts among today's midlife women experienced predictable life transitions in different historical times. In addition, individuals within birth cohorts differ in the timing, sequencing, spacing, and duration of such life transitions as completing schooling, starting a family, and establishing careers.

Schooling, working, and family life can be thought of as multiple careers, developing at different rates within the individual's life-span. Midlife represents a period in the unrolling of the multiple careers that stems from the multiple roles enacted by women. The midlife period brings a series of life transitions that may include changes or disruptions in family life, changes in labor force participation, and alterations in emphasis or priority among women's multiple roles.

JUDY LONG • Department of Sociology, Syracuse University, Syracuse, New York 13210. KAREN L. PORTER • Maxwell School, Health Studies Program, 712 Ostrom Avenue, Syracuse, New York 13210.

Our particular interest in this chapter is with how women's roles affect their economic viability at midlife and after. Occupational and marital careers, in particular, are major determinants of a woman's economic situation both at midlife and in old age. Many women who are now in midlife will face poverty in old age, given their current employment and marital history and the existing public programs available to aid them. There is clearly a role for public policy in ensuring the future well-being of today's midlife women. Public programs must be responsive to the diverse needs of distinct subpopulations within the midlife category. Innovations and modifications in public policy are indicated on the basis of analysis of the needs of current midlife women.

Existing public programs appear to be informed by faulty social science. Distortions in social science theorizing and research on older women are reflected in the provisions and rationales of programs on which many women will depend in old age. The shortcomings of current social science perspectives on older women must also be corrected if they are to be the basis of a rational and equitable social policy.

The latter half of the female life cycle has been too little studied. Perhaps as a consequence, midlife has more often been treated as a terminus than as a transition. An overemphasis on women's family roles has led to characterizations of midlife as a time of loss and diminishment for women. Current research contests the pervasive images of midlife women as losers and has-beens. The focus on women's family roles has led to a neglect of economic outcomes for women. When employment of women who are in midlife today is analyzed, it is usually in terms of "jobs" rather than "careers." Many questions concerning women's experience in the labor market have not been investigated. Among the most critical are the questions of long-run economic outcomes for employed women.

At present, of a total female population of 116 million, slightly more than 36 million (or 31%) are between the ages of 35 and 64 (U.S. Bureau of the Census, 1981). Midlife women, as a share of the population, can be expected to increase in the future as a result of both the size of the younger birth cohorts and gains in life expectancy. The life expectancies at birth for women born in 1920, 1930, and 1940 are 55, 62, and 65 years, respectively (U.S. Bureau of the Census, 1976). Women aged 45 in 1978 can now expect to live to age 80 (U.S. Bureau of the Census, 1981). According to the most conservative census projections, by the year 2000 the number of midlife women between the ages of 35 and 64 will have increased to slightly more than 50 million, approximately 42% of the entire female population (U.S. Bureau of the Census, 1978).

Each birth cohort ages in a unique way, as it lives through a distinct history. Nevertheless, women who are now in midlife shared certain experiences that distinguish their life trajectories from those of women now in their 20s or early 30s. Available options in life-styles, as well as the timing, spacing, sequence, and duration of major life transitions, are major factors determining the situation of women at midlife.

Most of the women now in midlife married. When they reached nubility at or after the Second World War, the marriage rate reached a record high. Between 1945 and 1947, an average of 143 first marriages were taking place for every 1000 single women aged 14 to 44. Since 1947, the marriage rate has declined steadily and the divorce rate, declining until the 1963–65 period, has risen steadily since. Between 1970 and 1978, the number of never-married women between the ages of 25 and 34 increased by 111%, the number of divorced women of the same ages who had not remarried rose by 170%, while the number of married women climbed only 17% (U.S. Bureau of the Census, 1978). The result is an increase in the number of single older women in the 1980s.

Most of today's midlife women remain married, however. In 1980, of all women aged 35 to 64, 77% were married either in a first and only marriage or by remarriage after widowhood or divorce. Another 9% were divorced, 5% single, and 9% widowed (U.S. Bureau of the Census, 1981).

Most of today's midlife women bore children. Women now in their early 40s to early 50s married at earlier ages, gave birth to more children, began childbearing sooner, and completed childbearing in a span of just over 7 years, on the average, compared to their mothers and older sisters (Norton, 1980). The diminution of family responsibilities has implications for women's availability for labor force participation in midlife. The contraction of the child-intensive phase of family life, in the context of ever-increasing life expectancy, has implications for a woman's work expectancy at midlife, whatever her work history in previous periods.

Though normative disapproval of working mothers was strong during the years when today's midlife women had young children, the statistics show that labor-force participation of this group has never been negligible. At midcentury, the labor force participation rates for women aged 20 to 24 and 25 to 34 were among the highest of all groups of women (46 and 34%, respectively; U.S. Bureau of the Census, 1976). Moreover, the greatest increases in labor force participation since World War II have been among mothers with school-age children. Currently, 66% of the women aged 35 to 44, 60% of the women aged 45 to 54, and 42% of the women aged 55 to 64 are employed in the civilian labor force (U.S. Bureau of the Census, 1981). Estimates of work-life expectancy indicate that the labor force attachment of women at midlife and after exceeds that of men (Laws, 1979). Though midlife women are the fastest-growing segment in the female labor force, the poverty rates for women at midlife (aged 35 to 44—11%; 45 to 54—9%; 55 to 59—11%; and 60 to 64—13%) are rather high compared with the rates for men of the same ages (8%, 7%, 6%, and 8%, respectively; U.S. Bureau of the Census, 1982). A wage differential between the sexes persists. Women who exhibit labor-force participation patterns different from those of men receive penalties in the form of lower wages for comparable jobs. Differences in labor force histories among midlife women place them in different positions with respect to economic viability in later life.

A study by Neugarten and Brown-Rezanka (1978) illustrates the heterogeneity of the midlife population. The authors compare demographic features and life outcomes of three adjacent cohorts of women. The cohort exiting midlife contains a disproportionate number of women who remained single until age 30 or older, and many married women who delayed childbearing until their late 20s or remained childless altogether. The cohort entering midlife married earlier and had more children, on the average, than the preceding cohort. The cohort that was to enter midlife by the end of the 1980s exhibited lower fertility expectations and higher educational rates than either previous cohort.

Today it makes sense to ask what the latter half of life holds for women, in terms of work rewards, success, satisfaction, and economic security. It is revealing and significant that these questions have only rarely been asked. Though social scientists have, in recent years, taken cognizance of women's work roles, discussion has for the most part assumed that women have jobs, and men careers. Consequently, success, level of rewards, and commitment are rarely the focus of research on women's employment. Conversely, women in the first half of life have been discussed primarily in terms of family roles. Only recently has the second half of the female life-span been examined in detail. Yet current work has made it clear that many aspects of women's lives at midlife are problematic. Among the most notable features of midlife is an economic vulnerability that derives directly from the combination of work and family history.

With changing marital status and childbearing patterns, more and more women are finding themselves alone in midlife. Changes in family roles and the timing and spacing of births have resulted in longer periods of time after the youngest child leaves home and before retirement age: It tends to be assumed that income is accumulating during this time. For the married woman, midlife may be a period of income accumulation. But for the woman who has lost her spouse, the risk of poverty is great.

The ideal of economic self-sufficiency among women was not part of the sex-role script when today's midlife women were being socialized for their adult roles. More to the point, the sex-role prescriptions for the marital relationship required the husband to support his wife, and often to deal with all financial matters. The sexual division of labor minimized women's financial responsibilities. One consequence is that most women are poorly prepared to support themselves, and to compete in the job market when separated from their husband's income. Women at midlife who are widowed, separated, or divorced are at risk of poverty.

As we seek to assess the condition of women at midlife, and to predict their future well-being, three strands of social science theory and research have contributions to make: the literature on occupations and careers, the work on "dual roles," and the tradition of the study of the life-course. In each of these are to be found omissions and distortions that limit their applicability to the situation of midlife women today. New orientations and new research are required in order to realize the potential benefits of these three perspectives.

Research on occupational roles and the research on the articulation of work and family roles have a common basis in role theory. Research on careers and the life-course share a common focus on transitions among statuses over time. Nevertheless, these traditions, which have potentially so much to contribute to each other, have developed in parallel, with very little intercommunication or complementarity. In part, this outcome can be traced to the different subject populations studied under each focus. Ideally, theories of roles, careers, or the life-course should be generic in form, capable of explaining variations in terms of the same general principles. In fact, however, most of the research on careers has focused on men. Research on "dual roles" has until recently dealt exclusively with women. Much of the life-course research has focused on transitions among what used to be called "stages of the family life cycle," which were widely assumed to have their primary impact on women. Role theory is generic in form but rests upon research in which men's work experience predominates. Thus, theory and research that bear on midlife women are substantially sex-segregated, thereby imposing regrettable limits on social science contributions to date.

In this chapter, we will attempt to integrate the contributions from the literature on occupations and careers, role theory, and the life-course perspective. We will indicate directions for future research to carry forward the understanding of midlife women. In addition, a rational social policy relates to the economic vulnerability of midlife women based on their roles will be provided.

Occupations and Careers: "Generic Theory"

The world of work, and social science portraits of it, is dominated by imagery, vocabulary, normative judgments, and timetables that are masculine in culture and framed to the experience of males (Derr, 1980).

Each of these elements carries a freight of evaluation (which is generally not subjected to analysis), so that vocabulary, imagery, and timetables that describe men are considered dominant and normal, and those that characterize women are considered deviant.[1] Such judgments, unconscious though they are, constitute a normative climate in which the occupational efforts of midlife women are received. Public policy and social science theory appear to be colored with the same normative slant, and do injustice to midlife women in similar ways.

Theories of vocational development set the tone for the normative manner of participation in the labor force. A good deal of convergence is apparent in commonly cited models of career choice and career commitment. They picture a world in which the young person moves upward in an educational structure that contains information about possible occupational options. Social and familial networks contain role models, sponsors, and advisors. Opportunities for role rehearsal, for summer or part-time work may be made available. Education, its content and direction, is assumed to be instrumental for future occupational attainment. Adults' ambitions are often projected onto the young person; they feel involved and have a stake in future success that will reflect upon them. A unified atmosphere of expectation, support, and benevolent anxiety about future occupational success hovers throughout the school years, if not before. Occupational choices themselves reflect success or failure before occupational role enactment—the occupational career *per se*—begins.

The normative timetable for careers assumes entry into the work force and the establishment of a career as a task of early adulthood. For men, it is the primary task, and violation of the timetable tends to be seen as a reflection on the individual and a threat to ultimate career success. Occupational success is assumed to follow a parabola of increasing rank and reward throughout early and middle adulthood, peaking and then reaching a plateau that may be maintained through late adulthood to retirement. The presumed isomorphism of this occupational script and the human life-span has been attacked by Sarason (1977).[2]

---

[1] The usage of the terms *dominant* and *deviant* is taken from Laws (1975).

[2] Nevertheless, the unconscious sexism of this normative model continues to be perpetuated in current work on careers. For Karp and Yoels (1981), the chronological life and work life are virtually coterminus, illustrating the essence of "career" as an ordered progression of ages or stages. Their unexamined assumptions about the nature of the occupational career include the following: that it involves an individual for the entire period from approximately age 18 to age 65; that it requires an early start; and that it is always "regular," i.e., upwardly mobile in a steady, predictable fashion. When it is not regular, it is deviant. The discussion of why women were excluded from their analysis is relegated to a single *footnote*.

It has now become commonplace to criticize these theories for their lack of applicability to women. The critique has been instrumental in stimulating inquiry into the processes by which young women develop occupational intentions (Laws, 1979) and choose adult life-styles (see Angrist and Almquist, 1975). Undoubtedly, the critique has undergirded the great increase in detailed studies of women's occupational lives that have appeared in the last decade.

The availability of such a body of data permits comparisons between the occupational experiences of women and men. These, in turn, shed new light on the theories and allow us to identify more clearly the substructure of male cultural experience on which the theories are constructed. Among the dimensions that enhance the fit of theories of occupational careers and male experience are the following: (1) It is clear that the theories assume continuity between childhood and adulthood, between school life and work life. (2) The career and the demands of the occupational role take clear priority over other roles and commitments. (3) The peers who monitor and the superiors who reward occupational performance are men. Careers that follow this script are normal, and these features of a career are assumed to be requisite for success.

These elements seem to be part of the structure of careers, and of career success. In the occupational world, for example, the most prestigious and best-paid occupations are those in which the concentration of males is very high, especially in the upper ranks. It is understood that spectacular careers require sacrifices, particularly in the early years. For the professions, this means extended schooling. For business and the professions, it means that the time demands of the job may be double the standard work week. Compartmentalization of work and personal life may be impossible. In addition to long hours, career commitment requires open-ended and flexible availability to the demands of the work or the employer. Lower priority plans such as recreation, or activities centered on self or family, may be canceled when duty calls. Throughout the world of work, the highly significant distinction between exempt and nonexempt employees is understood to mean that the former do not get paid for overtime. When we are speaking of careers (as contrasted with jobs), it is understood that *any* organization or employer possesses the characteristics of the "greedy institutions" analyzed by Coser (1974).

These dimensions of the career script operate not only in the expectations of recruits and those who supervise and reward them but in institutional arrangements as well. Researchers have written about the impact on women of entering and trying to function in work settings that are predominately and traditionally male (Bayes and Newton, 1978; Bernard, 1964; Harragan, 1977; Kanter, 1977a, 1977b; Laws, 1975; Laws and Tangri, 1979; Lorber, 1975; Wolman and Frank, 1972).

For the most part, these writers have neglected the role of prior socialization—sex-role socialization, in essence—in rendering such environments intelligible and conquerable. Yet for each of the dimensions of the career script discussed above, evidence is available that shows the link to sex-role socialization. The experiences of females and males diverge long before high school students seek vocational counseling, and long before individuals encounter the first day on the job.

Both girls and boys acquire detailed cognitive maps of the sex-segregated labor market early, and can render them for the social researcher by the time they are in the second grade; not only do boys and girls project different future occupations, but girls project marriage and family life, while boys do not even mention them (Looft, 1971). A difference in expectations regarding occupational planning is apparent in even second-graders. Females envision their future lives in terms of dual roles. Familial roles enter their calculations even when they are explicitly being queried about future occupational roles. Marital and familial roles do not loom so large in the future planning of school-age boys. Evidence that young girls expect to give priority to family obligations can be found very early. Later, even when occupational aspirations are being articulated, there is some awareness that the exigencies of marriage may interfere with occupational intentions (Davis, 1964; Mahajah, 1966).[3] Research demonstrating that it does so is plentiful (Mulvey, 1963; Tangri, 1972; Harmon, 1969; Levitt, 1971).

Even in the absence of awareness, discontinuities occur in the female life-span. Research on sex-role socialization indicates that boys are more rigorously sanctioned for sex-role conformity than are girls, at preschool and schoolage. Until puberty, girls enjoy greater license for androgyny than boys. At puberty, however, new restrictions are placed on girls. For college-going youth, the student role may offer a moratorium on adult sex roles. For the female student, this may mean support for serious academic commitment and career preparation. However, at some point the sex-role norm according priority to family roles is applied, and the student, dismayed, finds that parents are no longer interested in what she is learning and achieving, but only in her social life (Komarovsky, 1946).

The expectation of marriage brings with it the expectation of discontinuity in labor force participation. Although current data show a clear trend for women's labor-force attachment to converge with that of men

---

[3]Data collected in 1980 from kindergarten and fourth-grade boys and girls by Grace Baruch and Rosalind Barnett indicated that with respect to occupational aspirations, boys made more traditionally sex-typed and more prestigious choices than did girls, and these differences were more pronounced among the older group (fourth-graders).

(Kreps and Clark, 1975), it is still considered normal for women to remain at home with young children, perhaps reentering the labor force when the children are in school full time. For women now at midlife, the force of this norm was even stronger than it is at present. (For a compilation of public-opinion data on employment of mothers during the years when midlife women were in their childbearing years, see Oppenheimer, 1970, p. 45 ff.)

Intermittent labor force participation, as both norm and behavior, illustrates the priority that family responsibilities are supposed to have for women. This priority, the converse of that which is normative for men, is imputed *even where it does not apply*. Women in the labor force are treated *as though* they are mothers with unremitting and overriding responsibility for children who have not yet achieved basic competence. Sawhill (1973) has demonstrated that sex differentials in earnings, often attributed to women's intermittent labor force participation, persist in lifetime earnings curves *even of women with no intermittency*. Studies of male managers' attitudes toward women in management show that they believe women would refuse transfers, increased responsibilities, and extra time demands—elements consistent with the male career script. In these studies, the attitudes are not connected with the respondents' experience with females in management (Rosen and Jerdee, 1974a). Lorber (1975) has pointed out that male colleagues and superiors feel a concern for women's loyalty as organization members that is linked to their putative status as mothers. That is to say, the norm of dual role enactment and priority of family responsibilities suffices to create in men the *expectation* that women colleagues are of a different motivational type than themselves.

The difference between women and men in expectations for the share of responsibility they will take for their home and children appears to be established early in the process of sex-role socialization. As we have seen, dual role expectations are in evidence very early in girls. Boys, on the other hand, are sanctioned for exhibiting any "contrasex" attributes or interests, among which nurturing ranks high. Interestingly, it is men who sanction sex-role behavior, particularly in boys. A strong negative connection is established between the self and anything that is sex-typed as feminine. A reaction of "not me" in response to "feminine" spheres affects males' occupational choices and, indeed, their orientation toward spouse and family roles in relation to their work role in adulthood. As a result of sex-role socialization, it seems likely that males grow up with stronger boundaries dividing them from girls than the girls experience, and greater psychological distance from females than females feel toward males. This discrepancy will affect women's occupational mobility at any age. Although their own expectations are likely to correspond to the male career script, their bosses will have great difficulty in applying the male career model to women (Laws, 1975; Nieva and Gutek, 1980).

The analysis of sex-role socialization suggests dimensions that underlie and affect the interactions of women and men in mutually contingent work roles in their adult years. Even where work roles are symmetrical or complementary, women and men are likely to have different expectations of each other, as a function of sex-role socialization. Available literature suggests that sex-role scripts may be more definitive in men's treatment of their female colleagues than the reverse. In many work organizations, both women and men confront a situation in which the normal incumbent of their occupational role is male and a female incumbent is anomalous. The impact of this situation on female and male is likely to be quite different.

Part of this difference results from sex differences in earlier socialization, for immersion in male work groups and peer groups, headed by male authority figures, is a component of male sex-role socialization. Harragan (1977), in describing the corporate work environment, emphasizes the importance of team sports and the armed forces as models for work life and as training grounds for participation in a world of work organized along similar principles. Team sports, in particular, provide another source of continuity from school to work for many men who are now adults and for very few women of the same birth cohorts. For women who are now at midlife, compulsory and desultory gym class was their only involvement in athletics during the school years, and provided little in the way of models for adult work life. Bernard (1978) has commented on how different the organizational environment is for female and male, where the latter is secure in being backed up by his peers and the former becomes increasingly aware that she is in alien territory. Laws (1975) holds that individuals who are in the structural niche of the "token woman" do not initially perceive much difference between themselves and male peers, and assume that gender is irrelevant for the latter, too. They are concentrating on the task; they define themselves, in the work context, in terms of their skills and credentials. The irony is that both the token woman and her majority peer are focusing on what is unusual about her: For the woman, it is her achievements and abilities, and for the man, it is her gender. The different contexts in which they have grown up account for a difference in perception that is unlikely ever to be discussed or analyzed.

The literature on careers, then, is of limited relevance for midlife women—or midlife men (see Sarason, 1977; Brim, 1975; Weick, 1976)—in its present form. Both theory and research need to be developed in the direction of incorporating the multiple roles of workers and the varying trajectories of work and other roles over the life-span. It will be of primary importance, if outcomes for midlife women are to be understood, to study the sex structuring of work roles and the world of work.

"DUAL ROLES" AND ROLE CONFLICT

Sociology, as the study of the doings of men, reflects an emphasis on "public" life and public deeds as more important, more challenging, and altogether more worthy than the study of private life. The relative prestige of the study of social stratification and the study of marriage and the family, or the sociology of science versus the sociology of sex roles, tells that story.

It is in this context that we must understand the characteristics of the sociology of occupations and careers. Two characteristics of particular relevance to the study of women at midlife are the neglect of family roles and the normative status of a *single role* vision of work and success. As the preceding section made clear, workers (particularly in the professions, from which models of work and careers appear to be drawn) are viewed as though they occupy only one role or (what is normatively the same) as though only one role matters. This "myth of monism" (Laws, 1976) means that one role is normal and "dual roles" are deviant. When we examine the literature on dual roles for its contributions to the study of women at midlife, we must bear this in mind.

On no other basis can we understand the fact that the term dual roles, with the tradition of analysis peculiar to it, is used with reference only to women, even though a superficial recognition of men's roles is to be found in the literature. This recognition does not enter into discussion of men's occupational role enactment and careers, however. Men's dual roles do not officially exist. In contrast, women do not officially exist in discussions of careers except in the context of dual roles.

The study of role conflict has been an enduring concern of role theory in its generic form. However, research attempting to study the causes of and defenses against role conflict as set forth in theory has focused on men (Ritt, 1971; Ritzer, 1969; Rizzo *et al.*, 1970). Research on role conflict in women, on the other hand, has an *ad hoc* quality and ordinarily tests no systematic theory. Thus, the work on men neglects their multiple roles, while the work on women remains outside the mainstream of role theory.

Role Conflict in the World of Work: Generic Theory

A strong theme in the study of people at work has been the problem of role conflict. A number of different forms or aspects of role conflict have been discussed over the years, although not all have received empirical confirmation. Role conflict may arise from incompatible expectations associated with two different roles occupied by an individual, or from contradictory expectations that are part of the same role, or from lack of congruence between the role and the person (or role incumbent). Role ambiguity and role overload are also discussed as sources of role strain, the former referring to problems arising in knowing how to behave, due to inadequate specification of role expectations, and the latter to an excess of demands over time available for role enactment, although the demands themselves are not incompatible. Role diversity, or the number of different role relationships in which a person is involved, is also mentioned as a source of strain (Snoek, 1966). A distinction is sometimes made between objective role conflict and subjective role conflict. The term *role strain* is often used in the sense of subjective role strain. Indications are that the distinction between objective role conflict (the existence of the conditions listed above) and subjective role conflict (a psychological phenomenon) is one that should be observed more frequently in the study of role conflict.

Goode (1960) holds that role strain, or felt difficulty in fulfilling role obligations, is a normal condition and not a crisis or a disaster. It is a direct consequence of two related facts. Multiple role occupancy ensures that there will be contradictory demands on the person—that is, interrole conflict—at least some of the time. A second factor probably increases the occurrence of role conflict: By implication, role partners rush in to fill this vacuum, and the role pressures they generate are the direct source of conflict for the focal person. *The importance of role partners as a source of role conflict has been consistently underestimated in theory and research.* Yet, as we shall see, role partners are particularly critical in women's experience in the world of work.

As role strain is normal, so are the maneuvers by which role incumbents lessen, neutralize, or redefine the role expectations that, mediated by role partners, induce role strain. Mechanisms of role articulation include (1) compartmentalization of roles, (2) delegation of role performances, (3) elimination of roles, and (4) role accumulation (Goode, 1960). It is possible that various styles in enacting roles also constitute strategies for reducing role conflict—as, for example, Goffman's (1961) notion of role distancing.

The use of strategies of role articulation (Coser and Rokoff, 1971) is taken for granted, and evidence of their utilization has been found in studies of men in industry (Pugh, 1966; Ritzer, 1969) and stockbrokers, among others (Evan and Levin, 1966). Indeed, adeptness in role articulation appears to be one of the skills required by the work role. Strategies for reducing role strain are discussed in the vocabulary of games as rule-governed exchanges in which players can appreciate skillful moves, even when these do not advance their own side (cf. Spreitzer, Snyder, and Larson, 1979). Goode (1960) and others who followed employ an elaborate economic metaphor in discussing the active negotiation of the role incumbent in seeking to establish a "role bargain" with his role partners. Given the fundamental reality of role strain resulting from multiple role incumbency, the individual cannot satisfy all role expectations and hence bargains for the best deal he can make (Goode, 1960). In terms of the dimensions later developed by Sieber (1974), the individual tries to gain the maximum role rights in combination with the minimum role obligations. One of the most important issues as yet unaddressed in the role theory corpus is the bargaining positions of women and men *qua* women and men, and their bargaining positions vis-à-vis each other.

Although there is consensus on the range of strategies available to the individual suffering from role stress, there is little research as yet that sheds light on the factors that determine which strategy the individual selects. It seems likely that situational and personal characteristics have some influence. In addition, the source of role pressures—whether time pressure, simultaneous competing demands, or role partners—might indicate what response is most likely to be selected. Ritzer (1969) found that male personnel managers selected different strategies for reducing role conflict, depending on the relative power of themselves and their role partners. Independent, unilateral action was the most preferred response, but compromise or conformity was the choice if the role partner was more powerful than the focal person. Among men, withdrawal was the least favored response. The issue of relative power of women and men has become a ubiquitous issue in research on women and men in business and the professions (cf. Laws and Tangri, 1979) and will surely need to be addressed in research and policy bearing on careers of women at midlife and after.

Another issue that deserves the attention of researchers is the question of differential outcomes resulting from strategies for reduction of role conflict. Hall (1972) found that of three fundamental strategies for conflict reduction—structural role redefinition, personal role redefinition, and reaction role behavior—the first resulted in substantially greater satisfaction in a study of female college graduates. Findings of this study also indicated that various strategies may be differentially available to women who are situated differently in life.

Reduction of Role Conflict in Employed Women

The applicability of the generic theory and findings concerning role conflict to the situation and experience of midlife women must be carefully assessed. Though in principle a general theory is capable of subsuming the special cases of female and male, in practice, in social science, it is more common for the theory to be based on the normal case (male) and to require modification for the analysis of "deviant cases," that is, of women. Assumptions that do not apply to females cause the theory to fit this case poorly. In the literature on role conflict, these assumptions deal with power and parity. Substantial differences in power and peer status that have their roots in sex roles make the management of role conflict in the workplace more problematic for women than for men. This can easily be seen for the basic strategies enumerated by Goode (1960).

COMPARTMENTALIZATION OF ROLES. The effectiveness of compartmentalization as a means of reducing role conflict relies on a prior condition that Goode takes for granted: the existence of specified times and locales for role enactment. For most men, the work day is "off limits" to family demands, permitting compartmentalization. In addition, a principle of priority also separates the sets of role demands as well as the locales reserved for role enactment. A professor may work at home if his or her study is off limits and work time is uninterruptible. One limitation on the efficacy or availability of compartmentalization as a means to stress reduction is the specificity versus diffuseness of the role involved. A "master status" such as gender transcends specific locales and activities and elicits role demands transsituationally. These role demands may well disrupt enactment of occupational roles, in spite of the best efforts of women workers to employ the mechanism of compartmentalization to reduce role stress. Many women have reported that others treat their work as interruptible without qualification—a carry-over from the way the role of mother is defined in our culture.

DELEGATION OF ROLE RESPONSIBILITIES. Goode suggests that attributes or performances that are central to the role in question may not be delegated, but others may be. When we look at employed women in their dual roles, there seems almost a qualitative difference between the way familial roles and work roles are regarded by society at large. Traditional sex-role expectations for women have a sacred quality that contrasts greatly with the robustly secular tone of discussions of work roles. Wife, mother, and housewife roles do not seem to lend themselves to analysis of central and peripheral expectations. Expectations are diffuse, as may be seen in the instance above, in which the mothering figure is expected to be always there and always available. A certain amount of bias may be detected when social scientists seek to analyze housework as a job (Oakley, 1974) or when employed mothers assert that what is important is quality, not quantity of time with their children.

Public opinion research has tracked attitudes toward women's extrafamilial role enactment (evidently a problematic reality) for better than 30 years. The tone of censure that pervades laypersons' attitudes has not been absent from social scientists' discussions of "working wives," "latchkey children," and "broken homes." The persistence of the "maternal deprivation" shibboleth in both lay and professional circles is testimony to the normative status of full-time involvement of women in family roles. This normative climate severely limits employed women's ability to delegate role responsibilities as a means of reducing role conflict.

ELIMINATION OF ROLES. In the traditional sex-role script, work roles are expendable for women, but family roles are not. A woman who chooses work to the exclusion of family roles is still treated as a denatured female. At present, the climate of opinion in the United States seems punitive toward women who choose marriage-only as a life-style option. Marriage-cum-*some* employment (but not a career in the sense discussed earlier) is the expected pattern today (Pleck, 1977). Yet where elimination of roles is used to reduce role conflict in women, it seems more likely to lead to abandoning or reducing commitment to work roles rather than family roles. Epstein (1970) has suggested that women are rewarded for resolving any work–family conflict in this direction. The existence of this cultural pattern has implications for the careers of midlife women. They are likely to have intermittent labor-force participation as a feature of their work history before midlife, and they may be vulnerable to pressures to eliminate newly acquired work roles if family pressures are still strong.

ROLE ACCUMULATION. Goode suggested that taking on additional role obligations (accumulating roles) has the advantage for the focal person that role partners will adjust (reduce) their expectations in the light of the focal person's new obligations. In this way, role accumulation results in reduction of role strain.

Sieber (1974) has extended this analysis, challenging the perspective that has become conventional, that multiple role occupancy inevitably exposes the individual to role strain, which in turn results in decrements in role performance and in personal adjustment. Sieber, to the contrary, argues that role accumulation, rather like capital accumulation, presents a net gain rather than a penalty: The individual acquires privileges, rights, or resources by taking on new roles that may, within limits, be used to profit the individual as well as the role incumbent. The new acquisitions may be used to facilitate goals of the person. Sieber discusses four sorts of gains the individual may realize through role accumulation: role privileges, enhanced status security, resources for status enhancement, and gratification of ego and personality.

Sieber assumes that role accumulation leads to an ever-increasing surplus of role privileges over role obligations, since he makes the prior assumption that individuals strike role bargains having this feature. He dismisses in one parenthetical phrase the "exploitive" role relationships where obligations exceed privileges. He does not question who the role partners may be who accept an excess of obligations over privileges, complementary with the generic "he" of Sieber's analysis.

Role privileges include those aspects of the role that ordinarily act as inducements for the individual to enact it—e.g., legitimate authority. In addition, role incumbents gain "liberties" that do not involve the role partner. Some of the "liberties" one can gain via role accumulation seem more accessible to men than to women. The reduction of visibility has already been discussed; theoretical consensus seems to be that it is more difficult for a woman than for a man to escape surveillance in the occupational world, where she is viewed as a deviant by virtue of her "master status." The extension of authority without formal authorization is another such liberty. Research indicating the difficulties women have in exercising their legitimate authority suggests that extension may be an unlikely payoff for women at present (Bayes and Newton, 1978; Sterling and Owen, 1982).

Sieber suggests that role accumulation is a means to "status security," in the sense of offering compensatory success in one area in case of difficulties in another. There is, indeed, some evidence that work serves this function for women who are less than perfectly happy in their marriages (Spreitzer *et al.*, 1979; Rapoport and Rapoport, 1969). However, the interchangeability of successes must surely be conditioned by the priority the individual gives them, and this, in turn, by the normative forces that operate so powerfully to give preference to women's family roles.

Role accumulation also provides gains in the form of status enhancement of the role incumbent. Sieber uses the example of useful introductions and use of equipment and other resources of the employer, or the accumulation of status resources that can translate into power across different spheres. Insofar as status enhancement rests upon the facilitative operation of male networks, this payoff for role accumulation may be unavailable to women (Hoferek and Sarnowski, 1981; Albrecht, 1976). A number of writers have noted the difficulty women have in gaining access to or making use of such networks in business and the professions (Epstein, 1970; Laws and Tangri, 1979; Laws, 1980; Lorber, 1975). Female networks are not usually available in these work sites, because of the sex ratios that obtain in management ranks and in the professions. In addition, a woman's transferral of resources across institutional spheres is less likely if her access to those spheres is problematic in itself. To the extent that spheres of "public" activity remain socially masculine, women are unlikely to parlay resources acquired via the work role into, for example, the political scene.

Sieber also notes personal growth and ego gratification payoffs to be gained from multiple role occupancy: e.g., gains in sophistication, appreciation for one's own competence. A good deal of research evidence comparing housewives with employed women suggests that the latter report gratification through work and higher self-esteem (Birnbaum, 1971; Baruch, Chapter 6, this volume). However, there is no reason to attribute these effects to multiple role occupancy; indeed, these studies do not measure the extent of role accumulation in the two groups. These studies straightforwardly reflect the rewards available from working in the public world of paid employment. Women who do not occupy family roles report, without distortion, even greater levels of reward or satisfaction in many such studies (Birnbaum, 1971).

Although researchers commonly refer to "dual roles" in such comparisons, the effect of role accumulation remains a hypothesis for future research. The facile interpretation in terms of dual roles results from a familiar bias that is operating here: Women who occupy both work and family roles are assumed to have engaged in role accumulation, since a single role—housewifery—remains the unacknowledged norm in thinking about women. It is the position of the present authors that the reverse is the case: Housewife-only is an impoverished life-style, and multiple role occupancy is normal. The observed differences between employed women and housebound wives are better accounted for by this formulation than by the more conventional one.

Sieber's (1974) formulation of the benefits of role accumulation has been much quoted but, as yet, little researched. A number of limitations are apparent when we seek to apply Sieber's formulation to the situation of midlife women. First, there is a circularity in Sieber's argument, for all its appeal: He assumes that gains outweigh strains in role accumulation in terms of the excess of gratifications over strains. Another blind spot in Sieber's formulation is that it refers (and presumably applies) only to roles in formal organizations. Thus, the role privileges he lists as profits to be realized by role accumulation (due process, collective bargaining, and protection from physical abuse or arbitrary firing) are not available to those in wife and mother roles.

There are many reasons for doubting the applicability of Sieber's generic theory to women, not the least of them his failure to try out the analysis on any instances involving women. In discussing roles and role settings, however, Sieber clearly has the parameters of male experience in mind. When he discusses gratifications in excess of performance rewards, for example, will the proposition hold for members of a category that is subject to wage discrimination? The level of performance rewards assumed "normal" by this analysis is a far-off goal, not baseline, for the female role incumbent in most occupations. The value of Sieber's notion of role accumulation for understanding midlife women's prospects, therefore, remains to be demonstrated by future research. Given the reformulations made necessary by taking into account women's experiences in the work role, appropriate modifications of Sieber's predictions would be necessary. Nevertheless, when appropriately "grounded" in women's experience, the idea of role accumulation still has a contribution to make to a generic role theory.

To date, only the most elemental prediction from role accumulation has received empirical test. Spreitzer et al., (1979) tested the central proposition of Sieber's formulation with data from a national probability sample. They examined the relationship of multiple roles to a global sense of personal well-being. The analysis involved adults of preretirement age showing different configurations of the following roles: spouse, parent, worker, friend, and church member. Results showed a moderate absolute relationship between number of roles enacted and global well-being. This was moderated by satisfaction with the distinct role spheres: When only women who expressed satisfaction with their roles were included in the analysis, they showed a higher degree of global satisfaction than the comparable group of men.

The Spreitzer et al. data demonstrate another positive consequence of role accumulation: Satisfaction associated with one sphere may compensate psychologically for dissatisfaction in another. Spreitzer et al. did not analyze all possible comparisons, but they reported cross-tabulations of satisfaction/dissatisfaction with other roles when the respondent was satisfied or dissatisfied in the marital role. In this analysis, the picture is far more optimistic for men, in the sense that the compensation or compartmentalization mechanism seemed to work much better for men than for women. When overall happiness was compared for men with unsatisfactory marital roles, in all comparisons men satisfied in the other role (parent, work, friend, church) showed higher global satisfaction than men unsatisfied in the other role. For women, however, the mechanism broke down notably for the parent role, though the pattern appeared for the other roles. Either the spouse and parent roles are not so readily separable for women in this sample as for men, or spouse and parent roles mean different things and operate under different constraints for women and men. Research from other sources offers support for both these possibilities.

When satisfaction in the work role is the pivot for the analysis, both women and men show a regular compensation/compartmentalization effect in all comparisons (Spreitzer et al., 1979). It is surprising, given the implications of the normative priority of marriage over work for women, the degree to which satisfaction with the job appears to improve one's marriage. In this sample, the power of the "dual roles" to affect global life satisfaction appears stronger for women than for men: 48% of women experiencing satisfaction in both work and marriage roles express high overall happiness in life, as compared with only 40% of men.

ROLE DISTANCE. Goffman's (1961) notion of "role distance" may figure as a coping mechanism differentially employed by women in a dual role situation that is in fact a double bind. Goffman's dramaturgical concept refers to a posture that conveys "disdainful detachment" of the performer from his role. Specifically, the role incumbent acts in such a way as to deny a virtual self implied in the role. It is evident that the self expected in many occupational roles is a male person, possessed of many masculine attributes. Women role incumbents may engage in behaviors that symbolically deny the culturally masculine dimensions of their occupational roles. Or they may behave in ways that attempt to negate or neutralize their femaleness in the occupational role setting.

Women may engage in role distancing as a way of warding off social control maneuvers by role partners. One strategy may be to enact symbolically some aspect of "femininity," denying thereby any contradiction between the feminine self and the "masculine" role. Another may be to disclaim the priority that the role connotes in the life of the male role incumbent by self-limiting commitment through part-time work or modest ambitions. "Cognitive feminization" of occupations traditionally associated with cultural maleness can be accomplished, for example, by emphasizing healing, rather than authority or income, if the woman is a physician. However, role distancing in women has been little studied to date.

Coser's (1966) thinking about role distancing emphasizes the normative dimension. Role distancing is a behavior that occurs when there is a question as to the legitimacy of the role incumbency (or where the incumbency is transitory). It is a defensive strategy, an attempt to ward off a challenge to the legitimacy of role incumbency, or the driving of a wedge between self and role. Stebbins (1967) adds to the analysis in stressing the importance of significant others (role partners, in our terms) in providing support and validation for a challenged role. The other side of this analysis, of course, is the role partners as a source of invalidation and a stimulus requiring defensive coping. The issue of legitimacy, and the evaluation of the role incumbent as communicated through role pressures, is a crucial strand in understanding women's dual role enactment. In communicating role pressures and hence creating role conflict for women, role partners play a decisive and heretofore neglected part.

Role Conflict and Coping in Women's Dual Roles

The third resource for thinking about multiple role enactment by women is the curious literature on *women's dual roles*. The term is restricted to women who "add on" roles in paid employment, the fundamental (and "normal") roles being wife/mother/housewife. Men's work role is not added on; hence, men do not have *dual roles*, with all the freight of normative reaction that term entails. The lack of symmetry in vocabulary and analysis is a signal that the work on role conflict in women is not a subset of the generic role theory or a complement to the empirical tradition of work on role conflict in the work settings of men. Rather, the work on women's dual roles is a ghettoized literature, replete with the limitations and dangers of such intellectual segregation. Connections with popular stereotypes of women—though unacknowledged—appear closer than those with the propositions of generic role theory or with the comparable literature on men in work roles. What marks the research on this topic is the assumption that "dual roles" are unmanageable, leading inevitably to disabling role conflict. Thus, negative outcomes are assumed when women work outside the home. Explicitly, they and their role partners are expected to suffer from this unnatural state of affairs. This appears to be a normative judgment rather than a scientific one, and research on role conflict in women exhibits little attempt to discover or explain variation in the occurrence or severity of role conflict. With rare exceptions, the well-known mechanisms of management of role conflict are not investigated in the research. The woman who is enacting "multiple roles" appears cut off from support, 'tricks of the trade', and mechanisms of role articulation on which her male peers matter-of-factly rely. Another peculiarity of this research is that the "dual role" woman is assumed to suffer an internalized, psychological form of role conflict (guilt?) that is different from that experienced by ordinary multiple role occupants in the ordinary role conflict with which they routinely cope.

In several studies of working wives and mothers (Nevill and Damico, 1972; Hall and Gordon, 1973; Gordon and Hall, 1974; Lashuk and Kurian, 1977; Holahan and Gilbert, 1979), the authors assumed difficulties for a woman attempting to manage both a family and employment. Walberg (1968) looked for person–role conflict in practice teachers. Ziebarth (1972) sought evidence for three distinct types of "feminine role conflict." In general, in such studies, concern is with predicting not the occurrence of conflict but rather its frequency and/or intensity, contingent upon such independent variables as hours worked per week, quality of the work experience, education, marital status, and spousal support. The hypotheses offered by Lashuk and Kurian (1977) and Holahan and Gilbert (1979) exemplify the "internal" nature of conflict assumed to afflict women. Lashuk and Kurian expected employed wives and mothers to experience greater "negative internal effects" such as anxiety, tension, and feelings of inadequacy about the wife–mother role than their full-time housewife counterparts. Holahan and Gilbert expected that employed wives and mothers who perceived their employment as a "career" would suffer more role conflict than those who perceived their employment as "only a job." But in both studies, contrary to the authors' expectations, the hypotheses were disconfirmed. The female respondents, in fact, reported less or no conflict, the more roles they assumed.

Other studies indicate that housewives report more role conflict than women employed outside the home (Baruch, Segal, and Hendrick, 1968). It is possible that conflict between self and role is felt more by women who have not dared to seek expression of some of their talents and skills outside the home. Certainly, there is evidence that women who choose "housewife-only" as a career are women who cannot face the conflict they have been told exists between career and family (Watley and Kaplan, 1971; Birnbaum, 1971). Certainly, many of the compensations that ease role conflict are not available to women who do not work outside the home (Epstein, 1970; Spreitzer *et al.*, 1979; Rapoport and Rapoport, 1969; Gannon and Hendrickson, 1973).

The empirical existence of a distinctively feminine response to role conflict remains to be established. It does not appear when it "ought to," given the underlying assumptions of the dual role conflict literature. More extensive comparisons among women and between women and men are needed in order to ascertain whether there are specifiable conditions under which role conflict has psychological sequelae. At present, we are in danger of calling any role conflict experienced by a female person "psychological." This sort of prejudgment resembles the "motivational deficit" theories that once prevailed about the achievement of black Americans. In careless science like this, it is possible to find discussions of phenomena whose existence remains unsubstantiated. A "blame the victim" tone accompanies the neglect of structural and historical influences on the phenomenon of interest. A description of the *status quo* may be achieved but fall short of causal explanation. Unfortunately, such formulations, whether verified or not, can find their way into popular media and parlance and become self-fulfilling prophecies.

Many of the shortcomings of the research on role conflict in women can be seen in an influential article by Coser and Rokoff (1971). While focusing on women, these authors neglect the implied comparison with men. Indeed, they seem to assume that women are qualitatively different from men. The assumed differences resemble the normative script for women's priorities: Home responsibilities take precedence over work responsibilities. Coser and Rokoff seem to assume an invariant relationship between family and work responsibilities in women; they neither seek variance in this relationship nor seek to explain variance. Coser and Rokoff assert baldly that mechanisms of role articulation available to men—mechanisms that are part of the equipment, standard issue for persons in occupational roles—cannot be employed by women. Disappointingly, Coser and Rokoff fail to analyze the dynamics of gender as they affect the enactment of family and work roles by women and men, and the gender-related assumptions of work and family contexts that affect the definition of work and family roles. They hint that women are prevented from enacting their occupational roles in the normal way, and are confined to a deviant style that is, by definition, ineffective. However, Coser and Rokoff do not develop this allusion to the normative context of dual role enactment. Their failure to analyze the institutional context of occupational role enactment leads them to two errors. In not specifying what structural variables determine individual outcomes, they cut themselves (and their hapless subjects) off from the appropriate analyses of variation and links to generic role theory. They then retreat to a psychological formulation—always uncomfortable, and usually untenable, for sociologists. By default, it seems, Coser and Rokoff locate the problem in the individual woman and reach conclusions that are both static and pessimistic.

The work of Coser and Rokoff has been influential in shaping research on "role conflict" in employed women. Regrettably, the conclusions of this theoretical work have carried so much conviction for some researchers that they have insisted on seeing "intrapsychic role conflict" where their respondents report none (See, for example, Hall and Gordon, 1973). So influential a theoretical paper might very well have the effect of inhibiting research on role bargaining, coping, and innovation among women occupying multiple roles. It may contribute to a posture of pessimism in the literature on women's dual roles, and may create a static image of an eminently dynamic process.

Findings from research on dual careers that reveals the effective use of compartmentalization, and from the family time use studies that show both elimination and delegation of some role functions, apparently result from inadequate socialization of researchers. Researchers who did not know their role theory were able to discover important phenomena that, according to theory, did not exist. Certainly, much more remains to be learned. The existence of multiple roles in an ongoing time stream points toward commitments, rates of development, and priorities that change over time, rather than remaining fixed.

Role Partners and Role Conflict in Women

The existence of sex-role scripts that contain negative evaluations of women's extrafamilial roles is not sufficient, in itself, to produce role conflict in employed women. Indeed, the findings of Gordon and Hall (1974) suggest that even conscious awareness of traditional sex-role scripts does not induce role conflict in working women in and of itself. Pressures for sex-role conformity, like all role pressures, must be directly mediated in a relationship. Role pressures that induce role conflict in multiple-role women can be brought to bear by female relatives, authority figures, peers, or the proverbial mother-in-law. However, although research to date has dealt little with this process, there is evidence that such role pressures are exerted by husbands and by male co-workers. Examined closely, the data indicate that subjective role conflict, with or without disruption of role performance, can be instigated in women by role partners who challenge the legitimacy of dual role enactment or the adequacy of role performance. One can attack a woman's femininity or her competence; one can assert that one who is feminine cannot be competent, or that the female achiever is deficient as a female. One can portray the achieving woman as a ruthless individual whose pathetic family pays the price for her monstrous ambition.

Husbands are particularly efficacious in inducing role conflict in employed women or in neutralizing it (Rapoport and Rapoport, 1971; Weil, 1961; Feldman, 1973; Mahajah, 1966). "Dual career" wives commonly express gratitude that their husbands approve of their careers. However, the emotional support derived from approval may not be accompanied by help with the burdens of dual role responsibilities, and indeed, wives with professional careers report role overload (Rapoport and Rapoport, 1969), In one sample of college-educated women, professional women report more symptoms than a comparable group of wives without dual roles (Powell and Reznikoff, 1976).

Evidence exists, then, for two seemingly contradictory effects of multiple roles. Some studies show the negative effects of role stress and some the positive effects of enrichment or role accumulation. Clearly, more work needs to be done in order to clarify conditions under which multiple roles lead to positive and to negative outcomes for the role incumbents. Barnett and Baruch (1981) have found evidence for both positive and negative effects of women's multiple role occupancy. They found, in a study of 238 women aged 35 to 55, that feelings of role strain were related to the number of roles a woman occupied. Employed women did not report significantly more role strain than did women who worked only in the home. When the roles of wife, mother, and paid worker were examined for their relationship to role strain, only the mother was found to bear a significant relationship. Barnett and Baruch also found the number of roles a woman occupied significantly related to two aspects of personal well-being: mastery and pleasure.

Research on women's life-style planning indicates that they are aware of a potential conflict between the ambitions toward which their abilities lead them and the destination for which the culture intends them (Davis, 1964; Feldman, 1973). There is substantial evidence that boyfriends and, indeed, all potential husbands, have a power over younger women's choices and plans with regard to dual role life-styles that parallels the influence of husbands over wives. Typical data show that an overwhelming majority of college women prefer a dual role lifestyle, show high career commitment, intend little or no interruption of labor force activity with the advent of children—and would abandon it all, if a future husband disapproved of a working wife.

Current studies of college men (the presumptive future role partners of college women) indicate some support for dual roles in women (Komarovsky, 1973) and increased interest in family roles for men (Rossi, 1980). However, there is no empirical evidence at the present writing for a change in behaviors corresponding to such attitudes. Indeed, Komarovsky's (1973) data show men's attitudes to be much more conservative than those reported by college women in other studies. This corresponds to earlier findings by Siegel and Haas (1963) that men disapproved of employment of mothers to a greater extent than did women. Nelson and Goldman (1969) found that although public attitudes toward employment of women have become liberalized over time, men reject employment as an option for their *own* wives.

Interestingly, it is the sex role *attitudes* of women and men that permit the latter to go on the offensive and the former to become defensive, rather than the objective conditions of multiple role occupancy. Sense of time pressure and role overload are part of the objective role stress (Rapoport and Rapoport, 1969), which remains "external" until a finger of blame is pointed. We may speculate that most women are quite accustomed to dealing with too many things to do and too little time, but few are skilled at rejecting blame. It is the cultural script, specifying domestic concerns as the "one role" appropriate for women (Bernard, 1972b), that permits women to be blamed for enacting multiple roles. This script, coexisting with other cultural themes such as equal opportunity and individualistic achievement, constitutes an ever-present potentiality for conflict. Existing research suggests that both women and men are aware of the existence of the achievement versus femininity formulation (cf. Monahan, Kuhn, and Shaver, 1974). The consequences of the knowledge are different for women and men. However, only women can be impaled and disrupted by the conflict. Possessing the knowledge that most women are vulnerable to this latent conflict between achievement and femininity gives men a weapon to use against women who are invading new occupational turf.

From research on women entering traditionally "masculine" occupations (e.g., the construction trades, steel production, business management), it is increasingly clear that induced conflict between sex-role expectations and work goals may be used as a form of social control of women. Ridicule, sexual challenge, isolation, and seduction are a few of the means documented in research to date (Wolman and Frank, 1972; Mayes, 1976). Out-and-out harassment has been reported in many situations where women are entering traditionally male-dominated occupations. Sexual harassment and sexual hazing are frequently used to intimidate women recruits and throw them off balance (Laws and Tangri, 1979). This research makes it clear that some form of sexual harassment or hazing is part of the working conditions of many, if not most, women currently in paid employment. This factor clearly constitutes a job stress and can be expected to have effects on women's outcomes in the job market. Kahn, Wolfe, Quinn, and Snoek (1964) found that high role conflict was related to reduced job satisfaction and increased job-related tension. Being subjected to conflicting role expectations reduces career satisfaction and happiness for women (Hall and Gordon, 1973).

This material on occupational stress of women needs to be incorporated into the tradition of research on occupational stress, which, regrettably, has understudied women (Kahn *et al.*, 1964; Haynes, Levine, and Scotch, 1978). Haynes and Feinleib (1980) make a start with an analysis of the incidence and antecedents of coronary heart disease in women, comparing employed women and housewives. Their data show a relationship between role overload and heart disease in women: Number of children and marital status, as well as employment, contributed to elevated rates of coronary disease in their sample. Single women had the lowest rate of coronary disease. Among women, marriage and family responsibilities predicted to coronary disease, although employment *per se* did not.

Interestingly, it was not the "demanding" professional jobs that carried most job stress but rather the clerical occupations, in which women, locked in by necessity, suffered lack of occupational mobility and lack of support from their bosses, and suppressed their anger. When heavy family responsibilities are added, the risk of heart disease among women in clerical occupations is considerably increased.

The Haynes and Feinleib data suggest that relationships with two important role partners—husbands and bosses—are a factor in occupational stress leading to coronary disease in women. These authors do not, however, systematically assess role relationships as a factor in occupational stress of women. The connection between role partners' behavior and role conflict in employed women needs to be thoroughly researched. The corpus of research on occupational stress is in need of updating to include and reflect the research on women's experience in the world of work.

Sex Structuring of Roles

The sex structuring of work roles is a question that is only now recieving attention from researchers. Past research on "women's occupations" has pointed out continuities between women's work in the home and women's work in the labor market. Underlying this analysis can be discerned a rudimentary sketch of the feminine sex-role script, with a focus on the activities that correspond in the two work environments. The analysis can be extended, however, to show correspondences in *ways of performing work activities*, even where the activities may be different from those found in women's home tasks. In terms of roles and role expectations, we can say work roles and working relationships become colored by characteristics expected of women *qua* women. Of course, men's work roles and working sytles can be analyzed in the same way, as we have suggested at several points in this chapter.[4]

An aspect of sex structuring that has not been investigated to date is the way in which role expectations are adjusted for females and males in the same occupational roles. A fundamental asymmetry in role definitions of women and men in the "same" job are embedded in role expectations and role relationships that are decisively different.

On the basis of research in sex roles, it appears that women and men in the same jobs experience differences with respect to power relations, peer relations, and benefits to self and others. Much of this difference can be summarized, in terms of Sieber's (1974) analysis, by the propositions that (1) men's roles and role relationships are structured in terms of an excess of role privileges over obligations, and (2) women's roles and role relationships are structured in terms of an excess of role obligations over role privileges. The "complementarity" implied by these formulations has very different consequences for women and men in their work roles.

A number of researchers have observed that women in predominately male work settings are responded to by others in terms of a very restricted set of roles strongly marked by sex-role expectations (cf. Kanter, 1977b). Of these, the dominant one is Mother. When women are dealt with as Mother, they are characterized (and treated) as giving

[4]The fact that this is rarely done is due more to the psychology of the dominant and deviant than to any inherent difficulty in the analysis. (cf. Laws, 1975).

without counting the cost, as ever-available. Their diffuse willingness to facilitate and support others, and the goal attainment of others, is contrasted with a contractual mentality. Self-interest and personal ambition do not feature in Mother's makeup. A willingness to expend time and energy on others' personal problems is expected of Mother. This kind of investment is ordinarily not reciprocated: Mother does not receive nurturance. Mother can be relied on to take care of any (and many) details. The "office wife" is one who performs many small personal services that are beneath the attention of the boss but contribute to smooth maintenance and smooth achievement sequences. Although the secretary most often functions as the "office wife," most women with professional credentials have had the experience of being expected or asked to perform Motherly functions in the office.

The casting of female colleagues into stereotypical feminine sex roles not only influences the relationships between pairs of women and men in the workplace but also prejudices the woman's chances of being included in peer relations. Observational studies of interacting work groups show that normal processes of competition, coalition formation, and cooperation exclude women (Wolman and Frank, 1972; Mayes, 1976). The sole or token woman is isolated, and her contributions are distorted (Laws, 1975; Kanter, 1977b; Taylor and Fiske, 1976). Emphasizing sex roles has the effect of polarizing women and men, and of further isolating women, in situations where the sex ratios are heavily skewed (Grimm and Stern, 1974). Women's access to peer networks and to sponsorship that facilitates career success is further compromised by this often unrecognized factor.

Masculine sex roles, too, can be discerned in the work setting. The literature on role expectations for those in management positions is particularly rich in characterizations of masculinity: Men in their organizational roles are expected to exhibit decisiveness, authoritativeness, expertise, or the posture of knowledgeability: firmness. They receive deference. They delegate work. They evaluate. They chew out their subordinates. They make their subordinates shape up.

Power and the exercise of power are major dimensions underlying the sex structuring of occupational roles. The research on women in management shows that men perceive a contradiction between the attributes of women and those required for success in management (Bass, Krusell, and Alexander, 1971; Rosen and Jerdee, 1974a). Although studies have repeatedly shown that women and men recruits to management have the same characteristics (Day and Stogdill, 1972; Terborg, 1977), the perception that women cannot command—and in particular, cannot command men—persists (Bartol and Butterfield, 1976). The power dimension clearly enters into consideration of the use of persuasion and negotiation, as in the discussion of role bargains (Merton, 1968; Sieber, 1974). If women cannot credibly exercise power, their bargaining position is diminished and the ratio of role privileges to role obligations that they can wring from role partners is accordingly reduced.

The frank pursuit of self-interest is consonant with male sex-role scripts, in the occupational sphere as in others; it is dissonant with images of femininity. Bluffing and bargaining are skills that prevail and pay off in male games, including occupational games (Harragan, 1977). In light of the cultural penalties for the exercise of power by women, women may indeed have difficulty playing these games with the agility and verve that is called for.

The sentimental image of the home as haven from the stresses of the occupational world has a misplaced focus. It is not the home but the homebody to whom the expectations attach. As women have moved into the labor market in increasing number, we find that the asymmetry of spousal roles in the home moves with them.

Midlife women are workers, wives, mothers, daughters, and domestic workers. In each sphere, they are surrounded by role partners whose roles are complementary to their own. In each sphere, it can be seen that the role expectations for the female role incumbent are framed to an excess of obligations over privileges. This becomes clearer as we examine specific role partnerships.

Female and male partners in marriage can be referred to by the identical term, but their privileges and obligations are asymmetrical by law and custom. In some localities, law and custom are at variance; for example, custom holds that a husband should support his wife and minor children, but laws currently hold that each spouse is responsible for the other's debts. Husbands have rights of sexual access to their wives, but the law does not recognize a similar right of wives or an obligation of husbands.

Ironically, research indicates that women and men seek the same benefits in marriage—nurturance, intimacy, emotional support—and thrive when they encounter them (Kotlar, 1962). However, men expect these attributes in a spouse, as a function of sex roles (or feminine nature), but women are aware that these attributes contradict the masculinity their spouses are supposed to embody.

Male and female parents, similarly, can be designated by the same term, but research makes it evident that virtually all the parenting in the United States is done by mothers. The enormous child-care burden is assumed by mothers, and only a trivial amount of it is shared with spouse, relatives, or paid help. There is some evidence that fathers, when they share in child care at all, by and large limit their contribution to routine custodial activities or "playing with" their children (Lamb,

1976). Guidance, the inculcation of values, coaching, nursing, and teaching are among the parental responsibilities that seem to follow an "on-call" kind of schedule rather than occurring conveniently, say, on Sunday afternoons. The asymmetrical role demands on parents extend into late life rather than being limited to the period when children are legally dependent. The same asymmetry can be found in other kin relations maintained by the marital pair, as with the care of aged parents by daughters (and daughters-in-law) rather than sons. Many women find the role obligations of the daughter increasing in midlife as aged parents come to require care.

The asymmetry in household work is well documented at present (Laws, 1979; Robinson and Converse, 1966). Detailed studies of family time budgets make it clear that a rising standard of living has imposed increased burdens on housewives. Husbands and children bear only a trivial share of the work generated by their joint households, and do not take a significantly larger share as the children grow older or the mother's total work week is increased by paid work (Walker, 1970).

"Dual Roles"/Multiple Roles

As individual roles are structured differently for women and men, so too are their "dual roles" and the multiple role system that is the context of all adults in our society. We have pointed out the way in which sex-role scripts prescribe a different normative weighting of work and family roles for women and men. Women's "dual roles" often mean adding the inflated demands of a male-style (single-role) career to those of a wife's domestic duties, which in themselves frequently add up to a work week twice as long as the paid work week. When Baird (1967) identified structural sources of role stress for individuals beginning graduate school, he found that extra-academic roles, and particularly marital and family responsibilities, exacerbated role stress. Family roles, of course, make far heavier demands on women than on men. Feldman (1973), too, found that graduate women's productivity (publications) was impeded by marriage, while men's was enhanced.

If the general principle of sex structuring of roles holds, role accumulation—such as may be involved in kin bonds, office in professional associations, committee work, and the like—may well mean increasing the total role obligations enormously, and increasing the relative excess of obligations over role privileges still more. Role overload would be the predicted result. Continuing and chronic stress from overwork might be expected to result in substantial increases in occupational health problems for employed women.

Sex differences found by Spreitzer *et al.* (1979) reflect the facts of women's multiple role incumbency as contrasted with that of men.[5] When women reporting marriage/work combinations were compared with women reporting marriage/work/family, the percentage reporting a high degree of happiness was substantially lower (38% as compared with 44% with an additional role). For men, the difference was only 2 percentage points (37% as compared with 35%). The addition of friend and church roles did not detract in a comparable way from global happiness, suggesting that these roles are less demanding than work and family roles. The Spreitzer *et al.* data confirm the problem of role overload in women documented in the time-use studies.

Data showing husbands' (increasing) leisure relative to their work week, and wives' (vanishing) leisure relative to their double work day, succinctly tell the story of asymmetry in dual roles of women and men (Kreps and Clark, 1975). In the light of these trends, it is not surprising that the wives—and only the wives—in Rapoport and Rapoport's (1969) study of dual career families complained of role overload. The inescapable conclusion is that "dual roles" and multiple roles make greater demands on women than on men. Beyond the regular "marriage tax" of heavy home obligations, however, women pay an additional penalty. Its consequences are felt at midlife and later, in the form of economic vulnerability. The period of the life-course when family demands are greatest often coincides with the high investments required by the establishment of a career. The "dual roles" of men are engineered to enhance career investment, while the role expectations for women are designed to enhance their partners' and not their own career success. It is to be expected that many midlife women's careers reflect this rather typical prior experience. At this point in their lives, they have already suffered the penalties of having chosen the approved life-course for their gender: Very few women have built up the equity in the work world and the contingent social benefits that their male peers enjoy.

When women seek to compensate for their earlier work history by retraining or reentering at midlife, however, they feel the sting of the normative judgments of the world they seek to enter. As students, as apprentices, or as colleagues, they meet a subtle prejudice to the effect that if they had possessed the requisite talent and motivation, they would, of course, have followed different (and incidentally, male) priorities in their 20s and 30s. Teachers and fellow apprentices make it clear that little contribution can be expected from such "late bloomers" or "late starters."

[5]Speitzer *et al.* did not attempt to study the lack of symmetry between women's and men's work and marital roles (or other roles). However, the authors note the importance of differential commitment to roles—or priorities, as discussed here—and suggest a focus on this issue in future research.

Midlife women find it difficult to make a "new" start even when they must or want to do so. Others will not let them; they carry their life histories with them. In order to understand their situation, it is not enough to know what roles they occupy or aspire to in the present moment. Rather, the life they have lived, with its transitions and changes, colors their present and their future. The situation of midlife women calls for a life-course perspective.

Women and the Life-Course

Life-course research has consistently included women, and a great deal of it has focused on transitions in the family life-cycle that are widely assumed to affect women disproportionately. One of the earliest traditions in life-course research subsumes the so-called family life-cycle studies. In this tradition, the family as the unit of analysis is assumed to mature over its life-span with the accomplishment of successive "developmental tasks" (Duvall, 1957). These developmental tasks define the normative requirements for the family throughout the life cycle. Developmental tasks may be individually or socially prompted and include such sets of activities as reproduction, socialization, status attainment, and physical maintenance (Hill and Mattessich, 1979). The family life cycle comprises an orderly progression of life events such as establishment of the family by marriage, birth of the first child, entrance of the first child into school, departure of the last child from the parental home, retirement, and widowhood.

The conceptual thrust of the life-cycle perspective lies in its treatment of the family as a semiclosed system of interrelated positions (i.e., wife/mother, husband/father, sister/daughter) that evolves over time. Each position is occupied by a family member who performs multiple roles. As a result of the inclusion of a time dimension, the family is not perceived as a static entity, but rather a dynamic one with a past, present, and future conceptualized as sequential stages of development. New stages are initiated with change in the system of positions or in the content of any role(s).

Despite the advantages of a life-course perspective (primarily its way of viewing family development longitudinally), there are certain deficiencies, particularly in older work (see Hill and Mattessich, 1979, for an extensive review). Several assumptions made in connection with the way family is defined render this perspective inadequate for studying individuals or any family configuration other than the nuclear one. To begin with, family life-cycle theorists assumed that a family will follow a "predictable natural history" (Hill and Hansen, 1960). Deviations from this normal life cycle were sometimes categorized not only as atypical, random, and disruptive, but also as ultimately unnatural (Rodgers, 1973). Thus, for example, the female-headed family, by virtue of its failure to fulfill the cultural mandate that a family have a male and a female head, was thought weak and incapable of accomplishing further developmental tasks in the family life cycle.

Because the unit of analysis is the family and the family members are expected to perform their roles normatively, individual development tends to be glossed over in the life-cycle perspective. Development occurs in the family only because of individual maturation, yet personality development and individual growth are underrepresented in the family life-cycle vocabulary.[6] Rather, we find that the members growing and working in unison are seen to produce family outcomes, not individual outcomes. The household or family is reified in order to be viewed processually or developmentally (Elder, 1980/1981). The heterogeneity in the population of midlife women and their households is particularly ill-served by the unitary model of family development.

As Elder (1977) has pointed out, the life-cycle model does not offer a precise definition of change or development over time—but merely records a plus or a minus in the configuration of the family. It does not make use of all possible information on the economic careers and work lives of adult family members. The family development stages are not capable of charting the life-course of an individual, or her career path, or the career paths of several adult family members simultaneously. The model usually offered delineates stages in relation to compositional change in the family only, as when a baby is born or a member leaves the household.

To a certain extent, the family was understood as a group capable of development in and of itself. Yet family members develop in spheres other than the family. Women, especially, have been underestimated in the family development literature because of this familial determinism. From this perspective, it appears that women's "developmental tasks" have required that they promote the growth and well-being of others at the expense of their own development. Although a woman may have enacted only her family roles to the exclusion of all others in early adulthood, at midlife as family demands slack off, she is capable of launching a delayed career in spheres other than the family. At this point in her life-course, a woman may complete an education or begin one, train for a new job or seek a promotion, join a volunteer association or found one. A midlife woman is much more than her familial roles,

---

[6]Hill and Mattessich (1979) recognize the need for convergence between family development theory and life-span developmental psychology in remedying this problem and suggest ways in which the convergence might occur.

more than "just a wife" or "just a mother." The multiple roles of a midlife woman constitute her biography, each role contributing to her development.

Another area of life-course research focuses on differences between birth cohorts in the incidence, timing, sequence, spacing, and duration of major life events, such as school-leaving or the birth of a first child. One question for such inquiries concerns the impact and consequences of normative expectations on the timing of life transitions. A second question concerns the impact and consequences of social change on the variation and timing of traditional life-cycle events across successive birth cohorts (Glick, 1957; Uhlenberg, 1974). The social concept of "on-time" transitions and the pressure on the individual to follow the social schedule for life transitions have intrigued researchers in this tradition (cf. Modell, Furstenberg, and Herschberg, 1976). One further question deals with the impact of nonnormative events on traditional life-cycle patterns. Norton (1980) studied the relationship of divorce to standard life-cycle measures such as age at first marriage, birth of first child, birth of last child, and end of child-rearing for successive birth cohorts of women who had ever borne children.

Current work in the life-course perspective is open-ended, nonjudgmental, and better equipped to question the effects of certain sequences and timing of life events beyond the familial ones on the economic well-being of women in their middle and later years (Elder, 1977, 1981; Riley, 1971, 1979; Brim, 1980; Brim and Ryff, 1980; Featherman, 1981). Principles of current life-course theory include the following:

1. The life-course is structured by major life events—events such as completion of training, entry into the labor market, marriage, divorce, widowhood, birth of a child, departure of the last child from the home, reentry into employment, retirement—which require role transitions resulting in permanent changes in the individual's life. Brim (1980) describes these as "triggers for personal change and development." At each of these transitions, a new period in an individual's life is initiated. No single period may be adequately understood apart from antecedent or consequent periods.

2. Cohort membership locates an individual within the life-course. A birth cohort refers to a group of people born at approximately the same time. They share either birth year or birth period. As Riley (1979) warns, the term *cohort* should not be confused with *generation,* used to describe individuals of similar ages within a kinship context. An individual's age supplies approximate knowledge about one's biological, psychological, and social experiences.

3. The stages of development implied in the life-course process are neither fixed nor immutable. Successive birth cohorts do not experience

the same life patterns due to social change and environmental variation. As history unfolds, it influences and shapes the life-course of entire cohorts of individuals differently because each cohort lives through it in unique ways.

4. An individual's social roles undergo changes several times over the life-course and are said to follow careers. An individual's life-course may be conceptualized as a convergence of career lines or trajectories that follow a series of age- and sex-differentiated roles across several spheres—educational, familial, occupational.

5. The life-course covers the entire life-span. As an individual ages, there is an interactive effect involving the biological, psychological, and social processes of life.

An individual's life-course is made up of interlocking strands of careers rooted in multiple roles. Multiple role occupancy is not associated with a particular stage in the life-course but continues throughout the life-span. The various combinations of marriage, parenthood, and employment across time suggest the diverse trajectories possible for women at midlife. By paying attention to multiple roles and careers through time, the life-course perspective offers an understanding of the individual not only in a familial context but also in the contexts of marriage, fertility, and employment. Too often one context has been singled out at the neglect of others. For midlife women, the impact of the "empty nest," losing a spouse, entering the labor market, or finishing a college degree is not isolated from other spheres and other careers. In this chapter, we are most concerned with the impact of changes in multiple roles at midlife (occupational, marital, parental, and domestic) on women's economic well-being in later years.

The normative order and timing of life events judges individuals "on time" if their role behavior accords with the cultural prescriptions for their age/sex category and "off time" if their role behavior does not. The consequences of the nonnormative incidence, sequence, spacing, timing, and duration of life events are yet to be widely researched (Norton, 1980). Although we know that conformity to traditional timetables is eroding, women now in midlife were subjected to those traditional timetables and lived lives "on time" for the most part. Ironically, for a midlife woman, a lifetime of "on-time" events such as marriage and childbearing early in adulthood means being vulnerable to economic declines throughout the latter half of the life-span. Being "off time," for women, as in completing a college degree, entering an occupation early in the work life, and postponing marriage and childbearing so as to advance in the career, usually predicts to economic security in later years.

Women who are now at midlife may well have chosen their adult life-styles at a period when women's options were more restricted than at any other time in this century. In their mothers' and grandmothers' generations, there were more never-married women and more women who never bore children. The variability in educational attainment was greater, and substantially higher educational levels were attained by women who did not marry. The characteristics of midlife women's four major careers—occupational, marital, parental, and domestic—are important for determining the needs of future research and policy on women in their later years.

The Marital Career at Midlife

Simone de Beauvoir (1974) has argued that most women marry, have married, or suffer from not marrying. The cultural mandate holds that marriage is of the utmost importance for the well-being of women. By midlife, however, a wife's chances of being divorced, separated, or widowed are high and climbing higher. At any given time, divorced women outnumber divorced men of all ages due to the higher remarriage rate among the latter. Younger divorced people are more likely to remarry than older ones; hence, those who stay divorced tend to be older and female. Women outlive men more often, and more widowers remarry than widows; hence, those who remain widowed are predominately older and female. The premature death of a spouse or the dissolution of a marriage may leave a middle-aged wife in dire social and economic straits, not because she has "lost" the role of wife, as the literature would word it, but because, in a more fundamental sense, the cultural stipulation of female dependence in marriage leaves her financially hard-pressed, occupationally inexperienced, and ill-equipped for independence.

The literature supplies some evidence to contradict the assumption that well-being for women requires an intact marriage (Bart, 1971; Bernard, 1972a; Brown, Feldberg, Fox, and Kohen, 1976). Bart (1971), in a study of depression of middle-aged women being treated in mental hospitals, concluded that if a woman's sense of worth derives from her own accomplishments, as in initiating or expanding an occupational role, she is less vulnerable to breakdown when other salient roles contract or disappear—for example, when a husband dies or children leave home.

For those who remain married throughout midlife, the changes experienced in the wife role appear potentially liberating. Brim (1975) acknowledges that at midlife, wives may be moving toward a genuine growth in self-esteem and self-actualization. Other studies have shown that women at midlife tend to be more eager to strike out on their own than perhaps in their earlier years of marriage (cf. Rubin, 1979). It is at this time in the life-course that the opportunities for involvement with extrafamilial activities increase for many women. Well-being seems to be a function of having multiple roles and multiple options rather than being "just a wife."

The Parental Career at Midlife

Occupying the role of mother produces lasting effects over the lifecourse that influence many aspects of a woman's life. Using retrospective data collected from a nationally representative sample of midlife women, Borker, Loughlin, and Rudolph (1979) found that the age at which a woman became a mother for the first time determined, to a considerable extent, her socioeconomic status in later life. The authors found that women who became mothers early suffered lower earnings at midlife relative to those who did not, primarily as a result of their lower educational levels. Studies of teenage mothers and the rate actually completing high school or its equivalent corroborate these findings (Moore, Hofferth, Caldwell, and Waite, 1979).

A life-course perspective defines midlife for mothers, not principally by chronological age but by the experience of a major life event: the launching of the last child into the adult world (Neugarten, 1968). This event initiates the so-called "empty nest" stage, a stage during which the mother, married or not, experiences an attenuation of childrearing obligations. The menopause and the "empty nest" are typically associated with the female at midlife as crises. The view that marriage and children are essential ingredients for a full and healthy life for a woman is based on a biological determinism that links mind and body more closely for women than for men (Barnett and Baruch, 1978). Against this view, Troll and Turner (1978) argue that the majority of midlife women, having identified themselves with other interests, do not experience severe trauma upon the departure of the last child from the home. Most midlife mothers, they claim, positively anticipate the freedom from child-rearing responsibilities and the opportunities to pursue their own interests and to spend more time with peers. Mothers who view mothering as an episode rather than a lifelong occupation, it appears, are better able to facilitate their own as well as their children's development. However, mothers who have dedicated their entire lives to mothering were found in one study to be plagued by adjustment problems when their children left home (Bart, 1971). The effects of the emptying nest, of course, depend in part on the degree of independence achieved by maturing offspring. Present trends indicate that many midlife women take on substantial responsibility for care of grandchildren. Current economic factors mean that many young adults who have left home return for longer or shorter periods to live under the parental roof.

There is an image of the postparental woman in our society as a "former achiever" (Mayer, 1969). This image is based on a definition of woman as "just a mother" and a definition of female achievement as reproduction of the species. When the duties associated with motherhood are no longer required, as when a midlife woman watches her last child depart the parental home, that certain social recognition she received as reproducer of the species changes emphasis: An "active" mother becomes a "former" mother. Retiring from active motherhood can potentially detract from a woman's economic well-being as well: Her eligibility for public assistance such as Aid to Families with Dependent Children or survivor's benefits (if she is widowed with dependent children) ceases when her children reach age 18. At this time, a woman's opportunities to receive job training and career placement are in short supply. Her experiences and skills, accrued while mothering and homemaking, are unrecognized or underestimated. In general, mothers who wish to enter or return to the public world as active participants find the going difficult and few places or persons willing to offer assistance such as training, career placement, or support.

The Domestic Career at Midlife

Upon reaching midlife, women do not find too many drastic changes in the content of their domestic role. Perhaps with children gone, the work load decreases, but it never disappears altogether. Indeed, sometimes the middle-aged housewife's work load is increased by the presence in her home of elderly parents who can no longer care for themselves. No matter what her age, the housewife is still expected to meet the needs of the remaining household members and to perform the domestic tasks until she is no longer capable. She continues to have multiple role responsibilities.

The Occupational Career at Midlife

Of all women currently in the labor force, the 35- to 64-year-olds have consumed the highest doses of a segregated sexual division of labor in the home and the labor force. Their labor force histories reflect this exposure to the cultural prescriptions for womanhood. Essentially four patterns are distinguishable for midlife women's labor force histories, these being rank-ordered from most to least prevalent (Parnes, Jusenius, Blau, Nestel, Shortlidge, and Sandell, 1975; Howe, 1982):

1. Long intermissions between times in the labor force: Usually a job is held until marriage or the birth of the first child, followed by a protracted absence during the child-rearing years and reentry after children are launched.

2. Short intermissions between times in the labor force, usually to have a child or meet a family exigency.
3. No labor force experience as an adult whatsoever: Usually marriage and motherhood occupy the woman full time.
4. Continuous labor force employment, until recently an option exercised mainly by never-married women.

Is outside employment beneficial for a midlife woman's well-being? We have reviewed evidence indicating that employment enhances a woman's well-being by providing wages with which to maintain a standard of living, social status as an incentive to upward mobility, and a sense of personal competence that contributes to self-esteem. However, it is well documented that female employment is paid less and carries lower social status than most male occupations. Employment tends to afford some self-esteem for women, usually more than is accrued in a housewife-only existence, but its rewards are less when the job is dead-end, tedious, or otherwise demeaning.

Nonetheless, in light of present trends, the role of labor force participant is an extremely important one for women of every age. A skyrocketing cost of living is encouraging replacement of the husband-as-provider with the dual-earner marriage. In addition, a growing segment of highly educated, professional career women in dual-career families are exhibiting new patterns of family living. Divorce and widowhood force many women to head their households single-handedly. Midlife women, in particular, are entering or returning to the labor force for financial reasons, personal aspirations, or some combination of both. Whereas the midlife male is thought to experience a "time squeeze," a realization that time is running out on his career ambitions, the midlife female is thought to be experiencing a "time gap," a realization that she has many years left before retirement age with perhaps no husband, no children at home, and no means of supporting herself socially and/or economically (Cohen, 1979).

It appears that employment will loom large in the futures of most midlife women, whatever has been their life-course to this point. For most, the life-course they have lived has not been sufficient to assure them of economic self-sufficiency in later life. There will be an urgent need for social programs to meet some of their needs. These programs, in turn, must be grounded in an adequate social theory.

FUTURE DIRECTIONS FOR THEORY AND RESEARCH

Recognition of the fundamental reality of multiple roles could stimulate an enormously fruitful reorientation in role theory and could generate research that will provide for more adequate bases for policy formulation. New research in role theory needs to incorporate a time dimension, such as inheres in the life-course perspective, and give particular attention to the dynamic character of role demands, role bargains, and role enactment as multiple careers unfold over the life-span.

A greater variety of life transitions—and their timing, spacing, and sequencing—are now "expected" than was the case in past generations. In future, we can expect more research on the unexpected transitions: career change, downward mobility in occupations, remarriages, reentries, and exits. We can expect more research on nonunitary career lines, and a more acute analysis of continuities and discontinuities in the individual's multiple careers. The time dimension will be taken for granted, and we will see research not solely on occupational planning but on planning for multiple roles over the life span. The payoffs of various strategies—including alternative sequencing and timing of education, employment, and family formation—need to be calculated. It is clear from the situation at present that planners and legislators are unaware of the negative consequences of certain prevalent patterns of education/marriage/employment. "Social accounting" needs to be informed, to a greater degree than is the case at present, of the outcomes of the various paths women take to midlife. It is to be hoped that in the future, as a result of research that demonstrates these causal paths, women will be enabled to make choices that do not doom them to penury in midlife.

A focus on the economic situation of women at midlife and beyond underscores the need for studies of outcomes. It is essential that the paths to various midlife outcomes be charted. These paths must further be related to choices that women make, and to choices that women perceive. Some authors have pointed out that "economic rationality" based on differential earning power of spouses dictates that it be the wife's career that is interrupted by family moves, or her job options that are limited by where the household is located. From other studies we learn of the effects of family responsibilities on women's occupational achievements. Studies of "dual career" marriages tell us that wives consciously subordinate their careers to those of their husbands. This strategy may have different outcomes in the short run—particularly where marital harmony is given priority—and the long run, where a woman's economic viability is at stake should the marriage terminate. A major shortcoming of the "dual role" research is that it seems to assume a single and lifelong marriage. Very few studies contain a time dimension extended enough to permit the assessment of long-term economic outcomes of different strategies. Yet this is the kind of research that is most needed.

Current research has underestimated the importance of employment and employment history for women's future. Indeed, research on "dual roles" evidences a genteel neglect of the economic dimension. New research on women's multiple roles needs to focus more on the salable and transferable skills and experience women gain from employment, and less on their husbands' marital satisfaction. Above all, there needs to be considerably more work on developing predictive models that chart women's paths to the economic outcomes of midlife.

Unacknowledged normative perspectives have distorted existing research on women's multiple roles and options. "Regular" careers, composed of "on-time" life transitions, have been viewed as more respectable. "Off-time" transitions are viewed as deviant, giving rise to imputations of personal irresponsibility or immaturity. However, an emphasis on outcomes of differing pathways should produce rather different judgments. Some "off-time" transitions may be detrimental to women's economic self-sufficiency in later life (for example, very early childbearing), while others, equally "deviant," may enhance later economic status (for example, "late" marriage contigent upon educational and career goals).

In specifying future directions for research, we are stressing the need for sustained study of women's multiple roles, with an emphasis on outcomes over longer periods of time. A major thrust must be increased study of women in their work roles. In the course of our review, we have raised many issues that call for comparisons of women and men in the work world.

Many pressing questions involve the outcomes of multiple role enactment for women and men. Under what conditions does one enjoy the benefits of role accumulation? Under what conditions does role conflict occur? Specifically, what elements in the organization, setting, or staffing of employment facilitate coping strategies of what types? Are there ranks, occupations, or employers that facilitate the acquisition or exercise of methods of status articulation? And for the range of organization variables to which our attention is directed, we can ask: How are women and men distributed over these opportunities?.

The study of women's role partners in the world of work deserves much more attention than it has received to date. One focus for needed research is the question of women's peers in the workplace, and the related, crucial factor of sex composition of the work group. Past research has shown positive effects of both peers and superiors on the career success of men, but the picture will be more complex for women. When women in sex-typical occupations are studied, the role of peers tends to be overlooked competely. Research on women in sex-atypical occupations suggests negative influences of male peers on women's career progress. The picture will be equally complex with respect to women's superiors in the workplace. Researchers have raised issues concerning mentoring and role modeling for long-term occupational success of women, stressing the importance of support and coaching by superiors in the organizational structure. Most accounts note the paucity of women at higher ranks as an impediment to career facilitation for women, but have not systematically examined the role of male superiors. When researchers document negative attitudes toward female careers in men at high organizational ranks, they do not analyze the implications in terms of role relationships and face-to-face interaction.

Co-workers, particularly men, are not inert elements of industrial design in women's work contexts. Rather, they engage women actively and, as we have seen, actively impede women's role enactment and career advancement in some instances. The importance of role partners in deliberately inducing role conflict surfaced first in accounts of women's experiences on the job. By this means, a new and significant type of role conflict was brought to the attention of the social science fraternity. The effects of this factor, previously overlooked by researchers interested in occupational mental health, are important for the study of job stress, in both the short run and the long run. More research is needed on the ways in which women's performance in the work role is impeded and on the ways long-term outcomes, such as labor force attachment, are affected.

It appears that in her role as worker, a wife has an invisible role partner, in addition to peers and superiors on the job. Although research has documented the importance of husband's attitude in a woman's initial decision to embrace employment, his continuing influence is rarely taken into account. Systematic research on the interactions of obligations and privileges associated with work and family roles for women and men is called for.

One critical variable that appears in both work and family role relationships is power. Current evidence seems consistent with the proposition that the acquisition of role privileges in the work organization is facilitated by possessing and wielding credible power. Being perceived and reacted to as credible wielders of power appears to be problematic for women. Yet the effective use of power contributes to career advancement in many ways. As only one example, when one has the power to command desired outcomes for subordinates, their loyalty is strengthened, and the individual's power position is enhanced as grateful former subordinates move up in the organizational hierarchy. Lack of career mobility, as much as intermittent labor force participation, produces poor economic outcomes for women in midlife.

Another focus for researchers is the connection between role stress in women workers and aspects of the organizational context that are susceptible to change. Both the stressors and the need for change have been neglected topics during decades when the norm was the male breadwinner–full-time housewife household. Current interest in the economic status of the midlife woman has led us to reevaluate that path, whose effects are disastrous in the event of marital dissolution. Similarly suspect are the script and associated employment career that define wives' employment as incidental and episodic. When women (and their wages) are viewed as dispensable, public concern about their conditions of employment is minimal. As a result of past definitions of the situation, substantial gaps in both policy and research are evident.

Today it is apparent that continuous labor force participation enhances women's midlife economic outcomes. Women's experiences in the labor market are given increasing importance, and researchers are increasingly drawn to the study of factors that drive women from employment or compromise their productivity. There has been too little research on job satisfaction among women, and its long-term effects on productivity, mobility, and labor force attachment. When we make the linkages between low labor force participation and economic trouble in midlife, we are forced to examine fundamental questions about what paid work offers women of any age. Program policy and planning must also attack these basic issues.

FUTURE DIRECTIONS FOR POLICY

Midlife women are a heterogeneous group, exhibiting varying degrees of economic viability and vulnerability. Although they represent a wide range in educational attainment, labor force experience, occupational prestige, marital and family status, and health, they share the need to achieve economic security. For most women, economic security in the latter half of the life-span is often uncertain. Older women are joining the ranks of the poverty-stricken faster than any other group in this country: The poverty rate for women over age 65 is almost twice the rate for men of the same ages (U.S. Bureau of the Census, 1982). A sound economic future can be obtained through a well-paying job with ample benefits and a pension plan, a husband with the same, or both. At midlife, the proportion of women holding well-paying jobs that provide benefits is small, while the chance that they may experience the loss of a husband is large. Employed women, married or not, have better chances for economic survival at midlife and later than women who are unemployed. Women without their own earnings *and* without husbands fare the worst.

Social security entitlement programs such as the Old Age, Survivor's, Disability, and Health Insurance (OASDHI) program are supposed to provide benefits to persons in need of income and to provide insurance against economic disruptions resulting from disability, retirement, or the death of an income-producing spouse. Midlife women without incomes or with meager incomes have only these programs to turn to at midlife and in later years. Some 60% of older single women collect their major source of income from social security (Miller, 1982).

The system of entitlement programs known simply as "social security" was created with one role in mind for women, homemaker, and one for men, breadwinner. While Social Security has tried to keep pace with inflation, it has done relatively little to accommodate the changes in family roles and life-styles occurring since Social Security was established. The once-common pattern of lifelong marriage between a career homemaker and her breadwinning husband has been replaced by a growing diversity of marital, familial, and occupational roles of women and men over the life-course (U.S. Dept. of H.E.W., 1979; National Commission on Social Security, 1981; Cahn, 1978).

Despite the changing roles of women and men, the objectives of the Social Security entitlement programs remain much the same as they were at the programs' inception in the 1930s: Women are provided for mainly in their roles as workers' wives and mothers of workers' children. According to eligibility criteria and benefit formulae, women who do not have long and continuous labor force histories are entitled to benefits by virtue of their relationships to men and children. For example, under Social Security, men "earn" disability benefits and retirements benefits (if and when they need them) by paying taxes on their earnings. In most cases, women also "earn" disability and retirement benefits, not because they may be paying taxes on their own earnings and require such benefits but because they are related to disabled or retired men and qualify for benefits as "dependents" rather than "workers." Social Security pays a widow with dependent children a caretaker's allowance, but only until her children reach age 16. Social Security then does not supplement the widow's income again until she reaches age 60 (age 50 if she becomes disabled). (For a thorough description of federal programs and their treatment of women, see Griffiths, 1976; Kinsley, 1977; Gordon, 1979; Miller, 1982; Mudrick, 1983.)

The midlife woman who has never been employed is usually a career wife and homemaker. Her husband's pension and future retirement benefits will support the couple in their later years. Their monthly Social Security check will amount to the husband's full benefit plus an additional half for his wife. However, if the husband should die or the marriage dissolve before retirement age, financial security for the widow or divorcee is severely diminished. Private pensions and life insurance contribute to the widow's economic well-being in only a small percentage of cases. Survivor's Insurance provides relief in this situation, but only to midlife widows who are disabled or have dependent children. Employment remains the sole option for formerly married women without dependents before retirement age, yet the government provides little in the way of job placement and training to upgrade educational credentials or teach profitable skills for these women.

The midlife woman who has been continuously employed throughout adulthood is least likely to experience poverty at midlife or later. She is, however, treated unfairly in public program definitions. Continuously employed married women receive no return on *their own* contributions to the Social Security system unless their entitlement (on account of their own earnings record) is larger than half their husbands' full benefit. The same applies to divorced women whose marriages lasted at least 10 years and who have not remarried. As a result of these stipulations, married and divorced midlife women whose lifetime earnings are less than their husbands' or ex-husbands' (of 10 years or more) receive retirement benefits no larger than if they had never worked for pay. A widow who has continuous labor force experience must be entitled to a retirement benefit larger than her deceased husband's full benefit in order to collect on account of her own earnings record rather than as a surviving dependent.

The midlife woman employed intermittently throughout adulthood and who is no longer a wife or mother fares worst under the current set of public programs. Time out of the labor force reduces the number of years used to compute retirement benefits, resulting in lower benefits for women who have spent some portion of their adult years in child care and homemaking. A previously married midlife woman usually has lifetime earnings far below those of her former spouse. Her retirement benefit, if she was married for at least 10 years, reflects her former dependency status as a wife. She is not entitled to an additional benefit because of her tax contributions to the system for however many years she was employed. The same applies to a married woman. These dichotomous classifications mask the realities of women's multiple roles and, indeed, penalize them.

Midlife women who have not followed a traditional male occupational earnings career (a majority) and who are no longer wives and/or mothers of dependent children (an increasing percentage) fall through the holes in the "social safety net." There are no programs available to supply financial aid to the midlife career homemaker should she become disabled or unable to perform her domestic occupation. The survivors of a deceased career homemaker are not entitled to benefits, either. Should a midlife woman find herself widowed, divorced, or separated prior to retirement age, the risk of poverty is high, while the chance for employment is low if she is not already employed.

What, then, are the forms of assistance and support for midlife women in need of income? There exist no federal cash transfer entitlement programs that provide for women before retirement age unless they have dependent children, with the exception of disability insurance. However, disability insurance is not paid to career homemakers who become disabled or chronically ill. Even if needy midlife women receive cash transfers from disability insurance, the benefits are usually insufficient to boost the women out of poverty. Women with paid employment experience who become disabled and can prove recency of employment are entitled to benefits, but their dependents collect benefits only if the disabled woman can prove she is the primary wage-earner in the household. The Old Age, Survivor's, Disability, and Health Insurance program seems blind to the realities of women's employment rhythms. There is a considerable need for new programs as well as modifications to the current Social Security system.

Interest in the way women are treated under the Social Security system has grown in recent years. Task forces, national commissions, and congressional committees have been formed to examine the issues and offer proposals or recommendations for change (U.S. Dept. of H.E.W., 1979; National Commission on Social Security, 1981; Cahn, 1978). Three variations on the Social Security tax and benefit structure have received considerable attention. These three proposals offer the most practical solutions for revising the unwieldy Social Security system.

The first variation proposes an individually based benefit structure. This structure would resemble the current one, with the exception that survivors' and dependents' benefits would eventually be phased out. Women and men would be encouraged to enter paid employment as well as to share homemaking responsibilities. Without time spent in paid employment, a person would not be eligible for the forms of Social Security assistance available today.

The second variation proposes changes to accommodate homemakers who are, under the current system, not entitled to any benefits on account of their status as workers. Rather than deriving benefits from spouses, full-time homemakers would be credited for their years of service in the home. The credits would apply toward future retirement benefits, which the homemaker could collect at retirement age regardless of marital status. These credits would be financed through taxes on the homemaker or on the total household income.

The third variation proposes that the total income of a couple, regardless of the actual proportion contributed by each spouse, be shared equally in calculating credits toward benefits. Under this plan, full-time homemakers would receive the same benefits as their husbands while married, accumulating these credits throughout their marital career, and keeping them if the marriage should end.

These proposals are a first step in remedying the unfair treatment of women under Social Security. But while these plans recognize that women, regardless of the type and amount of work they have performed, need basic protection like men, they do not realize that women lack the opportunities to achieve economic security through their own efforts. Innovative and diverse support systems are required to address the needs of women at midlife and after. Programs must be established to accommodate successive groups of midlife women with varied educational, marital, and employment histories—women who desire to learn new skills to enter or reenter the job market, to engage in volunteer activities as leaders, teachers, and counselors, to complete high school or college degrees, and to enhance and transform multiple role experiences into socially valued, marketable credentials.

REFERENCES

Albrecht, A. Informal interaction patterns of professional women. In B. A. Stead (Ed.), *Women in management*. Englewood Cliffs, N.J.: Prentice-Hall, 1976.

Angrist, S., and Almquist, E. M. *Careers and contingencies: How college women juggle with gender*. Port Washington, N.Y.: Kennikat Press, 1975.

Baird, L. L. Role stress in graduate students. *Dissertation Abstracts*, 1967, *11-A*, 3929.

Barnett, R. C., and Baruch, G. K. Women in the middle years: A critique of research and theory. *Psychology of Women Quarterly*, 1978, *3*, 187–197.

Barnett, R. C., and Baruch, G. K. *Role strain, number of roles and psychological well-being*. Working Paper, Wellesley College Center for Research on Women, 1981.

Bart, P. Depression in middle aged women. In V. Gornick and B. K. Moran (Eds.), *Women in sexist society: Studies in power and powerlessness*. New York: Basic Books, 1971.

Bartol, K. M., and Butterfield, D. A. Sex effects in evaluating leaders. *Journal of Applied Psychology*, 1976, *61*, 446–454.

Baruch, R., Segal, S., and Hendrick, F. A. Constructs of career and family: A statistical analysis of thematic material. *Journal of Counseling Psychology*, 1968, *5*, 308–316.

Bass, B. M., Krusell, J., and Alexander, R. A. Male managers' attitudes toward working women. *American Behavioral Scientist*, 1971, *15*, 221–236.

Bayes, M., and Newton, P. M. Women in authority: A sociopsychological analysis. *Journal of Applied Behavioral Science*, 1978, *14*, 7–20.

Bernard, J. *Academic women*. University Park: Pennsylvania State University Press, 1964.

Bernard, J. *The future of marriage*. New York: World, 1972. (a)

Bernard, J. Changing family lifestyles: One role, two roles, shared roles. In L. K. Howe (Ed.), *The future of the family*. New York: Simon & Schuster, 1972. (b)

Bernard, J. Models for the relationship between the world of women and the world of men. In L. Kriesberg (Ed.), *Research in social movements, conflicts, and change* (Vol. 3). Greenwich, Conn.: JAI Press, 1978.

Birnbaum, J. A. *Life patterns, personality style, and self-esteem in gifted family oriented and career committed women*. Doctoral dissertation, State University of Michigan, Ann Arbor, 1971.

Borker, S. R., Loughlin, J., and Rudolph, C. S. The long-term effects of adolescent child-rearing: A retrospective analysis. *Journal of Social Service Research*, 1979, 2, 341–355.

Brim, O. G., Jr. Theories of the male mid-life crisis. *Counseling Psychologist*, 1975, 6, 2–9.

Brim, O. G., Jr. *Socialization in an unpredictable society*. Paper presented to the plenary session on family and socialization, American Sociological Association annual meeting, 1980.

Brim, O. G., Jr., and Ryff, C. D. On the properties of life events. In P. B. Baltes and O. G. Brim, Jr. (Eds.), *Life-span development and behavior* (Vol. 3). New York: Academic Press, 1980.

Brown, C. A., Feldberg, R., Fox, E. M., and Kohen, J. Divorce: Chance of a new lifetime. *Journal of Social Issues*, 1976, 32, 119–133.

Cahn, A. F. Highlights of eighteen papers on problems of midlife women. In U.S. Congress Select Committee on Aging, *Women in midlife—Security and fulfillment* (Part I). Washington, D.C.: U.S. Government Printing Office, 1978.

Cohen, J. F. Male roles in mid-life. *Family Coordinator*, 1979, 28, 465–471.

Coser, L. *Greedy institutions*. New York: Free Press, 1974.

Coser, R. L. Role distance, sociological ambivalence, and transitional status systems. *American Journal of Sociology*, 1966, 72, 173–187.

Coser, R. L., and Rokoff, G. Women in the occupational world: Social disruption and conflict. *Social Problems*, 1971, 18, 535–552.

Davis, E. Careers as concerns of blue-collar girls. In A. Shostak and W. Gomberg (Eds.), *Blue collar world: Studies of the American worker*. Englewood Cliffs, N.J.: Prentice-Hall, 1964.

Day, D. R., and Stogdill, R. M. Leader behavior of male and female supervisors: A comparative study. *Personnel Psychology*, 1972, 26, 353–360.

de Beauvoir, S. *The second sex*. New York: Vintage Books, 1974.

Derr, C. B. (Ed.). *Work, family and the career: New frontiers in theory and research*. New York: Praeger, 1980.

Duvall, E. M. *Family development*. New York: Lippincott, 1957.

Elder, G. H., Jr. Family history and the life course. *Journal of Family History*, 1977, 2, 279–304.

Elder, G. H., Jr. *History and the family: The discovery of complexity*. Ernest Burgess Award Lecture, Portland, Oregon, October 25, 1980. (Revised, March 1, 1981.)

Epstein, C. F. Encountering the male establishment: Sex status limits on women's careers in the professions. *American Journal of Sociology*, 1970, 75, 965–982.

Evan, W. M., and Levin, E. G. Status-set and role-set conflicts of the stockbroker: A problem in sociology. *Social Forces*, 1966, 45, 73–83.

Featherman, D. L. The life-span perspective in social science research. Social Science Research Council, January 15, 1981.

Feldman, S. D. Impediment or stimulant: Marital status and graduate education. *American Journal of Sociology*, 1973, 78, 982–994.

Gannon, M. J., and Hendrickson, D. H. Career orientation and job satisfaction among working wives. *Journal of Applied Psychology*, 1973, 57, 339–340.

Glick, P. *American families*. New York: Wiley, 1957.

Goffman, E. Role distance. In E. Goffman, *Encounters*. Indianapolis: Bobbs-Merrill, 1961.

Goode, W. J. A theory of role strain. *American Sociological Review*, 1960, 25, 483–496.

Gordon, F. E., and Hall, D. T. Self-image and stereotypes of femininity: Their relationship to women's role conflicts and coping. *Journal of Applied Psychology*, 1974, 59, 241–243.

Gordon, N. M. Institutional responses: The social security system. In R. E. Smith (Ed.), *The subtle revolution*. Washington, D.C.: Urban Institute, 1979.

Griffiths, M. W. How much is a woman worth? The American public policy. In J. R. Chapman (Ed.), *Economic independence for women* (Sage Yearbooks in Women's Policy Studies, Vol. 1). Beverly Hills: Sage, 1976.

Grimm, J. W., and Stern, R. N. Sex roles and internal labor market structures: The "female" semi-professions. *Social Problems*, 1974, *21*, 690–705.

Gross, N., McEachern, A., and Mason, W. Role conflict and its resolution. In B. Biddle and E. J. Thomas (Eds.), *Role theory: Concepts and research*. New York: Wiley, 1966.

Hall, D. T. A model of coping with role conflict: The role behavior of college women. *Administrative Science Quarterly*, 1972, *17*, 471–486.

Hall, D. T., and Gordon, F. E. Career choices of married women: Effects on conflict, role behavior, and satisfaction. *Journal of Applied Psychology*, 1973, *58*, 42–48.

Harmon, L. W. Predictive power over ten years of measured social service and scientific interests among college women. *Journal of Applied Psychology*, 1969, *53*, 193–198.

Harragan, B. L. *Games mother never taught you*. New York: Warner Books, 1977.

Haynes, S. G., and Feinleib, M. Women, work and coronary heart disease—Prospective findings from the Framingham Heart Study. *American Journal of Public Health*, 1980, *70*, 133–141.

Haynes, S. G., Levine, S., and Scotch, N. The relationship of psychosocial factors to coronary heart disease in the Framingham Heart Study I. Methods and risk factors. *American Journal of Epidemiology*, 1978, *107*, 362–383.

Hill, R., and Hansen, D. A. The identification of conceptual frameworks utilized in family study. *Marriage and Family Living*, 1960, *22*, 299–311.

Hill, R., and Mattessich, P. Family development theory and life-span development. In P. B. Baltes and O. G. Brim, Jr. (Eds.), *Life-span development and behavior* (Vol. 2). New York: Academic Press, 1979.

Hoferek, M., and Sarnowski, A. Feelings of loneliness of women medical students. *Journal of Medical Education*, 1981, *56*, 397–403.

Holahan, C. K., and Gilbert, L. A. Interrole conflict for working women: Careers versus jobs. *Journal of Applied Psychology*, 1979, *64*, 86–90.

Howe, L. K. The world of women's work. In J. P. Rosenfeld (Ed.), *Relationships: The marriage and family reader*. Glenview, Ill.: Scott, Foresman, 1982.

Kahn, R. L., Wolfe, D. M., Quinn, R. D., and Snoek, J. D. *Organizational stress: Studies in role conflict and ambiguity*. New York: Wiley, 1964.

Kanter, R. M. *Men and women of the corporation*. New York: Basic Books, 1977. (a)

Kanter, R. M. Some effects of proportions on group life: Skewed sex ratios and responses to token women. *American Journal of Sociology*, 1977, *82*, 965–900. (b)

Karp, D. A., and Yoels, W. C. Work, careers, and aging. *Qualitative Sociology*, 1981, *4*, 145–166.

Kinsley, S. Women's dependency and federal programs. In J. R. Chapman and M. Gates (Eds.), *Women into wives: The legal and economic impact of marriage* (Sage Yearbooks in Women's Policy Studies, Vol. 2). Beverly Hills: Sage, 1977.

Komarovsky, M. Cultural contradictions and sex roles. *American Journal of Sociology*, 1946, *52*, 184–189.

Komarovsky, M. Cultural contradictions and sex roles: The masculine case. *American Journal of Sociology*, 1973, *78*, 873–884.

Kotlar, S. Intrumental and expressive marital roles. *Sociology and Social Research*, 1962, *46*, 186–194.

Kreps, J., and Clark, R. *Sex, age and work: The changing composition of the labor force*. Baltimore: Johns Hopkins Press, 1975.

Lamb, M. E. *The role of the father in child development.* New York: Wiley, 1976.
Lashuk, M. W., and Kurian, G. Employment status, feminism, and symptoms of stress: The case of a Canadian prairie city. *Canadian Journal of Sociology,* 1977, 2, 195–204.
Laws, J. L. The psychology of tokenism: An analysis. *Sex Roles,* 1975, 1, 151–174.
Laws, J. L. Work aspirations of women: False leads and new starts. *Signs,* 1976, 1, 33–49.
Laws, J. L. Work motivation and work behavior of women: New perspectives. In J. A. Sherman and F. L. Denmark (Eds.), *The psychology of women: Future directions in research.* New York: Psychological Dimensions, 1978.
Laws, J. L. *The second x: Sex role and social role.* New York: Elsevier/North Holland, 1979.
Laws, J. L. *Problems of access and problems of success in women's career advancement.* Paper presented at the NIE Conference on Attitudinal and Behavioral Measurement in Social Processes/Women's Research, Washington, D.C., 1980.
Laws, J. L., and Tangri, S. S. *Institutional sexism: Or, why there is no conspiracy.* Paper presented at the American Psychological Association annual meeting, 1979.
Levitt, E. S. Vocational development of professional women: A review. *Journal of Vocational Behavior,* 1971, 1, 375–385.
Looft, W. R. Sex differences in the expression of vocational aspirations by elementary school children. *Developmental Psychology,* 1971, 5, 366.
Lorber, J. *Trust, loyalty and the place of women in the informal organization of work.* Paper presented at the American Sociological Association annual meeting, 1975.
Mahajah, A. Women's two roles: A study of role conflict. *Indian Journal of Social Work,* 1966, 26, 377–380.
Mayer, T. F. Middle age and occupational processes: An empirical essay. *Sociological Symposium,* 1969, 3, 89–106.
Mayes, S. S. *Women in positions of authority: An analysis of changing sex roles.* Paper presented at the American Sociological Association annual meeting, 1976.
Merton, R. K. *Social theory and social structure.* New York: Free Press, 1968.
Miller, D. C. *Social security and women's lives.* Paper presented at the National Conference on Social Welfare, Boston, Mass., 1982.
Modell, J., Furstenberg, F. F., Jr., and Herschberg, T. Social change and transitions to adulthood in historical perspective. *Journal of Family History,* 1976, 1, 7–32.
Monahan, L., Kuhn, D., and Shaver, P. Intrapsychic vs. cultural explanations of the fear of success motive. *Journal of Personality and Social Psychology,* 1974, 29, 60–64.
Moore, K. A., Hofferth, S., Caldwell, S. B., and Waite, L. J. *Teenage motherhood: Social and economic consequences.* Washington, D.C.: Urban Institute, 1979.
Mudrick, N. R. Disabled women. *Society,* 1983, 20: 51–55.
Mulvey, M. C. Psychological and sociological factors in prediction of career patterns of women. *Genetic Psychology Monographs,* 1963, 68, 309–386.
National Commission on Social Security. National commission on social security: Recommendations. *Social Security Bulletin,* 1981, 44, 3–13.
Nelson, H. Y., and Goldman, P. R. Attitudes of high school students toward the gainful employment of married women. *Family Coordinator,* 1969, 18, 251–255.
Neugarten, B. The awareness of middle age. In B. L. Neugarten (Ed.), *Middle age and aging.* Chicago: University of Chicago Press, 1968.
Neugarten, B. L., and Brown-Rezanka, L. Midlife women in the 1980's. In U.S. Congress Select Committee on Aging, *Women in midlife—Security and fulfillment* (Part I). Comm. Pub. No. 95–170. Washington, D.C.: U.S. Government Printing Office, 1978.
Nevill, D., and Damico, S. Role conflict in women as a function of marital status. *Human Relations,* 1972, 28, 487–498.
Nieva, V., and Gutek, B. Sex effects on evaluation. *Academy of Management Review,* 1980, 5, 267–276.

Norton, A. The influence of divorce on traditional life cycle measures. *Journal of Marriage and the Family*, 1980, 42, 63–69.
Oakley, A. *The sociology of housework*. New York: Pantheon, 1974.
Oppenheimer, V. K. *The female labor force in the United States: Demographic and economic factors governing its growth and changing composition*. University of California at Berkeley: Population Monograph, Series No. 5, 1970.
Parnes, H. S., Jusenius, C. L., Blau, F., Nestel, G., Shortlidge, R., Jr., and Sandell, S. *Dual careers: A longitudinal analysis of the labor market experience of women* (Vol. 4). Columbus: Ohio State University, Center for Human Resource Research, 1975.
Pearce, D. The feminization of poverty: Women, work, and welfare. In K. W. Feinstein (Ed.), *Working women and families* (Sage Yearbooks in Women's Policy Studies, Vol. 4). Beverly Hills: Sage, 1979.
Pleck, J. H. The work-family role system. *Social Problems*, 1977, 24, 417–427.
Powell, B., and Reznikoff, M. Role conflict and symptoms of psychological distress in college-educated women. *Journal of Consulting and Clinical Psychology*, 1976, 44, 473–479.
Pugh, D. Role activation conflict: A study of industrial inspection. *American Sociological Review*, 1966, 31, 835–842.
Rapoport, R., and Rapoport, R. N. The dual-career family: A variant pattern and social change. *Human Relations*, 1969, 22, 3–30.
Rapoport, and Rapoport, R. N. Early and later experiences as determinants of adult behavior: Married women's family and career patterns. *British Journal of Sociology*, 1971, 22, 16–30.
Riley, M. W. Social gerontology and the age stratification of society. *Gerontologist*, 1971, 11, 79–87.
Riley, M. W. Introduction: Life-course perspectives. In M. W. Riley (Ed.), *Aging from birth to death: Interdisciplinary perspectives*. Boulder, Colo.: Westview Press for the American Association for the Advancement of Science, 1979.
Ritt, L. G. The relationships between role conflict, satisfaction, and the dropout potential of college students. *Dissertation Abstracts International*, 1971, 31(11-B), 6910–6911.
Ritzer, G. Commitment, professionalism and role conflict resolution: The personnel manager. *Dissertation Abstracts*, 1969, 29, 4567A.
Rizzo, J. R., House, R. J., and Lirtzman, S. I. Role conflict and ambiguity in complex organizations. *Administrative Science Quarterly*, 1970, 15, 150–163.
Robinson, J. R., and Converse, P. *Basic tables of time budget data for the United States*. Ann Arbor: Survey Research Center, 1966.
Rodgers, R. H. *Family interaction and transaction: The developmental approach*. Englewood, N.J.: Prentice-Hall, 1973.
Rosen, B., and Jerdee, T. H. Influence of sex role stereotypes on personnel decisions. *Journal of Applied Psychology*, 1974, 59, 9–14. (a)
Rosen, B., and Jerdee, T. H. Sex stereotyping in the executive suite. *Harvard Business Review*, 1974, 52, 45–58. (b)
Rossi, A. S. Aging and parenthood in the middle years. In P. B. Baltes and O. G. Brim, Jr. (Eds.), *Life-span development and behavior* (Vol. 3). New York: Academic Press, 1980.
Rubin, L. B. *Women of a certain age: The midlife search for self*. New York: Harper & Row, 1979.
Sarason, S. B. *Work, aging, and social change: Professionals and the one life-one career imperative*. New York: Free Press, 1977.
Sawhill, I. The economics of discrimination against women: Some new findings. *Journal of Human Resources*, 1973, 8, 383–396.
Sieber, S. D. Toward a theory of role accumulation. *American Sociological Review*, 1974, 39, 567–578.

Siegel, A. E., and Haas, M. B. The working mother: A review of research. *Child Development*, 1963, *34*, 513–542.
Snoek, J. Role strain in diversified role sets. *American Journal of Sociology*, 1966, *71*, 363–372.
Spreitzer, E., Snyder, E. E., and Larson, D. L. Multiple roles and psychological well-being. *Sociological Focus*, 1979, *12*, 141–148.
Stebbins, R. A. A note on the concept of role distance. *American Journal of Sociology*, 1967, *73*, 247–250.
Stebbins, R. A. Role distance, role distance behaviour, and jazz musicians. *British Journal of Sociology*, 1969, *20*, 406–415.
Sterling, B. S., and Owen, J. W. Perceptions of demanding vs. reasoning male and female police officers. *Personality and Social Psychology Bulletin*, 1982, *8*, 336–340.
Tangri, S. Determinants of occupational role innovation among college women. *Journal of Social Issues*, 1972, *28*, 177–201.
Taylor, S., and Fiske, S. T. The token in a small group: Research findings and theoretical implications. In J. Sweeney (Ed.), *Psychology and politics: Collected papers*. New Haven: Yale University Press, 1976.
Terborg, J. R. Women in management: A research review. *Journal of Applied Psychology*, 1977, *62*(6), 647–664.
Troll, L. E., and Turner, J. Overcoming age-sex discrimination. In U.S. Congress Select Committee on Aging, *Women in midlife—Security and fulfillment* (Part I). Comm. Pub. No. 95–170. Washington, D.C.: U.S. Government Printing Office, 1978.
Uhlenberg, P. Cohort variations in family life cycle experiences of U.S. females. *Journal of Marriage and the Family*, 1974, *36*, 284–292.
U.S. Bureau of the Census. A statistical portrait of women in the U.S. *Current Population Reports*, Special Studies, Series P-23, No. 58, 1976.
U.S. Bureau of the Census. A statistical portrait of women in the U.S.: 1978. *Current Population Reports*, Special Studies, Series P-23, No. 100, 1978.
U.S. Bureau of the Census. *Statistical abstract of the U.S.: 1981* (102nd ed.) Washington, D.C., 1981.
U.S. Bureau of the Census. Characteristics of the population below the poverty level: 1980. *Current Population Reports*, Special Studies, Series P-60, No. 133, 1982.
U.S. Department of Health, Education, and Welfare. Social security and the changing roles of men and women. Washington: U.S. Government Printing Office, February 1969.
Walberg, H. J. Personality-role conflict and self-conceptions in urban practice teachers. *School Review*, 1968, *76*, 41–49.
Walker, K. *Time-use patterns for household work related to homemakers' employment*. Washington, D.C.: U.S. Department of Agricultural Research Service, 1970.
Watley, D. J., and Kaplan, R. Career or marriage? Aspirations and achievements of able young women. *Journal of Vocational Behavior*, 1971, *1*, 29–43.
Weick, K. E. Careers as eccentric predicates. *Executive*, 1976, Winter, 6–10.
Weil, M. W. An analysis of the factors influencing married women's actual or planned work participation. *American Sociological Review*, 1961, *26*, 91–96.
Wolman, C., and Frank, H. *The solo woman in a professional peer group*. Working paper 133. Philadelphia: Wharton School, University of Pennsylvania, 1972.
Woods, M. B. The unsupervised child of the working mother. *Developmental Psychology*, 1972, *6*, 14–25.
Ziebarth, C. A. Feminine role conflict: The influence of models and expectations of others. *Dissertation Abstracts International*, 1972, *33*(6-B), 2828.

Chapter 6

The Psychological Well-Being of Women in the Middle Years

Grace K. Baruch

This chapter addresses three questions with respect to the psychological well-being of women in the middle years. What is psychological well-being? How do midlife women vary in level of well-being? What are women's sources of psychological well-being? In other words, what is it, who has it, and how did they get it? Because answers to the last two questions depend upon how well-being is defined, the conceptualization and measurement of well-being are discussed first; findings are then presented that bear on variations and sources.

What is Psychological Well-Being?

The American College Dictionary defines well-being as "a *good or satisfactory* condition of existence" (italics added). This definition reflects an important point about well-being—that it may be assessed by objective or by subjective indices. To know whether a person's condition of existence is *good*, a researcher could objectively measure income, housing, and so on. One might argue, for example, that Caucasian women are higher in well-being than Hispanic women because they have larger income and larger homes and are hospitalized less often. Clearly, judgments and relative standards enter into this approach, but the judgments and standards are the researcher's.

To know whether a person's condition of existence is *satisfactory*, in contrast, you must ask the person; satisfaction is in the eye of the sub-

---

Grace K. Baruch • Wellesley College Center for Research on Women, Wellesley, Massachusetts 02181.

ject. A woman's degree of satisfaction with her home, for example, may be very different from what the researcher expects on the basis of an objective index of number of rooms. studies of psychological well-being, then, rely primarily on self-reports, on people's evaluations of their lives.

Satisfaction is by no means the only dimension of their lives that people are asked about. Until the late 1950s, most studies of psychological well-being focused on symptoms of mental illness; epidemiological studies reported the incidence in communities of psychiatric symptomatology, such as anxiety and depression (e.g., Srole, Langner, Michael, Opler, and Rennie 1962). In 1957, however a "quality of life" survey carried out by the Institute of Social Research at the University of Michigan went beyond this approach to investigate, in addition to symptomatology, aspects of "positive mental health," such as happiness, satisfaction, and coping styles (Gurin, Veroff, and Feld, 1960). This chapter draws heavily on this study, and on two other national surveys also done at the University of Michigan: a replication of the 1957 study carried out in 1976 and reported in *The Inner American* (Veroff, Douvan, and Kulka, 1981) and *The Quality of American Life* (Campbell, Converse, and Rodgers, 1976). Each study was based on a national probability sample of over 2000 subjects. (As is often the case, the numbers of minority women included in these and in other studies cited were usually not sufficient to permit fine-grained analyses.)

Despite a lack of agreement about what constitutes psychological well-being—about the specific components—researchers have consistently acknowledged that well-being is not "one thing" but rather is multidimensional and requires multiple measures (Andrews and Withey, 1974; Bryant and Veroff, 1982). There is consistent evidence, for example, that one's level of negative feelings and of positive feelings are relatively independent (Bradburn and Caplowitz, 1965). One may, for example, have high self-esteem but feel anxious and unhappy, as might be true of the mother of an acutely ill child, or the wife of a coronary patient.

In *The Quality of American Life*, Campbell *et al.* focused on two major components of well-being: happiness, defined as an affective, somewhat labile state, and satisfaction, a more stable, cognitively based appraisal of how one's life is turning out relative to one's expectations and aspirations. Happiness and satisfaction were treated as separate aspects of well-being, although they are correlated with each other at about the .50 level. The 1957 Gurin *et al.* study (1960) included, in addition to happiness and satisfaction, several measures of the self-concept, as did Veroff *et al.* (1981) in their 1976 replication. The latter study had an extremely broad array of 18 well-being indices, including happiness and satisfaction, current worries, "morale" about the future, and past feelings of an impending nervous breakdown.[1] The authors argue that the 18 indices measure distinct components of well-being and that analyzing the patterns and correlates of each index separately therefore stays closer to psychological reality than does combining indices. Nevertheless, it is extremely difficult to deal with so many different measures in conceptualizing the nature, patterns, and sources of well-being. For example, the answers to such questions as "How is a woman's age related to her well-being? or "How do women and men compare in level of well-being?" will differ depending upon the specific component selected for analysis. Moreover, many components, such as happiness and satisfaction, are typically measured by single-item scales, which are less reliable than composite measures. As Campbell stated in 1976, "We must begin to work seriously on problems of identifying the major dimensions of the experience of well-being."

Drawing on data from the 1957 and 1976 Michigan studies, Bryant and Veroff (1982) examined the underlying dimensions of well-being—seeking a structural model to reduce "conceptual chaos."

The authors examined separately data for men and for women collected in 1957 and in 1976. Using sophisticated factor-analytic techniques, they found empirical support for a proposed three-dimensional conceptual model of well-being (Their labels refer to the negative pole): (1) *unhappiness* (negative affect), (2) *strain* (symptomatology and worries), and (3) *personal inadequacy* (Poor self-concept). Women and men resembled each other in how their well-being was structured with respect to these three dimensions—that is, in how the components were clustered. Sex differences in structure were smaller than differences *within* each sex between the two time periods of 1957 and 1976. The unhappiness and personal inadequacy factors were independent of each other, while strain was moderately related to each. In other words, the level of a woman's self-esteem and her degree of happiness may be quite different; however, the extent of symptomatology she reports is related to each.

In a study of psychological well-being in women 35 to 55, carried out in 1979–1980, the author and Rosalind Barnett also examined the dimensions of well-being, using exploratory factor analysis (Baruch, Barnett, and Rivers, 1983).[2] The 238 subjects, all Caucasian, were ran-

---

[1]For a detailed description of the measures used in the three Michigan studies, the reader is referred to the three books cited.

[2]Exploratory factor analysis is distinguished from confirmatory factor analysis, which is used to test whether the data fit a proposed theoretical model. Exploratory factor analysis is a tool for investigating the dimensions underlying an array of indices: Results need to be replicated to determine whether they are generalizable or are the product of chance.

domly selected from a community in the Greater Boston metropolitan area. Four family-status groups were included: never-married, married without children, married with children, and divorced with children. All never-married and divorced women were employed; each of the two groups of married women was divided equally between employed and not employed. Six role-pattern groups of 45 each were thus formed.[3] Employed women were selected equally among those in high-, medium-, and low-prestige occupations (Siegel, 1971); nonemployed women were selected similarly according to the prestige of their husbands' occupations. Thus, certain groups were oversampled in relation to their presence in the general population. The study was designed to include women whose role patterns are of conceptual interest and of increasing social importance; results cannot be generalized to American women as a whole.

Eight measures of well-being were included: standard single-item scales measuring happiness, satisfaction, and optimism; the anxiety and depression subscales of the Hopkins Symptom Checklist (Derogatis, Lipman, Rickels, Uhlenhuth, and Covi, 1974); the Pearlin Mastery Scale (Pearlin and Schooler, 1978), measuring locus of control; the Rosenberg (1965) self-esteem scale; and a measure of self-concept developed for this study that assessed the balance of rewards and concerns (rewards minus concerns) women reported about themselves. The analysis yielded two major underlying dimensions or factors. The first factor was labeled *mastery*; scores contributing strongly to this factor were the two self-concept scales, locus of control, and the anxiety and depression subscales. Thus, a woman with a high sense of mastery evaluates herself positively, feels in control of her life, and has low levels of depression and anxiety. The second factor that emerged was labeled *pleasure*; scores contributing strongly to this factor were happiness, satisfaction, and optimism. Comparing these dimensions to Bryant and Veroff's, sense of mastery can be seen as combining personal inadequacy and strain; pleasure is analogous to their unhappiness factor.

This two-dimensional model, mastery and pleasure, is useful in thinking about certain puzzles and dilemmas with respect to the well-being of women. For example, the women Betty Friedan described in *The Feminine Mystique* (1963) reported deriving satisfaction from their attachment to husband and children, but they also reported feeling purposeless and worthless. They can be seen as doing well with respect to the pleasure dimension of well-being but not so well with respect to

---

[3]Despite screening over 6000 women, it was not possible to locate sufficient numbers of married, childless, nonemployed women. This role pattern is apparently becoming less viable, given current economic and social conditions.

their sense of mastery. In contrast, some career women who have struggled successfully to attain prestigious positions are portrayed by the media as asking resentfully: Where is the joy? Is this all there is to life? These women can be seen as having a strong sense of mastery but as feeling deficient in pleasure. As Freud's famous dictum on love and work suggests, different dimensions of well-being may have different sources. For mature women in our society today, it may often prove difficult to maintain a highly positive self-concept in the absence of socially valued work, and it can also be difficult to derive an adequate sense of enjoyment from a life in which intimate relationships are missing.

Who Has Well-Being?

Comparing Women and Men

A question repeatedly asked about the psychological well-being of women is: How do they compare with men? The answer, as has been noted, depends on how one defines well-being—on which component one examines. Studies consistently report that women have higher rates of psychiatric symptomatology, and especially of depression, than do men, although they are not less happy or satisfied; there is agreement that this difference in symptomatology is not primarily due to women's greater willingness to report symptoms (Radloff, 1975; Rosenfield, 1980). For example, Veroff *et al.* found that women report more difficulties in their lives, and more worries, than do men. Gurin *et al.* found that women had less positive self-concepts, as well as higher levels of symptomatology. In both studies, however, levels of *happiness* and *satisfaction* were similar; Campbell *et al.* also found no significant sex difference in overall life satisfaction.

The authors of *The Inner American*, speculating about the reasons for the sex differences in symptomatology, argue that women's role as nurturers responsible for the well-being of others—especially as primary caretakers of children—means living with uncertainty, lack of control, and other stressful conditions conducive to the development of symptomatology. The fate of others is uncontrollable and unpredictable; to feel responsible for it is risky. Rosenfield (1980) argues that power relations between women and men may be key variable in explaining women's higher roles of depression.

Other researchers point to the difference in women's and men's patterns of involvement in paid employment as critical to their relative psychological well-being. Gove and Tudor (1973) argue that men's participation in two domains of life—paid work and the family—provide a kind of buffer and well-being "insurance." According to their two-role theory, when life is going badly in one domain, a second valued role may provide compensatory satisfaction. This view is consistent with much recent theory and research on multiple roles (Marks, 1977; Sieber, 1974; Thoits, 1983), as is discussed below.

In a review of data from six large national surveys spanning 20 years, Kessler and McCrae (1981) report a decreasing gender gap between the sexes with respect to psychiatric symptomatology and find that women's increasing labor force participation appears to account for about 20% of the variance.[4] Why and how employment may function to increase women's well-being is discussed in the section on employment below.

Chronological Age

How one expects a woman's chronological age to influence her psychological well-being depends upon how one views the feminine role. Freud's well-known comparison of women and men illustrates the traditional view of age differences perhaps even more than of sex differences: "A man of about thirty strikes us as a youthful, somewhat unformed individual, whom we expect to make powerful use of the possibilities for development opened up to him by analysis. A woman of the same age, however, often frightens us by her psychical rigidity and unchangeability. . . . There are no paths open to further development. . . . [It is] as though, indeed, the difficult development to femininity had exhausted the possibilities of the person concerned."

In the traditional conception of femininity, physical attractiveness and involvement in motherhood and in heterosexual relations are central; a decline in well-being with age would seem almost inevitable. In this view, physiological changes in reproductive functioning, in appearance, and in a woman's role as mother should threaten a woman's core identity; women will differ mainly in their capacity to cope with this decline in their sources of well-being.

A contrasting view is that women's well-being, like that of men, is tied to their social identity and thus to how society views them; these in turn shape their self-concepts and their opportunities to obtain satisfaction in a variety of roles throughout their life-span. This view permits the prediction of positive as well as negative changes with age. If wom-

---

[4]A decreasing gender gap in symptomatology was also reported by Srole & Fischer (1980) in their 1978 replication of the Manhattan Mental Health (1957) survey. This study has been severely criticized for methodological problems, such as sample attrition (Dohrenwend, personal communication, 1982).

en's status rises within a society during the second half of a woman's life, for example, then her later years can bring greater well-being.

Findings of relevant studies seem to depend upon when the data were collected. Several studies carried out in the 1950s and 1960s showed women in the middle and later years to be particularly distressed. In 1958 Weiss and Samuelson reported that when asked, "What are the things you do that make you feel useful or important?" a rather substantial proportion of women in the older age groups said that "nothing made them feel useful and important." Lowenthal, Thurnher, and Chiriboga (1975), in their study of four age groups of men and women, described "post-parental" women as strikingly low in well-being—as wanting to grow but seeing no way to do so.

In contrast, when the 1957 Gurin et al. study (1960) was replicated in the 1970s, Veroff et al. (1981) reported that a decline in women's self-esteem with age found in 1950 was no longer evident. Overall, the authors of *The Inner American* conclude that older women were better off in 1976 than in 1957. Women in the Berkeley Growth Study who were rated as relatively autonomous seemed to experience a decline in well-being in their 40s, but when seen again while in their 50s, they were particularly high in well-being. Whether the difference in the social climate of the two time periods, rather than chronological age, explains the improvement is unclear (Livson, 1975).

With respect to satisfaction and happiness, women, like men, typically show increased levels of satisfaction, but a decline in happiness, with age. Campbell et al. (1976) suggests that one's life is an increasingly good "fit" as one grows older, resulting in greater satisfaction, but the intense emotions associated with feelings of happiness may become rarer.

MENOPAUSE AND THE EMPTY NEST

During their middle years, most women experience menopause, and mothers experience the empty nest. Earlier theory and research on menopause and the empty nest have been criticized for focusing on women primarily in their reproductive role, and for failing to consider that these events not only might be neutral but even might be experienced as positive (Barnett and Baruch, 1978; Long and Porter, Chapter 4, this volume). For example, Lowenthal et al. (1975), failing to find evidence of dread of the empty nest among the women in their sample who were facing that transition, concluded that the women's anxiety must be "too deep to be tapped." Yet reinterviews 5 years later confirmed the absence of traumatic effects.

The more women as individuals and as groups are confined to their maternal role, of course, the greater the negative impact such events as menopause and the empty nest are likely to have (Bart, 1971).

Opportunities to participate in other social roles and domains of life can give the cessation of the menses and the independence of one's children a positive meaning, facilitating involvement in paid work, enhancing sexuality (Luria and Meade, Chapter 17; this volume), permitting attention to other needs. As will be discussed in the section on motherhood, being at home with small children can be much more threatening to well-being than the empty nest, which, as Campbell points out (1976), "has a reputation that is not deserved."

THE MIDLIFE CRISIS AND OTHER AGE-LINKED CONCEPTUALIZATIONS OF THE MIDDLE YEARS

The concept of the midlife crisis has recently received wide attention. While many theorists hold the generally optimistic view that growth and change continue throughout life, theories of the middle years nevertheless typically exude a certain aura of gloom. They focus on the juxtaposition in the midlife individual of a growing sense of mortality and an awareness of limited possibilities for achieving one's goals; there is an emotional, as opposed to intellectual, recognition of the biological reality that one in fact does not live forever.

The concept of the midlife crisis is typically part of a theory of adult development in which an invariant sequence of stages linked to chronological age is postulated; the "crisis" then occurs at a predictable time. For example, Daniel Levinson's (Levinson, 1978) mapping of adult development, based on the study of 44 males age 35 to 45, gives special attention to the anxiety and depression that may accompany the tendency around age 40 to reevaluate one's achievements in the light of time left to live. Successful completion of the task of resolving this crisis is thought to lead to further personal growth, new directions, and other positive outcomes. If the crisis is not resolved, discontent and depression are likely to persist into old age.

The age-linked basis of Levinson's theory has been widely criticized, perhaps most effectively by Leonard Pearlin (1975). Pearlin points out that evidence for the existence of a midlife crisis cannot rest solely on studies of middle-aged subjects, for it is possible that the experiences they report may be equally common among 25-year-olds, or among 65-year-olds. In a large national survey of adults over 21, Pearlin and his colleagues found no evidence of a "piling up" in the middle years of anxiety, depression, or indeed of unique transitions and crises. The study of midlife women by the author and Rosalind Barnett found no differences in well-being associated with age among women 35 to 55. When we specifically asked the women about crises and turning points—their presence, their nature—no age-related patterns emerged.

To the extent that an "age and stage" view of adult development is flawed, so too is the concept of the midlife crisis. Another weakness in this concept is that the theoretical, clinical, and empirical bases for it were developed in studies of males, who were the patients, the subjects—and the researchers. Very little theory-based or theory-generating work has focused on women's middle years. Perhaps for this reason one biological sex difference is typically *ignored*—the differential life expectancy of men and women. A man of 45 who is concerned about the implications of having only 20 or so years to live is being realistic about his life expectancy. A woman of 45, who can expect to live perhaps 35 more years, is more likely to be concerned about living too long, with the specter of dependency and loneliness (Baruch, 1980). Most women now in their middle years, moreover, did not have expectations of astounding achievement in the adult world of work; therefore, few find their accomplishments falling short of expectations. Rather, many midlife women in occupations similar to those of Levinson's male subjects are amazed and delighted at achieving more than they imagined to be possible. In the absence of relatively imminent mortality and a sense of accomplishing less than one's dream, the midlife crisis loses its substance.

It may be that such crises are "age-coincidental." That is, certain cohorts have experienced, and will experience, particular influential events at similar ages, as Glenn points out in his work on the impact of the Great Depression (Glenn, 1975). Men born in the 1920s and 1930s, as were Levinson's subjects, were socialized to be achievers and breadwinners, and they may wonder as they turn 40 about the costs of their progress. Women of that era typically married and had children early, and thus found themselves increasingly free of child-rearing responsibilities as they neared 40. It may have seemed, therefore, that women had their own inevitable midlife crisis, characterized by concern about alternatives to their investment in child-rearing, followed by a burst of achievement-related fantasies and activities. But today's young women who remain active in careers throughout their lives are unlikely to experience the same issues at midlife. (Young men who were influenced by the 1960s to be less driven in their work roles are also likely to experience midlife differently from earlier cohorts.)

The likelihood that each cohort will have different normative patterns over the life-course gives rise to another perspective on chronological age and well-being—the on-time/off-time concept. As depicted by Neugarten (1970), Rossi (1980), and others (see Long and Porter, Chapter 5, this volume), it is not so much what happens to a woman at what age but whether it happens at the predicted or expected time that shapes its impact on her well-being. Unanticipated events are more likely to be stressful, and those occurring off time are more likely to be unanticipated. Thus, the latter should have a more negative effect on well-being. The classic example is widowhood, which should be more devastating at age 35 than at 60.

Many other factors, of course, influence a woman's ability to cope with negative events. The important point is that we learn much less about a woman's level of well-being from knowing her chronological age than from knowing how her life pattern fits that which is normative for her cohort (see Brooks-Gunn and Kirsh, Chapter 1, this volume).

Sources of Well-Being

For both women and men, income and education are consistently found to be positively associated with most measures of well-being. Beyond these, how do particular roles that women occupy affect their well-being? Why do these roles function as they do—what specific aspects are important? These questions address variations in women's well-being and the sources of these variations.

Employment

How a woman's employment status—the simple fact of being employed or not—affects her well-being depends upon which aspect of well-being is being examined. Symptomatology scores typically do not differ significantly between homemakers and employed women (Pearlin, 1975; Radloff, 1975). As for happiness, Veroff *et al.* found that housewives were slightly happier; however, among women 40 to 59 in intact first marriages, there were no differences (Serlin, 1980). Campbell *et al.* reported no differences in happiness or satisfaction associated with employment status, with one exception: Among college-educated housewives, employed women were higher. The authors suggest that when "able" women are confined to the homemaker role, they may be more distressed than women in general. For midlife women, self-esteem may be the aspect of well-being most enhanced by paid employment. Coleman and Antonucci (1983) reported that for midlife women included in the 1976 Michigan study, employment was the only significant predictor of self-esteem.

In our study of women 35 to 55, employed and nonemployed women did not differ in pleasure—the components of which are happiness, satisfaction, and optimism; marital status, rather than employment status, was associated with higher pleasure scores. Employed women were significantly higher in sense of mastery, however, indicating a more positive self-concept and lower levels of symptomatology. All four groups of employed women—never-married, married with children, married without children, and divorced—were higher in mastery than were the two groups of nonemployed women—married with children and married without children. Regardless of marital status, then, paid employment seems to have positive consequences for women's self-concept and possibly for the tendency to report psychiatric symptoms, but employment *per se* does not contribute significantly to happiness and satisfaction in the middle years.

In interpreting these patterns, several considerations are important. First, employed and nonemployed women tend to differ in marital status—non-employed women are most likely to be married. A confounding of effects of employment and marriage is thus inevitable unless marital status is controlled. Second, the effects of employment are likely to vary among cohorts, and also within the midlife range. How a woman experiences being a paid worker is influenced, for example, by her socialization and her values, such as whether she was brought up to believe that good wives and mothers stay home. Another reason that age groups may vary in how employment affects well-being is that for women with young children, combining roles may be more stressful than for women whose children are older and more independent.

A third consideration is that, compared with men, women are more constricted in the range of occupations they occupy and are less likely to be in high-prestige occupations. Any interpretation of the effects of employment on women's well-being should take this difference into account. The prestige of an occupation affects job conditions, which in turn affect well-being (Kessler, 1982). Among the employed women in our study, for example, occupational prestige was strongly related to sense of mastery. Since the nature of women's occupational status is changing, patterns now found are likely to differ when more women are employed in prestigious occupations.

As the data on occupational prestige suggest, it is important to consider the quality of a woman's experience within a role, and her attitude toward that role. When a woman's preference for being a homemaker versus being employed is taken into account, for example, homemakers who would prefer to be employed are consistently found to be lower in well-being than homemakers who prefer the role they occupy (Pearlin, 1975). (For employed women, role preference typically does not have a significant effect on well-being. Those who prefer not to be employed are not significantly lower in well-being than those who prefer their actual pattern of paid employment.)

The Psychological Benefits of Employment

There is increasing empirical evidence to support recent theoretical arguments that employment can function to enrich a woman's sense of identity and to provide other psychological rewards, even for women who must juggle many roles (Marks, 1977; Sieber, 1974; Thoits, 1983). For example, a study of English women showed that for those in stressful life circumstances who did not have confidantes, being employed seemed to protect against the occurrence of psychiatric symptoms; symptoms developed in 79% of such nonemployed women but in only 14% of the employed (Brown, Bhrolchain, and Harris, 1975). Campbell (1976) found that employed women reported more pleasures in their lives than did nonemployed women, and since the two groups did not differ in reports of negative aspects, employment was associated with a greater net balance of good over bad.

What particular components of employment may account for the positive effects that have been found? In the first stage of our study, 72 women were interviewed intensively about the rewarding and distressing aspects of the different roles they occupied. On the basis of these interviews, scales with equal numbers of "reward" and "concern" items were developed to assess women's experiences in employment, marriage, and similar factors. The 238 women in the survey stage then indicated to what extent each item was either rewarding or distressing. For example, in employment, rewards included a variety of tasks, a good income, and liking the boss. Concerns included having too much to do, job insecurity, and lack of opportunity for career growth. For each role, the balance between rewarding and distressing aspects could be assessed; this "balance score" constituted an index of the quality of a woman's experience in that role. The balance between rewards and concerns in employment was significantly and positively related to both sense of mastery and pleasure.

With the use of factor-analytic techniques, the underlying dimensions of the rewarding and distressing aspects of each role were also explored. For employment, the major reward factors were *challenge* and *social relationships*; the major concern factors were whether the job was *dull* and whether it was a *dead end*. Scores on these reward and concern factors were significantly related to both sense of mastery and pleasure, with the exception of social relationships, which did not affect mastery. In other words, the components of employment most likely to affect a woman's well-being are how challenging her job is and whether it is dull and dead-ended. Gratifying social relationships at work increase her happiness and satisfaction but not her self-esteem and sense of control.

What is it about the role of homemaker that affects well-being?

Scholars studying homemaking point to negative aspects such as the lack of standards for performance, the lack of objective feedback, the dependence for approval on husbands and children; there are no "entry requirements" (Gove and Tudor, 1973; Lopata, 1971; Oakley, 1974). Studies also show, however, that the freedom to plan one's own schedule—being able to structure and order one's tasks, or not do any at all—is very important to homemakers, especially if the jobs they have previously held, or the jobs they feel qualified to do, lack autonomy.

In our study, the relationship between well-being and the homemaker role was examined; the balance between the rewards and the concerns in the homemaker role was strongly related to a woman's sense of mastery and to her pleasure scores. Factor analyses indicated that the two major sources of distress for the homemakers in our sample were *boredom and isolation* and *not earning money*. The major rewards were the *satisfaction of "being there" for one's family*, the *freedom from supervision*, and the *opportunity to do tasks that fitted one's skills*. Interestingly, only the last factor was related to a woman's well-being; the more a woman felt rewarded by this, the greater her sense of mastery. Homemaking tasks that are a good "fit" may function like paid work as a source of self-esteem.

Marital Status

One of the most consistent findings in the literature on psychological well-being is that married women are happier and more satisfied than are those who are not married, whether the latter are never-married, divorced, or widowed (Baruch *et al.*, 1983; Depner, 1979; Campbell *et al.*, 1976; Glenn, 1975; Veroff *et al.*, 1981; Ward, 1979). In contrast, marriage is not associated with components of well-being other than happiness and satisfaction. For example, comparing never-married women over 30 with a matched sample of married women, Gigy (1980) found that never-married women were less happy, but their self-esteem was no lower, nor did they report more psychiatric symptomatology. In our study, married women were higher in pleasure, of which happiness and satisfaction are major components, but they were not higher in sense of mastery; that is, they did not have more positive self-concepts or lower levels of anxiety and depression.

In interpreting these patterns, several considerations are critical. First, married women are a different group now than earlier in our history. As is often pointed out, divorce is more accessible now, and women who are unhappily married are more likely to remove themselves from the ranks of the married. Moreover, marital status is less confounded with employment status than it once was; today's married women are more likely than formerly to be employed, and as we have seen, employment has a positive effect on several components of well-being. Thus, married women are now more self-selected with respect to both marital status and employment status.

A second point is that marriage is confounded with income—married women tend to have higher family incomes than do nonmarried women—and income is associated with well-being. Thus, one reason for the greater happiness and satisfaction of married women may be their access to money.

Third, marriage also provides access to a sexual partner. Whatever difficulties married women may experience in their sexual relationships, the availability of a sexual partner means a greater likelihood of sexual satisfaction, and sexual satisfaction is highly correlated with overall life satisfaction (see Luria and Meade, Chapter 17, this volume). While both money and sexual satisfaction can certainly be found outside marriage, they are usually more difficult to obtain, especially as women get older.

Beyond these considerations, what is it about being married, and about not being married, that may account for the patterns described?

In our study, factor analyses of the rewarding and distressing aspects of marriage indicated that the major reward was *feeling emotionally supported and appreciated*, and the major concern was *marital conflict*. The more a woman rated emotional support and appreciation as a rewarding part of her marriage, the higher her pleasure score and, to a lesser extent, her sense of mastery. Similarly, the greater her concern about marital conflict, the lower her pleasure and, to a lesser extent, her sense of mastery. The pattern of a greater effect of marital quality on pleasure is consistent with findings already presented. Moreover, the balance score of rewards and concerns in marriage was very strongly related to pleasure but was only weakly related to sense of mastery.

A second approach to understanding how marriage affects well-being is to ask what qualities of the *nonmarried* state are experienced as particularly difficult. Being nonmarried today may be less distressing than it once was: There is less stigma and thus less threat to a woman's self-concept (Veroff *et al.*, 1981). Nevertheless, for many midlife women, it is a struggle to derive sufficient enjoyment from a life pattern that does not provide a stable, "built-in" intimate relationship with another adult. Both for never-married women and for divorced women in our study, the central concern was *lack of an intimate relationship*. To the extent that a woman reported distress about this, her pleasure scores were lower. Her sense of mastery was not affected, however, consistent with the finding that among *married* women, rewards and concerns, and marriage "balance," affected pleasure more than sense of mastery.

A reasonable conclusion about marriage and well-being is that when a married woman is free to choose her employment status and to end an unhappy marriage, being married is likely to enhance her happiness and satisfaction. As a source of self-esteem and protection against anxiety and depression, marriage is of little help; here, a good job is the key.

PARENTAL STATUS

In sharp contrast to the patterns that emerged with respect to marriage and employment, studies consistently find no evidence that being a mother—parental status—enhances a woman's well-being (Barnett and Baruch, 1981; Campbell et al., 1976; Depner, 1979; Sears and Barbee, 1977; Veroff et al., 1981). As Depner states, "There is little evidence that the childless are yearning for a role which they do not have."

Reasoning that the benefits of having children might show up later in life, Glen and McLanahan (1981) studied women over 50, using national survey data. Finding no differences in happiness or satisfaction between mothers and childless women (with income and employment status controlled), the authors conclude: "The best evidence now available indicates that the present young adult should not choose to have children on the basis of expectations that parenthood will lead to psychological rewards in the later stages of life. The prospects for such rewards seem rather dim at best."

Childless women who fear—or are warned—that they'll be sorry "later" should also be aware that a study of widows aged 60–75 shows that even for these women, who would seem to be most in need of them, children had only very slight effects on life satisfaction and other indices of "morale" (Beckman and Houser, 1982). The authors state: "Even among widows over 60, the difference [having children] made to well-being was minute compared to the quality of overall social ties."

That such a seemingly profound difference in women's lives—that between having children and being childless—should be undetectable in its effects on well-being is counterintuitive and somewhat startling. Yet there is at least one obvious reason all too familiar to parents: Children can make one's life miserable as well as wonderful. If one groups together all women who happen to be mothers, those for whom it has worked out well may be balanced by those who have had more suffering than pleasure from their role. In *Occupation Housewife,* Helena Lopata (1971) argues that being a mother is made especially difficult in our culture by the lack of agreement on standards for the role, combined with the unrealistic expectation that one can mold a child to be whatever one wants. The authors of *The Inner American,* as was noted, attributed the lesser well-being of women compared to men to the difficulties and uncertainties of having primary responsibility for child-rearing, and to feeling responsible for how children turn out. Data reported by Long and Porter in this volume (Chapter 5) are relevant here: The hypothesis that a good experience in one role compensates for problems in other roles is generally supported, with one exception—for women, problems in the parent role are not compensated for by satisfaction at work.

What influences the quality of a woman's experience in her role as a mother? In a study of 68 women in western Massachusetts, aged 33–56, Rossi (1980) found that the combination of having a large family and being older—that is, having had children later in life—was likely to impair a woman's sense of well-being. This combination suggests a condition of too much work and too little energy. In our study of women 35 to 55, the balance between rewards and concerns of motherhood was significantly related to both mastery and pleasure. The major concern factor was *conflict with children;* the more a woman reported distress over conflict with children, the lower her pleasure score. For employed women only, mastery was also significantly lower. Perhaps employed women are more likely to blame themselves for problems with their children than are women at home, and thus to react with anxiety and loss of self-esteem.

OTHER SOCIAL ROLES

The set of roles most often studied for both women and men is the "traditional triad"—spouse, parent, worker. Yet these three do not encompass all the roles women occupy, nor are they always the most important. The role of sibling has the longest time-span, for example, and both sibling relationships and relationships with same-age peers who are not kin seem to enhance well-being in later years more than do relationships with children (Beckman and House, 1982; Glenn, 1975). The importance of such roles as friend, neighbor, and colleague to well-being is increasingly being documented, especially in the literature on stress, coping, and social ties (Pearlin, 1982). All these roles have both rewarding and distressing aspects that require further study.

An important role spanning many years is that of daughter, discussed in detail elsewhere in this volume (see Wood, Traupmann, and Hay, Chapter 8; Stueve and O'Donnell, Chapter 9). Despite Nancy Friday's grim portrait of conflict and anger between mother and adult daughter in *My Mother/Myself* (1977), recent research shows that for women in the middle years, the role is typically a source of intimacy and gratification, not primarily of obligations and difficulties (Baruch and Barnett, 1983; Fischer, 1981). During the intensive interview stage of our study, women often mentioned relationships with mothers as particularly rewarding parts of their lives. Based on these interviews, a scale measuring "maternal rapport" was developed for the survey stage. The higher women's maternal rapport scores, the higher both mastery and pleasure—with one exception: For divorced women, there was a negative relationship between maternal rapport and sense of mastery. Perhaps divorced women who are particularly close to their mothers feel somewhat more dependent than is comfortable and thus do not feel in control of their lives. Mothers of divorced women, as Barnett points out (Chapter 15, this volume), too often communicate disappointment and disapproval along with their support, and thus may undermine daughters' feelings of adequacy.

Combining Roles

Long and Porter (Chapter 5, this volume) point to a sex segregation in the literature on combining roles. The study of multiple roles is based on the lives of men and the multiplicity is viewed as beneficial, while "dual roles" is a woman's topic, implying a condition in which the role of paid worker is added to the normative condition of being a wife, mother, and homemaker. Ensuing conflict and guilt are assumed, resulting in impaired well-being.

A new version of the negative view of women's involvement in multiple roles is the concept of "the woman in the middle" (Brody, 1981)—the middle-aged woman who must cope simultaneously with the needs of elderly parents and of teenage children. If she is employed, her job is assumed to make her life even more difficult. As Stueve and O'Donnell (Chapter 8) indicate, however, periods of simultaneous heavy demands from both children and parents are in fact relatively rare, although when they do occur, life can indeed be difficult. Even then, however, a woman's job may be experienced more as a life-saver than as a last straw. In our study, a major concern women had in their role as daughter was the care of elderly parents. But only for nonemployed women was this concern significantly related to a measure of role strain, and only for nonemployed women did level of role strain have a negative impact on mastery and pleasure (Baruch and Barnett, 1981). That is, employed women could be very concerned about the care of elderly parents without experiencing severe role overload and conflict. If they did experience role strain, it did not necessarily impair their well-being. But as data from our intensive interviews suggested, nonemployed women often feel they must be endlessly available to others, and when they do feel resentful or overwhelmed about obligations such as those to parents, they feel they have failed.

It makes a great deal of difference in our concepts of women's lives whether involvement in a variety of roles is shown to bring mainly overload and conflict, or to yield more benefits than costs. The women lowest in mastery in our study were married, nonemployed, and childless, a finding consistent with the Long and Porter argument that if a woman's sole role is that of housewife, this represents a condition of underload that can impair well-being. Those lowest in pleasure were the never-married women, who also occupied only one of the major roles—paid worker. A reanalysis of community survey data by Thoits (1983) gives a support to the view that multiple roles can provide multiple sources of well-being; the number of roles respondents occupied, up to seven, increased well-being, assessed by a measure of symptomatology. Like placing one's eggs in many baskets, investing in several roles is likely to mean having several sources of stimulation, gratification, and social validation.

In our study, employed married women who had children were the highest in well-being, taking into account both mastery and pleasure scores, despite their busy lives. But like most women who are currently middle-aged, few had very young children. Mothers of young children who are building careers often find their multiple roles difficult to manage, although the strain lessens as children get older. If the age at which women bear children continues to rise, more midlife women will have young children, and this may affect the patterns of well-being of future cohorts. The consequences will depend in part upon social conditions, such as the availability of child care. For this reason, and for many others explored elsewhere in this volume, women in their middle years have an important stake in monitoring the social and economic climate of their society.

References

Andrews, F. M., and Withey, S. B. Developing measures of perceived life quality: Results from several national surveys. *Social Indicators Research*, 1974, *1*, 1–26.

Barnett, R. C., and Baruch, G. K. Women in the middle years: A critique of research and theory. *Psychology of Women Quarterly*, 1978, *3*, 187–197.

Bart, P. Depression in middle-aged women. In J. M. Bardwick (Ed.), *Psychology of women: A study of bio-cultural conflicts*. New York: Harper & Row, 1971.

Baruch, G. *Health-related concerns and psychological well-being of middle-aged women*. Paper presented at the meeting of the American Psychological Association, Montreal, 1980.

Baruch, G. K. and Barnett, R. C. *Who has multiple role strain: The woman in the middle revisited*. Paper presented at the meeting of the Gerontological Society, Toronto, 1981.

Baruch, G. K., and Barnett, R. C. Adult daughters' relationships with their mothers. *Journal of Marriage and the Family*, 1983, *45*, 601–606.

Baruch, G., Barnett, R., and Rivers, C. *Life prints: New patterns of love and work for today's women*. New York: McGraw-Hill, 1983.

Beckman, L. J., and Houser, B. B. The consequences of childlessness for the social-psychological well-being of older women. *Journal of Gerontology*, 1982, *37*, 243–250.

Bradburn, N. M., and Caplowitz, D. *Reports on happiness*. Chicago: Aldine, 1965.

Brody, E. "Women in the middle" and family help to older people. *Gerontologist*, 1981, *21*, 471–485.

Brown, G. W., Bhrolchain, M. N., and Harris, T. Social class and psychiatric disturbance among women in an urban population. *Sociology*, 1975, *9*, 225–253.

Bryant, F. B., and Veroff, J. The structure of psychological well-being: A sociohistorical analysis. *Journal of Personality and Social Psychology*, 1982, *43*, 653–673.

Campbell, A. Subjective measures of well-being. *American Psychologist*, 1976, *31*, 117–124.

Campbell, A., Converse, P. E., and Rodgers, W. L., *The quality of American life*. New York: Russell Sage, 1976.

Coleman, L. M., and Antonucci, T. C. Women's well-being at midlife. ISR Newsletter, Institute for Social Research, University of Michigan, Winter, 1982.

Depner, C. *The parental role and psychological well-being*. Paper presented at the meeting of the American Psychological Association, New York, 1979.

Derogatis, L. R., Lipman, R. S., Rickels, K., Uhlenhuth, E. H., and Covi, L. The Hopkins symptom checklist. In P. Pichot (Ed.), *Psychological measurements in psychopharmacology*. Paris: Karger, Basel, 1974.

Fischer, L. R. Transitions in the mother–daughter relationship. *Journal of Marriage and the Family*, 1981, *43*, 613–622.

Friedan, B. *The feminine mystique*. New York: Norton, 1963.

Freud, S. *New introductory lectures on psychoanalysis*. New York: Norton, 1965.

Friday, N. *My mother/myself*. New York: Delacorte Press, 1977.

Gigy, L. L. Self concept of single women. *Psychology of Women Quarterly*, 1980, *5*, 321–340.

Glenn, N. D. The contribution of marriage to the psychological well-being of males and females. *Journal of Marriage and the Family*, 1975, *37*, 544–600.

Glenn, N. D., and McLanahan, S. The effects of offspring on the psychological well-being of older adults. *Journal of Marriage and the Family*, 1981, *43*, 409–421.

Gove, W. R., and Tudor, J. Adult sex roles and mental illness. *American Journal of Sociology*, 1973, *78*, 812–835.

Gurin, G., Veroff, J., and Feld, S. *Americans view their mental health*. New York: Basic Books, 1960.

Kessler, R. C. The disaggregation of the relationship between socioeconomic status and psychological distress. *American Sociological Review*, 1982, *47*, 752–764.

Kessler, R. C., and McRae, J. A. Trends in the relationship between sex and psychological distress, 1957–1976. *American Sociological Review*, 1981, *46*, 443–452.

Levinson, D., Darrow, C. N., Klein, E. B., Levinson, M. H., and McKee, B. *The seasons of a man's life*. New York: Ballantine, 1978.

Livson, F. *Sex differences in personality in the middle adult years: A longitudinal study*. Paper presented at the meeting of the Gerontological Society, Louisville, 1975.

Lopata, H. *Occupation housewife*. New York: Oxford, 1971.

Lowenthal, M. F. Psychosocial variations across the adult life course: Frontiers for research and policy. *Gerontologist*, 1975, *15*, 6–12.

Lowenthal, M. F., Thurnher, M., and Chiriboga, D. *Four stages of life*. San Francisco: Jossey-Bass, 1975.

Marks, S. Multiple roles and role strain: Some notes on human energy, time and commitment. *American Sociological Review*, 1977, *41*, 921–936.

Neugarten, B. L. Dynamics of transition of middle age to old age. *Journal of Geriatric Psychiatry*, 1970, *4*, 71–87.

Oakley, A. *The sociology of housework.* New York: Pantheon, 1974.
Pearlin, L. Sex roles and depression. In N. Datan and L. H. Ginsberg (Eds.), *Life-span developmental psychology: Normative life crises.* New York: Academic Press, 1975.
Pearlin, L. *Social roles and personal stress.* Paper presented at the National Conference on Social Stress Research, Durham, N.H., October 1982.
Pearlin, L. I., and Schooler, C. The structure of coping. *Journal of Health and Social Behavior,* 1978, *19,* 2–21.
Radloff, L. Sex differences in depression. *Sex Roles,* 1975, *1,* 249–265.
Rosenberg, M. *Society and the adolescent self-image.* New Jersey: Princeton University Press, 1965.
Rosenfield, S. Sex differences in depression: Do women always have higher rates? *Journal of Health and Social Behavior,* 1980, *21,* 33–42.
Rossi, A. S. Life span theories in women's lives. *Signs,* 1980, *6,* 4–32.
Sears, P. S., and Barbee, A. H. Career and life satisfaction among Terman's gifted women. In J. Stanley, W. George, & C. Solano (Eds.), *The gifted and the creative: Fifty-year perspective.* Baltimore: Johns Hopkins University Press, 1977.
Serlin, E. Emptying the nest: Women in the launching stage. *In* D. McGuigan (Ed.), *Women's lives: New theory, research, and policy.* Ann Arbor: University of Michigan Press, 1980.
Sieber, S. Toward a theory of role accumulation. *American Sociological Review,* 1974, *39,* 567–578.
Siegel, P. M. *Prestige in the American occupational structure.* Unpublished doctoral dissertation, University of Chicago, 1971.
Srole, L., and Fischer, A. K. The midtown Manhattan longitudinal study vs. the mental paradise lost doctrine. *Archives of General Psychiatry,* 1980, *37,* 209–221.
Srole, L., Langner, T. S., Michael, S. T., Opler, M. K., and Rennie, T. *Mental health in the metropolis: The midtown study.* New York: McGraw-Hill, 1962.
Thoits, P. Multiple identities and psychological well-being: A reformation and test of the social isolation hypothesis. *American Sociological Review,* 1983, *48,* 174–187.
Veroff, J., Douvan, E., and Kulka, R. A. *The inner American: A self portrait from 1957–1976.* New York: Basic Books, 1981.
Ward, R. A. The never-married in later life. *Journal of Gerontology,* 1979, *34,* 861–869.
Weiss, R. S., and Samuelson, N. M. Social roles of American women: Their contribution to a sense of usefulness, and importance. *Journal of Marriage and the Family,* 1958, *20,* 358–366.

Chapter 7

Social Change and Equality
The Roles of Women and Economics

DIANE E. ALINGTON AND LILLIAN E. TROLL

MODERN MYTHOLOGY

In our hunger for progress, we tend to encourage media-propagated myths that shroud the reality of women's lives and discourage efforts to improve that reality. One of the most fundamental—and misleading—of the current myths is that the seeds of equality sown over many generations have at last flowered in response to the collective efforts of 20th-century women. We argue that the facts do not provide support for the belief that women have played a causal role as agents of change, and that it is important to correctly identify the antecedents of social change. Our thesis is that the recent changes are rooted in the economic needs of the nation, not in the sociopolitical needs of its women. Because of the external genesis of this change, its consequences are less permanent, less significant, and less beneficial than commonly claimed.

We propose that lasting change may occur when its source is the wellspring of human need, when it is inspired by human deprivation, and when its goal is the improvement of the human condition. A journey through the pages of women's history shows us how temporary change can be when its source is external, when it is inspired by institutional necessity and based on economic exigencies.

The winds of change have swept through women's worlds before, opening the doors of opportunity in response to economic conditions, only to close them again when conditions change. Historically, women's

---

DIANE E. ALINGTON • Centenary College, Hackettstown, New Jersey 07840. LILLIAN E. TROLL • Department of Psychology, Rutgers University, 39 Easton Avenue, New Brunswick, New Jersey 08903.

entries into and exits from the "outer world" are encouraged by appropriate mythology, propaganda, and legislation. Some doors have opened recently, but the status of women and of their achievements remains low relative to those of men. For this reason, the promise of equal opportunity is an empty one, for many women lack both the self-confidence and the social support required to open the most challenging doors. Arbitrary change has arbitrary consequences, which are beneficial in some instances, negative in others, illusory in some, and nonexistent in the remainder. As a result of this capriciousness, the world of women is often filled with conflict, inconsistency, and ambiguity, all of which can affect motivations and emotion, determining which doors women will open and how they will feel about their choices.

THE WINDS OF CHANGE

Over the centuries, courageous feminists have articulated the longings of women with seemingly little success. The current movement has survived so far because it has provided a convenient rationale for the cultural change that whirled women out of their kitchens into newly created "pink-collar" jobs—and into newly empty classrooms.[1] Now the winds are beginning to change again: A lengthy recession and rising unemployment are taking their toll, and the antifeminist rhetoric of the New Right is thriving in an increasingly fertile social climate.

Dollars and Sense

The history of women's education is rife with unmet needs, broken promises, and reluctant compromises. To the degree that economic and social pressures have fluctuated over time, so have the quality and quantity of education available to women. Feminist movements have had seemingly little influence on the actual course of events, although feminist principles have frequently been utilized by institutions in *post hoc* "explanations" whenever they have opened their doors to women.

A ROOM OF ONE'S OWN. Many examples of scholarly excellence were found in the medieval convent, where a number of women achieved international renown. In addition to providing a physical haven, a "room of one's own," the convent served two other important functions: It provided women with independence and with authority.

---

[1] After all, feminism is hardly a new concept. Christine de Pisan argued for sexual equality 500 years ago. Her opinions in regard to military tactics were more esteemed by Henry VIII than were her opinions in regard to the status of women, for he had her military treatise translated into English in her own lifetime. Interestingly, *La Cité des Dames* was translated into English last year, after being out of print for several centuries.

Simone de Beauvoir (1953) tells us: "Living in a convent made women independent of man: certain abbesses wielded great power. . . . From the mystical relation that bound them to God [they] acquired the authority necessary for successes which women usually lack . . . Queens by divine right and saints by their dazzling virtue were assured a social support that enabled them to act on an equality with men. For other women, in contrast, only a modest silence was called for" (p. 96).

According to Mozans (1913), women of that era were accorded this luxury because learning was, in general, held in disrepute: "the knights and barons of France and Germany were inclined to look upon reading and writing as unmanly and almost degrading accomplishments . . . [and some] regarded learning as having an effeminating effect on men. . ." (p. 277). We can hypothesize that the low status of learning was a function of the economic structure of that period; a man did not have to be able to read in order to wield either a plowshare or a sword.

A CHANGE OF HEART: THE NEXT 400 YEARS. With the advent of the Renaissance, learning became more valued by men, and women were excluded once again (Mozans, 1913). We can assume that the fledgling technology sired by the Renaissance was responsible for the increase in the status of learning; now reading and writing were becoming essential to the economic survival of Everyman. As a consequence of the revolutionary zeal of the Reformation, the convents of Europe were destroyed, resulting in "the absolute extinction of any systematic education of women for a long period" (Mozans, 1913, p. 41). In a cruelly ironic twist of fate, the convents that Henry VIII appropriated became the men's colleges of Oxford and Cambridge. It was to be nearly four centuries before a systematic education would be available to Western women—and five centuries before an egalitarian educational system would exist at last.

BACK TO THE DRAWING BOARD. Women's colleges appeared on the American scene toward the end of the 19th century, created in response to the universally exclusionary practices of the burgeoning colleges and professional schools of that era. The women's college was modeled on the only existing prototype, the medieval convent (Baker, 1976). Unlike the medieval convent, however, its clientele was limited to young women, and its curriculum was far from scholarly. Even so, its goals were noble, and its creation a monumental achievement, given the attitudes of the day. Small wonder that it failed to live up to the dreams of its founders. For despite its blueprint of planned obsolescence, when sexual equality would pronounce it unnecessary, the women's colleges did have "promises to keep" to at least a few generations of women. And the college broke its most important promise when it failed to prepare the students for successful careers. As Baker (1976) says:

> It was a triumph of consumerism . . . it was almost as if there existed a nonaggression pact: the women's colleges would provide educated wives but not professional competition for the men of Amherst, Yale . . . and the rest; in return, the men's institutions assumed a real but paternal interest in the Sisters, serving as sources for administrators, trustees, faculty and, not least, financial support as alumnae husbands (p. 11).

The last bastions of male educational privilege continued to resist coeducation until the 1970s, when the doors of the Ivy League were finally pushed ajar by the pressure of economic exigency. Partially responsible for the opening of the doors were the federal government's executive orders requiring affirmative action programs and supported by the threat of loss of billions of dollars of federal contracts. However, the primary economic pressure was internal, and its source was the admissions office. Both the quality and the quantity of the Ivy League applicant pool was decreasing, as many of the most able students chose coeducational public institutions (e.g., Baker, 1976). All the more reason, then, to move boldly ahead with coeducation, borrowing feminist rhetoric to justify their revolutionary about-face!

POMP AND CIRCUMSTANCES. The other interesting educational phenomenon of the 1970s was the sudden emergence of the "reentry" student (see Schossberg, Chapter 14, this volume). The fact is that by the mid-1970s, all educational institutions were looking toward mature women to solve the increasingly serious enrollment problems caused by the changing demography of the country. According to Niebuhr (1980), the crisis higher education has been facing is of a magnitude not seen since the Civil War. Apps (1980) predicted that 200–300 more colleges would close during this decade if current trends continued. His solution? "[It is time to eliminate] the longstanding, condescending 'toleration' [of adult students which comprise] a possible new clientele." Since that time, the adult student (usually female) has been recruited "agressively" (Bowen, 1980). The part-time reentry student is, in fact, saving the day; because of her presence, college enrollment is not suffering the dreaded decline.

The adult student is a familiar, if lonely, figure trudging across the landscape of women's history; she is not a creation of this women's movement. Traditional educations being unavailable to the historical counterparts of today's students, some women were self-taught while others were trained as assistants in adulthood by male relatives. Among the latter category are two astronomers, Caroline Herschel and Maria Kirch. The 27-year-old Herschel first began to assist her brother in his studies in 1777; her late start notwithstanding, her contributions were substantial. She discovered a number of nebulae (including Andromeda), and at 39 she became the first woman to detect a comet (Mozans,

1913 pp. 182–190; Osen, 1980, pp. 71–81). Kirch, whose discovery of a comet was never formally recognized, was also tutored in adulthood; she and her three sisters-in-law were trained as assistants by her astronomer husband (Mozans, 1913 p. 173).

The journey of other women was lonelier yet. Completely self-taught, Mary Sommerville discovered algebra in the pages of a fashion magazine at the age of 15 and was simply unable to acquire any mathematical books until she was in her 30s. As a consequence of her late start, academic recognition was not forthcoming until she reached her early 50s (Osen, 1980, p. 110). Sophie Germain, a self-taught founder of mathematical physics, learned differential calculus from the books in her father's library and began her serious work in her late 20s, ultimately attracting the notice of the great mathematicians of her era, including Poisson, Fourier, and Gauss (Osen, p. 90).

Today's adult student differs from her predecessors in two important ways. She is highly visible today, in part because she is the subject of a great deal of (self-serving) institutional publicity, claiming humanistic concern for the welfare of the midlife woman, and in part because she is no longer lonely; even Jihan Sadat and Joan Kennedy have joined the stampede for a midlife degree.

In addition, midlife students are no longer subjected to the overt condescension and second-class status from which her predecessors suffered as recently as a decade ago (see Schlossberg, Chapter 14, this volume). On the contrary, now that her presence has become an economic necessity, she is the new campus sweetheart, and admissions offices vie for her business with two seductive promises. They have kept their promise to provide her with necessary financial aid and auxiliary services, such as daycare; they have failed to keep their promise, however, for long-term career development. According to H.E.W. (1980), "educational institutions, anxious to have students, allow women to follow traditional career paths (leading to employment) at the low end of the pay scale . . . rather then design new models that will open real career opportunities for women."

How Equal is Equal?

Women have been whirled in and out of the paid work force as the revolving doors of opportunity have turned in response to the economic exigencies of war and peace. Their entries and their exits have been "encouraged" by means of the two-edged swords of legislation and propaganda—even feminist propaganda has been utilized when necessary.

ROSIE THE RIVETER IN WAR AND PEACE. The notable achievements of women during World War I proved to be short-lived, for women were forced out of their jobs by the Armistice in 1918. Berkin (1979) points out that this ousting was egalitarian: "Women streetcar conductors and women judges were removed with the same dispatch." It is probably no coincidence that the disintegration of the women's movement of that era occurred simultaneously with the return of the newly unemployed veterans from the battlefields of Europe.

The effects of World War II on the employment of women were similar to those of the earlier global conflict. During this period of manpower shortage, a new generation of women was lured into the workplace for the first time, and Rosie the Riveter became the symbol of 6 million women, many of them wives and mothers. Both Germany and the United States used propaganda extensively in their efforts to reach this untapped labor force. Despite government-sponsored polls indicating that women respond primarily to economic motivations, recruitment campaigns were based largely on patriotism and emotion, because the government feared that a stress on wages would produce inflation (Rupp, 1979). As a consequence, slogans stressed the protection of loved ones, the revenge of lost lives—and the ease of the work: "Millions of women find war work pleasant and as easy as running a sewing machine or using a vacuum cleaner." This statement proved to be true, at least as far as a top official at the Aberdeen Proving Grounds was concerned; the performance of his workers "justified his hunch that a determined gal can be just as handy on a firing range as over the kitchen stove" (Rupp, 1979).

A few years later, the wind changed direction once again. Postwar appeals to married women stressed patriotic duty and were reinforced by the "mythic imperative" (Janeway, 1971) that a woman's "place" was in the home. The widespread internalization of this propaganda ultimately culminated in the Feminine Mystique described by Friedan (1963).

On the chance that this propaganda proved ineffective, the government further "encouraged" early retirement through its overnight elimination of the support services it had provided for women when their cooperation was required for the war effort: Child-care centers, flexible shift jobs, and job sharing all disappeared from the scene in 1945 (Stellman, 1977, p. 20).

Still, nearly one-third of all women remained in the paid work force, even at the height of the Feminine Mystique, and their recalcitrance only reinforced earlier fears voiced by the Office of War information that women might not want to "go back where they belong" after the war (Rupp, 1979). This figure should not be surprising, for nearly 20% of all women were in the paid work force as long ago as 1890—and this figure is probably a gross underestimate, since farm wives were not counted (Stellman, 1977).

The fact is that the majority of women have always worked alongside men (Fisher, 1979). Even though many women were isolated from the mainstream of the marketplace when the middle-class home was "invented" some 300 years ago (Janeway, 1971), many others continued to engage in paid employment outside the home as a matter of necessity.

The persistence with which one-third or more of American women claim a niche in the paid work force, regardless of propaganda efforts and inadequate support systems, has led to the institution of "protective" legislation, which is demonstrably effective in protecting men's jobs, if not women's health. Stellman (1977, pp. 179–80) details some of the "perils of protection". Lawmakers "protect" women from holding high-paying industrial jobs—where they would have to carry heavy weights—but remain strangely silent about heavy lifting when it comes to hospital and restaurant workers, whose presence is essential and whose jobs are less remunerative. Similarly, women are barred from lead exposure—only in industrial jobs, not in the (lower-paying) pottery industry. Further, exposure to X rays is "optional" for pregnant workers in health care facilities (where women are essential), despite the fact that legislative concern generally focuses on the female reproductive system. In reference to this "fetus fetish," Stellman says there is "an aura of sanctity about the fertilized egg that apparently disappears when a child is born or matures into a working person" (pp. 179–80).

Legislation in this area is hypocritical at best, absurd at worst. Laws in regard to lead exposure are based on a 1902 study that found a sex difference in normal hemoglobin levels, leading the authors to the peculiar conclusion that women suffer from an insufficiency of iron, which makes them more susceptible to the toxic effects of lead (Stellman, 1977). This unjustified use of male norms in determining the standards for women's health is not unique; the sole American study of the effects of maternal employment during pregnancy documented the fathers' occupations—but not the mothers' (Stellman, 1977)!

Undeterred by myths, propaganda, and legislation, more and more women entered the work force, until by 1960 their numbers equaled those of the war years. Their ranks were increased largely by the many middle-class wives and mothers who were forsaking full-time homemaking for the office. What happened between 1945 and 1960? Current mythology would have us believe that the influx of married women into the marketplace was a consequence of the altered consciousness of the American homemaker (and her somewhat recalcitrant husband). It is widely believed that women simply rejected the "procreative imperative" (Harris, 1980). Inspired by the Civil Rights movement, the sexual revolution, and Betty Friedan's book (not necessarily in that order), they founded a Woman's Movement. Not only that, they made a collective decision to develop a self-actualizing life-style that was to include a meaningful career, a sensitive husband, and few (if any) children. In fact, some authors cite a deliberate increase in childlessness as a factor in the alteration of female employment patterns (Stellman, 1977),[2] even though increases in childlessness have not been found over the 20th century. Recent historical scholarship suggests that this scenario is almost entirely mythical, and that the factors that lured women away from home and hearth were economic in nature.

SLEEPING BEAUTY TO THE RESCUE. Harris (1980) cites the demand of the fledgling service-economy for "pink-collar" workers as a determining factor in the migration of married women into the corporation: "the white housewife was the service employers' Sleeping Beauty. Her qualifications were superb . . . she had been trained to take orders from men . . . she would accept temporary jobs, part-time jobs, jobs that would let her go home to cook or take care of the children . . . at the end of the 1960's [women were in] a niche specifically designed for the literate but inexpensive and docile workers who would accept 60% or less of what a man would want for the same job. . . . It is a great deception to believe that women went out and found jobs . . . these jobs found the women as often as women found the jobs."

The doors to the typing pool were flung open with enthusiasm. Doors to move lucrative enterprises remained firmly closed, however, until the might of the federal government succeeded in wedging them open far enough for a few hardy women to squeeze through. Title VII of the 1964 Civil Rights Act, incorrectly considered a triumph of feminist activism, forcibly opened the way for many women. People take Title VII for granted now, but perhaps they would be less complacent if they knew that sex was only added to this crucial piece of legislation in a bizarre attempt to block the passage of a bill that many legislators found abhorrent (Kanowitz, 1971).

Why did women migrate into the corporation just when they were needed most? Did the siren song of the women's movement lure them into seeking "liberation"? On the contrary, researchers attribute the phenomenon to the "life-cycle squeeze" experienced by many women of that generation. The children of suburbia's "pioneering" families were off to college—and a single paycheck could not be stretched far

---

[2]According to Stellman, "Birthrate data show that from at least 1910–1960, the majority of women gave birth to only one or two live-born children during their life-time . . . since 1960 . . . the vast majority of women are now mothers of at least two children and childlessness is rapidly disappearing" (1977, pp. 4–5).

enough to cover tuition (Harris, 1980; Rossi, 1980a). Inflation was raging, and women were helping to fan the fires themselves, as they fell prey to Madison Avenue pressures to buy new furniture and better appliances (Friedan, 1963).

We can find little evidence that changes in women's employment patterns circa 1960 reflected a fundamental revolution in the consciousness of the American woman. Rather, we suggest, the "Movement" was a consequence of the changing work patterns of women, not an antecedent; it provided women with a rationale for their changing behavior, and it provided the corporation with a rationale for its (somewhat limited) change of tune.

Clearly, the climate was such that a new woman's movement was bound to flourish. The benefits derived from women's working were such that their "liberation" received amused (but tolerant) support where it counted. As Harris (1980) states:

> Neither the interests of big business nor of the government lay as they once had in a united defense of the marital and procreative imperative. . . . In an age of nuclear arms, high birth-rates were no longer a military priority, while for government and business, the immediate assured benefits of employing women overshadowed the long-run penalties of a falling birth-rate.

The long-term risks of a little "consciousness raising" were perceived as minor, probably because the state of a woman's consciousness seems irrelevant in most important respects. Even today, N.O.W. supporters find it necessary to sport "59 cent" buttons in order to advance the cause of salary equality.[3] Even today, women have not yet succeeded in their efforts to break into the executive suite—or the union shop.

In fact, current recessionary times are not good for women or for their cause; pending congressional legislation that would limit their reproductive freedom is but the tip of the growing antifeminist iceberg. Historically, women's rights generally suffer as a consequence of economic recession, and we are seeing many inroads into recent gains. *Academe* (Gray, Nichols, and Schafer, 1981) documents the disparate effects of proposed cutbacks on women. Numerous programs that are facing budgetary cutbacks or elimination are those upon which women—especially midlife women—are disproportionately dependent (see

---

[3]It is almost laughable: The women of ancient Rome and 14th-century Toulouse were limited by law to earning 60% of a man's salary (Stellman, 1977; Shayner, personal communication, 1982). Modern women are now earning 60% of a man's salary and are doing it voluntarily. A little-known but interesting fact is that women with degrees from prestigious Ivy League institutions also earn about two-thirds the salary of their male classmates, despite the lack of a discernible difference in occupational choice (e.g., Harlan, 1976).

Long and Porter, Chapter 5, this volume). Not surprisingly, the cuts that are affecting women are being made willy-nilly, without regard to cost-effectiveness. A supported-work project for long-term AFDC recipients has been abruptly eliminated, even though the program was successful—and paid for itself (Masters and Maynard, 1981).

THE EMPRESS'S NEW CLOTHES

Having looked at the transient nature of externally imposed change, we turn now to look at its superficiality. The unique constellation of events of the 1960s and the 1970s was such that the appearance of change surrounds us. The economic needs of the middle-class woman, the corporate demand for service workers, and the (accidental) passage of Title VII all played a role in the degree to which new doors were opened to women—at least in theory.

In fact, many of the most interesting doors are quite safe from assault by the fair sex; on or off a pedestal, women simply have a lower status than men, and the changes we have seen in this century have done almost nothing to alter this fact. The battle against overt discrimination is progressing well, but the war against negative stereotypes is not faring so well, and there is no indication that the future looks any brighter (Steinberg and Shapiro, 1982).

Here we have a classic example of a self-fulfilling prophecy. Because women are undervalued by others, they lack the necessary self-confidence to open the most challenging doors. And because women's work is undervalued by others, their efforts to achieve are often frustrated by the lack of necessary social support; only a woman of the most uncommon promise is likely to find support in her home, school, and community.

The Nimble Fingers Syndrome

Although some researchers report progress in the status of women, others fail to find any difference in the degree to which people judge women as less competent than men (Etaugh and Kasley, 1981). Women are still considered unsuitable for responsible management positions (e.g., Steinberg and Shapiro, 1982) and have not, in fact, made much progress in achieving such positions. Women are still employed in an "occupational ghetto" (Diamond, 1981), holding 80% of the clerical jobs, 70% of retail sales clerk jobs, and 98% of the domestic service jobs (Rones and Leon, 1979); college graduates continue to restrict their career choices to teaching and nursing (Harmon, 1981).

Women are not perceived as leaders, and their leadership behavior is not perceived as such (Denmark, 1980); further, they are perceived as less influential and less powerful than males (Wiley and Eskilson, 1982). Typically, a woman's success is attributed to effort, while a man's success is attributed to ability (Riger and Galligan, 1980). Since pay raises are based on effort, and promotions on ability (Heilman and Guzzo, 1978), the negative consequences for women wishing to climb the corporate ladder are obvious.

Whatever the reasons, women and their work are universally undervalued in a most mysterious manner. According to American mythology, women make good typists because they have nimble fingers; Englishwomen, on the other hand, are not judged capable of tackling the typewriters at that august establishment, Lloyd's of London. Unlike their American counterparts, Soviet women are considered competent enough to handle a scalpel, for medicine is a relatively low-status occupation in the USSR. Soviet mythology also supports the employment of women as typists, as the second author discovered to her amusement—and chagrin. In Moscow for a conference, L.E.T. found it necessary to type a few extra notes for her scheduled address; she found it all but impossible to maintain her concentration in the face of repeated interruptions, as one person after another requested her secretarial services.

It is reasonable to assume that these negative perceptions of women must have an influence on their own feelings of competence and value relative to men, and the data we have support the notion that women internalize these negative biases in predictable ways. Females typically lack confidence in their ability to succeed (Crandall, 1969; Stake, 1979) and suffer undue anxiety in the face of competition (Sassen, 1980), especially when they are required to compete against males (Ingram, 1980). The 'Catch-22' in this instance is obvious when we observe the fact that many women fear the negative social consequences of success in male-dominated occupational fields (Vaughn and Wittig, 1979). Considering the situational and institutional barriers that feed the female sense of inadequacy whenever they are required to function in a "man's world," the wonder is that any women ever open the most challenging doors.

The 40-Hour Day

The superficiality of recent change is clear when we examine the facts surrounding women's efforts to combine family and career responsibilities. There is no indication that any change has occurred at all in the degree to which women carry the heavier burden in the home, whether or not they are also in the paid work force.[4] Women's work, in or out of the home, is simply accorded less status than men's. Perhaps because it is inherently less valuable, it is supposed to be less taxing. Whatever the reason, many researchers report that a wife's employment status has little or no effect on role sharing within a marriage. Despite the luxurious appearance of the modern kitchen, today's homemakers spend more time engaged in housework than did their grandmothers (Oakley, 1974). When a wife works, she must, of necessity, reduce the number of hours she devotes to housework (Beckman and Houser, 1979). Even so she needs a 40-hour day and a 300-hour week (Troll, 1982), for her employment does not affect the percentage of household chores for which she is responsible (McCullough, 1980; Nelson, 1977). Haas (1982) even had trouble finding any subjects for her study on egalitarian marriage. The nonegalitarian marriage is the norm, even when both members of the couple are physicians (Hendricks, 1980), and labor in the home remains divided in a traditional sex-role fashion among the marriages of full-time professionals (Beckman and Houser, 1979). British (female) psychiatrists interviewed by Brook (1981) chose their profession in large part because it was one that would permit them to work part time, enabling them to carry out their family responsibilities.

Cultural attitudes in regard to the status of women are extremely resistant to change (Steinberg and Shapiro, 1982). But until they are modified, the opening of doors to women remains largely an empty gesture; most women will have neither the interest in nor the energy for fighting a long, hard battle to achieve success in rewarding, male-dominated occupations.

The Bride Wore Black

Externally imposed change tends not only to be transient and superficial but also to be capricious. Doors have been flung open, but the barricades of prejudice remain to block women's entry; women recognize the difficulties of tackling new and challenging fields when their status is such that they really do have to be "more equal than equal" in order to succeed. And they recognize the difficulties in achieving suc-

---

[4]Fisher (1979) compares the work load of the modern American woman (45–70 hours per week) with that of "the Australian Aborigine women of the Pitjandjara described in 1933 (as having a life of arduous drudgery, sometimes consisting of as much as four to six hours a day—a work week of twenty-eight to forty-two hours). Which, if either, is the liberated woman, I leave to the reader to decide."

cess when the status of their work is such that their support system is barely adequate to support an effort that is merely "equal."

Let Them Eat Cake

Most women know that it is difficult for anyone but Wonder Woman[5] to "have her cake and eat it too." Most women still feel the necessity to set priorities and make choices. As recently as 1981, the *New York Times* described the tearful words of a young bridesmaid who could not escape the bouquet that had been hurled in her direction by the happy (and insistent) bride. The bridesmaid's words were illuminating in the degree to which they show the lack of progress women have made. "But I don't want to get married. . . . I want to go to law school!" (Gilinsky, 1981). If men felt the necessity to make such a choice, how many of them would have the courage and the willingness to choose law school?

Marriage and parenthood have negative effects on the professional status (Broschart, 1978) and salary (Birnbaum, 1979) of women because of their impact on labor-force participation. Hence, the "59-cent problem" is largely explained, for fewer years of participation mean less seniority and fewer promotions.

Tending the hearth in addition to minding the store has negative consequences for women—and for men, as well. Ferber and Huber (1979) report that a husband's tendency to hold office and to publish is decreased when his wife is also an academician. Clearly, it is not easy to manage a home without a full-time wife; adjustments are difficult and costly (Burke and Weir, 1976). Somebody is going to have to pay the piper; unfortunately it is usually the wife.

Mothers and Mentors

Successful men tend to have parents—and wives and mentors—who encourage them and support their efforts (e.g., Levinson, Darrow, Klein, Levinson, and McKee, 1978). We have no reason to believe that

---

[5]Today's would-be supermoms have some awesome predecessors whom they may be trying to emulate. According to Mozans (1913). Laura Bassi, who was a famous Italian physicist, was the "mother of twelve children [and] she never permitted her scientific and literary work to conflict with her domestic duties or to detract in the least from the singular affection which so closely united her to her husband and children. She was as much at home with the needle and the spindle as she was with her books and the apparatus in her laboratory. . . . She was living proof that cerebral development [of women] does not lead to race suicide. . . ."

men and women differ in the degree to which such encouragement and support is necessary, although there are clear differences in the degree to which they are available.

The experience of having a mother who works enhances a daughter's interest in—and commitment to—a career (e.g., Altman and Grossman, 1977), especially if the mother is fortunate enough to hold a relatively high-status position (Haber, 1980). Other researchers have found that a mother's attitudes toward work are important antecedents of achievement motivation, even if she is not in the work force herself. "Successful" students (in graduate and professional schools) often attribute their motivation to their mothers' attitudes; this attribution was made significantly more often by females than by males (Poumadere, 1978). "Successful" women (i.e., professionals) who organize their lifecourse (including time of marriage) around their career goals report greater maternal encouragement than that of their colleagues who fail to establish their priorities at an early age (Allen, 1980).

If a mother's attitudes are significant in the life of a young woman, a husband's attitudes are equally critical in later life. A husband's attitude toward his wife's working affects her propensity to enter the work force[6] (Perrucci and Targ, 1978), and it also affects the degree of job satisfaction she will achieve. Among 30–40-year-old women, a negative attitude on the part of the husband may be more detrimental to her satisfaction than the underutilization of her skills and the presence of preschool children in the home (Andrisani, 1978). Andrisani reports that 55–65% of all women in the sample perceived their husbands to have a negative attitude; their disapproval may ultimately have an impact on the women's performance and commitment (Scanzoni, 1979). According to Huston-Stein and Higgins-Trenk (1978), only 4–6% of husbands surveyed want their wives to work continuously and express any desire to adjust their lives to her working needs in any way, although they do want to have an intellectual companion!

Mothers and husbands are not the only influential figures in a woman's interpersonal world; a mentor may be crucial to achieving success for women as well as men (Denmark, 1980; Hennig and Jardin, 1976; Riger and Galligan, 1980; Stake and Levitz, 1979). Some researchers report that mentors who are male are necessary for success (e.g., Hennig and Jardin, 1976), but that may be due to the historic paucity of women mentors, for Goldstein (1979) found that recent Ph.D.'s of both sexes were much more productive if they had same-sex mentors. It

---

[6]Unless she has worked before. Previous experience with the intrinsic and extrinsic rewards of employment will overcome the disappearing attitudes of a husband, according to Hongvivatana (1976).

appears to many (e.g., Denmark, 1980; Wittig, 1979) that the current dearth of senior female academics is at least partially responsible for the dismal statistics in doctoral programs in psychology, where only 35% of the women complete the programs, as opposed to 70% of the men (Hirschberg and Itkin, 1978).

Progress—real change—will remain an elusive goal until women are routinely provided with the same support and encouragement as men—no more and no less. Until this support is forthcoming, we have no reason to believe that women will storm the doors of the executive suite. In the meantime, we can expect that many women will meet their needs for achievement in the time-honored ways, in the home and in the community and in traditional career areas (Troll, 1982a), for these means of satisfaction result in less frustration and conflict, even if they also result in fewer extrinsic rewards.

STARTING OVER

Much recent change is illusory, transient, and far from dramatically beneficial in the short run. But the changes we see today may have positive consequences for the long run, for their impact on the experience of women may result in gradual—but profound—intergenerational and interpersonal development, development of a type that is not responsive to externally imposed ideology.

Mothers and Daughters: Intergenerational Development

Troll (1975) has pointed out the striking similarities between the attitudes of different generations within a family. In her exploration of attitudes toward careers and achievement, Troll found some generational shifts consistent with the changes in women's education and job-market participation. Each younger generation showed less conventional sex-role orientation and moralism, but greater cognitive complexity, feelings of control, and overall motivation to achieve. However, women in the same family tend to resemble each other more than they resemble other women of their own generation. A grandmother with high achievement motivation tends to have a daughter and a granddaughter who are also highly achievement-oriented. It is possible, in other words, to view high achievement motivation as a family theme (Troll, 1980).

As Troll and Bengtson (1982) have pointed out, social and historical forces serve as moderator variables in family lineage transmission. Transmission is tempered when social forces are inconsistent with family values and is enhanced when they are consistent. However, family themes tend to be rather stable; as Hill, Foote, Aldous, Carlson, and MacDonald (1970) state, "While rapid pace of social change encourages new ways of expressing old values, it is largely old values that are expressed"

It appears that changes in family themes occur as a function of the family's experience within the culture, rather than as a function of cultural values and ideology *per se*. For this reason, the fact that more and more women are working today as a consequence of personal misfortune, economic necessity, or individual preference has far-reaching consequences. Today's working women are discovering the intrinsic and extrinsic rewards of the paid work force (Hongvivatana, 1976), and they are discovering the frustrations of having skills that are undervalued, underutilized, and, all too often, underdeveloped. Their employment seems to "liberate" their attitudes (Molm, 1978; Olsen, 1980). Women report that they embraced feminist principles after going to work, not before. We can expect that the increasing dissatisfaction of today's working women (Andrisani, 1978) will begin to modify family themes such that boys and girls will grow up with the realization that things could—and should—be different. We can see signs that important changes are occurring in terms of family themes; Harmon (1981) reports that the daughters she surveyed mirrored their mother's attitudes toward work in every respect—except that 98% of them expected that they would always work, with minimal time off in order to raise their children.

Late Bloomers: Interpersonal Development

Women's history is filled with stories about women for whom life began at 40—or thereabouts (see Heilbrun, Chapter 3, this volume). "Grandma" Moses' late start was somewhat excessive—at age 78—but the fact that her serious work began late is not atypical for her sex. The "late bloomer syndrome" seems to be a consequence of several different factors. In some cases, personal misfortune serves as a catalyst to new types of achievement. Margery Hurst, one of the world's only self-made female millionaires, founded the original temporary help agency in London after being deserted by her husband. Divorced women are disproportionately represented among the ranks of adult students, and they are noticeably more committed, as students and as workers, than any other group (Huston-Stein and Higgins-Trenk, 1978; Maslin, 1978; Schlossberg, Chapter 14, this volume).

One can assume that divorced women may be more disillusioned with the Cinderalla myth than any other group. In addition, however, the fact that they are self-supporting again may have pointed them with newfound motivation. Motivation rooted in the need for survival may be the crucial factor enabling these women to overcome earlier inhibitions and hesistancy. For, as Hoffman (1978) states, the roles of wife and mother mean that "they have an alternative to professional success and can opt out when the going gets rough. A full-scale achievement effort involves painful periods of effort and many a man would drop out if that alternative were as readily available as it is to women."

In addition, midlife achievement in women, married or not, may be a function of the fact that their family responsibilities have been reduced. The Eagleton Institute of Politics (1978) published a study on women in public office; almost without exception these women were older than their male counterparts at their time of entry into politics. In almost all cases their children were over 18—and in almost all cases they were married to supportive husbands, whose aid they claimed was essential to their success.

An extraordinary number of women who have achieved a place in the history books have achieved their eminence late in life—often because they did not have the opportunity to indulge their passions for personal achievement earlier.[7] Since the number of "world class" mathematicians among women prior to this century is only slightly higher than the number of Supreme Court judges in our own time, it is astonishing to discover that three of them achieved their renown for work they had done in their late 30s. As we have already noted, Mary Somerville, Caroline Herschel, and Maria Kirch all achieved recognition for work accomplished in their 30s and long afterward, at an age when their male counterparts were resting on the laurels of youthful creativity.

As any woman knows, midlife is not without stress. But many women survive the trials of the "sandwich generation" with equanimity, and many report more confidence, freedom, and autonomy in the postmenopausal years (Rossi, 1980a; Baruch, Chapter 6, this volume). Most women report relief at the "empty nest" (Artson, 1978) and are, in fact, happy to have the time to engage in their own interests.

Finally, midlife achievement in women may be, in part, a consequence of the personality change that many researchers believe is universal at this time. Sex-role reversals have been found among women of

---

[7]Some female achievements occur early but are recognized late; Sophie Germain died (aged 55) before the University of Gottingen could award her the honorary doctorate recommended by Gauss (Olsen, 1980; p. 91). Caroline Herschel was more fortunate, for she lived long enough to experience recognition; she was elected an honorary member of the Royal Academy Society at 85 and was awarded a gold medal by the King of Prussia when she was 96 (Olsen, 1980, p. 80). Probably more women should have followed the path taken by Miranda Stuart, a.k.a. James Barry. As "James" she/he entered medical school as "Dr. Barry" she/he ultimately became the surgeon inspector-general to the British army, her secret safe until her death (Macksey and Macksey, 1975, p. 144).

45–55 years of age in the United States (Neugarten and Gutmann, 1980) and in many other cultures (Brown, 1982). Gutmann (1975) found a shift from nurturance to dominance among women, and Lowenthal, Thurnher, and Chiriboga, (1975) found an increase in assertive independence. Regardless of the source of these personality changes, they do seem to occur with remarkable consistency; undoubtedly they play a role in the achievement-oriented behavior that women display in midlife. Although the data are cross-sectional, hence open to different interpretations, two studies suggest that the need for achievement in women increases with age (Vanzant, 1980) and becomes a more useful predictor as women grow older and their familial responsibilities decrease (Faver, 1982).

Brave New World

When we pause long enough to appraise our current situation realistically, we will be able to plan our future more intelligently. We must take media claims of progress with a grain of salt; the press, after all, proclaimed that equality had been achieved after the passage of the 19th Amendment, even as the Women's Movement was disintegrating before their eyes.

True progress may occur in the days ahead in response to the articulated dissatisfaction of women who continue to experience frustration in the paid work force and exhaustion in their efforts to cope with two full-time careers.

The legacy that this generation of mothers leaves to their daughters—and sons—may mean a better life ahead for men and women of all ages. Change that is inspired by human experience and the collective wishes of individual people will be more meaningful and more lasting than change that has been imposed from without. In the legacy left by this generation of mothers to their children may lie the genesis of true progress.

REFERENCES

Allen, S. Professional women and marriage. *Dissertation Abstracts International*, 1980, *41B*, 4736.

Altman, S. L., and Grossman, F. K. Women's career plans and maternal employment. *Psychology of Women Quarterly*, 1977, *1*, 365–376.

Andrisani, P. J. Job satisfaction among working women. *Signs: Journal of Women and Culture*, 1978; *3*, 588–607.

Apps, J. W. Six influences in adult education in the 1980's. *Lifelong Learning: The Adult Years* 3(10) 4–7, 30 June, 1980.

Artson, B. Mid-life women: Homemakers, volunteers, professionals. *Dissertation Abstracts International*, 1978, *39B*, 3481.

Baker, L. *I'm Radcliffe, fly me! The seven sisters and the failure of women's education.* New York: MacMillan, 1976.

Beckman, L. J., and Houser, B. B. The more you have, the more you do: The relationship between wife's employment, sex-role attitudes, and household behavior. *Psychology of Women Quarterly*, 1979, 4, 160–174.

Berkin, C. R. Not separate, not equal. In C. R. Berkin and M. B. Norton (Eds.), *Women of America: A history.* Boston: Houghton Mifflin, 1979.

Betz, N., and Hackett, G. The relationship of career-related self-efficacy expectations to perceived career options in college men and women. *Journal of Counseling Psychology*, 1981, 28, 399–410.

Birnbaum, M. H. Is there sex bias in salaries of psychologists? *American Psychologist* 1979, 34, 719–720.

Bowen, H. R. Adult learning, higher education, and the economics of unused capacity. *In* Chandler, B. J. (Ed.). *Standard Education Almanac.* Chicago: Marquis Academic Media, 1980.

Brook, P. The choice of career or consultant psychiatrists. *British Journal of Psychiatry*, 1981, 138, 326–328.

Broschart, K. R. Family status and professional achievement: A study of women doctorates. *Journal of Marriage and the Family*, 1978, 40, 71–77.

Brown, J. K. Cross-cultural perspectives on middle-aged women. *Current Anthropology*, 1982, 23, 143–156.

Bruns-Hillman, M. Traditional and nontraditional female achievers: Factors which may account for divergent modes of expression of achievement motivation. *Dissertation Abstracts International*, 1980, 40B, 5460.

Burke, R. J., and Weir, T. Relationship of wives' employment status to husband, wife, and pair satisfaction and performance. *Journal of Marriage and the Family*, 1976, 38, 279–287.

Crandall, V. C. Sex differences in expectancy of intellectual and academic reinforcement. In C. Smith (Ed.), *Achievement-related motives in children.* New York: Russell Sage, 1969.

de Beauvoir, S. *The second sex.* New York: Knopf, 1953.

Denmark, F. L. Psyche: From rocking the cradle to rocking the boat. *American Psychologist*, 1980, 35, 1057–1065.

Diamond, E. E. Sex-typical and sex-atypical interests of Kuder Occupational Interest Survey criterion groups: Implications for counseling. *Journal Counseling Psychology*, 1981, 28, 229–242.

Eagleton Institute of Politics: The Center for the American Woman and Politics. *Women in public office: A biographical directory and statistical analysis.* Metuchen, N.J.: Scarecrow Press, 1978.

Etaugh, C., and Kasley, H. C. Evaluating competence: Effects of sex, marital status, and parental status. *Psychology of Women Quarterly.* 1981, 6, 196–203.

Faver, C. A. Achievement orientation, attainment values, and women's employment. *Journal of Vocational Behavior*, 1982, 20, 67–80.

Ferber, M., and Huber, J. Husbands, wives, and careers. *Journal of Marriage and the Family*, 1979, 41, 315–325.

Fisher, E. *Women's creation: Sexual evolution and the shaping of society.* New York: McGraw-Hill, 1979.

Friedan, B. *The feminine mystique.* New York: Dell, 1963.

Gilinsky, R. M. A cloudless June day . . . *New York Times*, June 6, 1981.

Goldstein, E. Effect of same-sex and cross-sex role models on the subsequent academic productivity of scholars. *American Psychologist*, 1979, 34, 407–410.

Gray, M. W., Nichols, I. A., and Schafer, A. T. The impact of the 1982 federal budget on women in higher education. *Academe*, 1981, 67(4), 202–204.

Gutmann, D. Parenthood: Key to the comparative psychology of the life cycle? In N. Datan and L. Ginsberg (Eds.), *Life-span developmental psychology*. New York: Academic Press, 1975. Pp. 167–184.

Haas, L. Determinants of role-sharing behavior: A study of egalitarian couples. *Sex Roles*, 1982, *8*, 747–760.

Haber, S. Cognitive support for the career choices of college women. *Sex Roles*, 1980, *6*, 129–138.

Hare-Mustin, R. T., and Broderick, P. C. The myth of motherhood: A study of attitudes toward motherhood. *Psychology of Women Quarterly*, 1979, *4*, 114–128.

Harlan, A. *Career differences among male and female managers*. Paper presented at the National Academy of Management, Kansas City, Mo., 1976.

Harmon, L. W. The life and career plans of young adult college women: A follow-up study. *Journal of Counseling Psychology*, 1981, *28*, 416–427.

Harris, M. Why it's not the same old America. *Psychology Today*, August 1980, pp. 23–51.

Hendricks, J. G. Career-family management of women and men physicians. *Dissertation Abstracts International*, 1980, *41A*, 1792.

Heilman, M. E. and Guzzo, R. A. Perceived cause of work success as a mediator of sex discrimination in organizations. *Organizational Behavior and Human Performance*. 21(3): 346–357, 1978.

Hennig, M., and Jardin, A. *The managerial woman*. New York: Doubleday, 1976.

Hill, R. N., Foote, J., Aldous, R., Carlson, R., and MacDonald, R. *Family development in three generations*. Cambridge, Mass.: Schenkman, 1970.

Hirschberg, N., and Itkin, S. Graduate student success in psychology. *American Psychologist*, 1978, *33*, 1083–1093.

Hongvivatana, T. Employment decisions of married women. *Dissertation Abstracts International*, 1976, *38A*, 2923.

Huston-Stein, A., and Higgins-Trenk, A. Development of females from childhood through adulthood: Career and feminine role orientations. In P. E. Baltes (Ed.), *Life-span development and behavior* (Vol. 1). New York: Academic Press, 1978. Pp. 258–298.

Ingram, R. P. The effects of locus of control and sex-role preferences on the achievement orientation of females. *Dissertation Abstracts International*, 1980, *41A*, 4337.

Janeway, E. *Man's world, woman's place: A study in social mythology*. New York: Dell, 1971.

Kanowitz, L. Title VII of the 1964 Civil Rights Act. In N. Reeves (Ed.), *Womankind: Beyond the stereotypes*. New York: Aldine/Atherton, 1971.

Levinson, D. J., Darrow, C. N. Klein, E. B., Levinson, M. H., and McKee, B. *The seasons of a man's life*. New York: Knopf, 1978.

Lowenthal, M. F., Thurnher, M., and Chiriboga, D. *Four stages of life: A comparative study of women and men facing transitions*. San Francisco: Jossey-Bass, 1975.

Macksey, J., and Macksey, K. *Book of women's achievements*. New York: Stein & Day, 1975.

Maslin, A. Older undergraduate women at an urban university: A typology of motives, ego development, sextypedness, and attitudes toward women's role. *Dissertation Abstracts International*, 1978, *39A*, 2067.

Masters, S. H., and Maynard, R. *The impact of supported work on long-term recipients of AFDC benefits: Vol. 3 of the final report on the supported work evaluation*. New York: Manpower Demonstration Research Corporation, 1981.

McClelland, D. C. *The achieving society*. New York: Free Press, 1961.

McCullough, J. L. Contribution to household tasks by Utah husbands and wives. *Dissertation Abstracts International*, 1980, *41A*, 4313.

Miller, D. V., and Philliber, W. M. The derivation of status benefits from occupational attainments of working wives. *Journal of Marriage and the Family*, 1978, *40*, 63–69.

Molm, L. D. Sex role attitudes and the employment of married women: The direction of causality. *Sociology Quarterly*, 1978, *19*, 522–533.

Mozans, H. J. *Woman in science*. Cambridge, Mass.: M.I.T. Press, 1913.

Nelson, E. N. Women's work—Household alienation. *Humboldt Journal of Social Relations,* 1977, *5,* 90–117.

Neugarten, B. L., and Gutmann, D. L. Age-sex roles and personality in middle age: A thematic apperception study. In B. L. Neugarten and Associates, *Personality in middle and late life.* New York: Arno Press, 1980.

Niebuhr, H., Jr. A renewal strategy for higher education. *Continuing Higher Education,* 1980, *28*(2): 2–9.

Oakley, A. *Woman's work: The housewife past and present.* New York: Pantheon, 1974.

Olsen, S. M. Sixteen middle-class mothers view the women's movement: Its ideological relevance and psychological effects. *Dissertation Abstracts International,* 1980, *41B,*

Osen, L. M. (1974) *Women in mathematics.* Cambridge: MIT Press.

Perrucci, C. C., and Targ, D. B. Early work orientation and later situational factors as elements of work commitment among worried women college graduates. *Sociology Quarterly,* 1978, *19,* 266–280.

Poumadere, J. I. Combining family and professional responsibilities: A study of graduate and professional students' plans. *Dissertation Abstracts International,* 1978, *39B,* 6203.

Riger, S., and Galligan, P. Women in management: An exploration of competing paradigms. *American Psychologist,* 1980, *35,* 902–910.

Rones, P. L., and Leon, C. Employment and unemployment during 1978: An analysis (Special Labor Force Report, No. 218). Washington, D.C.: Bureau of Labor Statistics, 1979.

Rossi, A. Life-span theories and women's lives. *Signs: Journal of Women in Culture and Society,* 1980, *6*(1), 4–32. (a)

Rossi, A. S. Aging and parenthood in the middle years. In P. B. Baltes and O. G. Brim, Jr. (Eds.), *Life-span development and behavior.* New York: Academic Press, 1980. (b)

Rupp, L. J. Woman's place is in the war: Propaganda and public opinion in the United States and Germany, 1939–1945. In C. R. Berkin and M. B. Norton (Eds.), *Women of America: A history.* Boston: Houghton Mifflin, 1979.

Sassen, G. Success anxiety in women: A constructivist interpretation of its social significance. *Harvard Education Review,* 1980, *50,* 13–24.

Scanzoni, J. Sex-role influences on married women's status attainments. *Journal of Marriage and the Family,* 1979, *41,* 793–800.

Stake, J. E. The ability/performance dimension of self-esteem: Implications for women's achievement behavior. *Psychology of Women Quarterly,* 1979, *3,* 365–377.

Stake, J. E., and Levitz, E. Career goals of college women and men and perceived achievement-related encouragement. *Psychology of Women Quarterly,* 1979, *4,* 151–159.

Steinberg, R., and Shapiro, S. Sex differences in personality traits of female and male Master of Business Administration students. *Journal of Applied Psychology,* 1982, *67,* 306–310.

Stellman, J. M. *Women's work, women's health: Myths and realities.* New York: Pantheon, 1977.

Troll, L. E. *Development in early and middle adulthood.* Monterey, Calif.: Brooks/Cole, 1975.

Troll, L. E. Intergenerational relations in later life. In N. Datan and N. Lohman (Eds.), *Transitions of aging.* New York: Academic Press, 1980.

Troll, L. E. *Continuations: Development after 20.* Monterey, Calif: Brooks/Cole, 1982. (a)

Troll, L. E. *Being called an eminent woman psychologist.* A.P.A. address, Washington, D.C., 1982. (b)

Troll, L., and Bengtson, V. Generations in the family. In W. Burr, R. Hill, F. Nye, and I. Reiss (Eds.), *Contemporary theories about the family* (Vol. 1). New York: Free Press, 1979.

Troll, L. E., and Bengtson, V. L. Intergenerational relations throughout the life span. In B. B. Wolman, G. Sticker, S. J. Ellman, P. Keith-Spiegel, and D. S. Palermo (Eds.), *Handbook of developmental psychology.* Englewood Cliffs, N.J. Prentice-Hall, 1982.

Troll, L. E., Neugarten, B. L., and Kraines, R. J. Similarities in values and other personality characteristics in college students and their parents. *Merrill-Palmer Quarterly*, 1969, *15*, 323–336.

U.S. Department of Health, Education, and Welfare, Education Division. *Lifelong Learning and Public Policy*. A report prepared by the Lifelong Learning Project. Washington, D.C. *In* Chandler, B. J. (Ed.). *Standard Education Almanac*. Chicago: Marquis Academic Media, 1980.

Vanzant, L. R. Achievement motivation, sex-role, self-acceptance, and mentor relationship of professional females. *Dissertation Abstracts International*, 1980, *41A*, 4248.

Vaughn, L. S., and Wittig, M. A. Occupational competence, and role overload as evaluation determinants of successful women. *Journal of Applied Social Psychology*, 1979, *10*, 398–415.

Wiley, M. G., and Eskilson, A. Coping in the corporation. *Journal of Applied Social Psychology*, 1982, *12*, 1–11.

Wittig, M. A. Graduate student success: Sex or situation? *American Psychologist*, 1979, *34*, 798.

Yorkis, K. L. Marital status, parenting, and pursuit of graduate degrees: Their relationship to and effect on the careers of women administrators in institutions of higher education. *Dissertation Abstracts International*, 1981, *41A*, 4932.

Chapter 8

The Daughter of Aging Parents

Ann Stueve and Lydia O'Donnell

Introduction

Demographic changes since the turn of the century have reshaped the contours of the parent–child relationship, considerably increasing the span of years in which children and their parents meet and interact as adults. Sixty-five-year-old mothers and fathers typically look back not only on long and shared relationships with their sons and daughters but also look forward to shared futures lasting, on the average, 15 years or more. In contrast to previous generations, when children often experienced the death of a parent during their formative or young adult years, contemporary men and women in midlife and beyond are having to define and negotiate what it means to be a son or daughter when one has children, or even grandchildren, of one's own.

Over the past several decades, researchers, service providers, and the public have become increasingly interested in how adult children negotiate this relationship and how they respond when parents need help. In large part their interest reflects the dramatic and well-documented increase in the number of elderly parents and a growing recognition of the important role children, and daughters in particular, continue to play in the lives of the old. There is considerable research, for example, on the kinds and levels of support needy parents receive from offspring (e.g., Cantor, 1979; Shanas, 1979a, 1979b, 1980) and on the kinds of problems children encounter when they attempt to care for seriously ill or disoriented parents at home (e.g., Archbold, 1978; Isaacs, Livingstone, and Neville, 1972; Lowenthal, 1964). While such pressing

---

Ann Stueve • 23 Hamilton Avenue, Ossining, New York. Lydia O'Donnell • Wellesley College Center for Research on Women, Wellesley, Massachusetts 02181.

and practical issues clearly merit attention, what has been overlooked is how children experience the long period of years during which parents are old but often healthy, and how they differ in the ways they frame their commitments to elderly kin. In this chapter, we examine the adult child–elderly parent relationship from the vantage point of daughters and look at how women in different social and life-cycle positions vary in the ways they respond to the adult–daughter role. To do so, we draw from our own research, which entailed interviews with 81 daughters of elderly parents, as well as from relevant literature on the parent–child tie.

Focusing on the Mother–Daughter Relationship

While sons, of course, also have elderly parents, the parent–child relationship in later life is of particular concern to women. Whereas demographic trends call attention to the elderly parent–adult child bond, sex-specific social changes focus our attention on the mother–daughter tie. First, women tend to outlive men; as a result, there are more elderly mothers than elderly fathers. As Treas (1977) documents, this situation is relatively recent. At the turn of the century, there were approximately 102 men 65 years and older for every 100 women. Thirty years later, the numbers of older men and older women were roughly equal. By 1960, however, a gap had emerged, and there were only 83 older men for every 100 women. By 1975 the gap had widened still further: For every 100 elderly women there were only 69 elderly men. These statistics mean not only that there are more elderly mothers than elderly fathers alive today but also that older women are more likely to be widowed and living alone. Whereas most elderly fathers can expect to live out their lives in the company of a spouse and to draw on the support and help that spouses routinely provide, elderly women are not so fortunate. In 1978 three-fourths of all men between 65 and 74 years of age were married and living with their spouses, compared to less than one-half of all similarly aged women; the disparity was even more pronounced among those 75 years and older, with 68% of all men married compared to only 22% percent of all women (Soldo, 1980). Not surprisingly, when women—and men for that matter—lose a spouse, they typically turn to their children, especially their daughters, to provide a wide range of material, social, and emotional supports (Lopata, 1979; Shanas, 1979a, 1979b, 1980). Indeed, many daughters pinpoint the death of a mother or father as the time when their relationship with the surviving parent changed and intensified, in part because they saw their newly widowed parent as more needy but also because the death of one parent provides a jarring reminder that parent–child relationships do not last forever.

While demographic changes draw attention to elderly mothers, there are also reasons to focus on daughters. In our culture, it is women who perform most of the work entailed in managing and nurturing a family and binding members of different generations together. For example, it is women in their dual roles as mothers and grandmothers who help out when grandchildren are born and who act as baby-sitters during the subsequent years. Similarly, it is typically women who, as daughters, tend to elderly parents when they are sick, provide transportation to and from doctors' offices, and are on call for any emergency. It is also women who, as daughters, wives, mothers, and sisters, make arrangements for visits, encourage phone calls, worry about whether their parents are lonely, and generally keep tabs on whether husbands, sons, and brothers maintain appropriate contact with older generations. Moreover, this kin-keeping work has recently been called into question by the increasing labor force participation of midlife daughters and, more generally, by the cross-flow of ideas and rhetoric about women's proper roles and the value of putting the needs of family members ahead of one's own aspirations and goals. Finally, unless differences in the life expectancies of men and women narrow appreciably, it is daughters, more than sons, who are likely to become tomorrow's elderly parents and, thus, to make demands on their children for help and support in old age. It is for these reasons that much of the research, as well as our own, focuses on daughters' responses to aging parents.

Dealing with Complexity in Parent–Child Ties

A recurring theme in much of the literature on adult development centers on the complexity and diversity of life paths and careers among older adults (Hagestad, 1981). With each passing year individuals become increasingly different from one another in terms of the life experiences they have accumulated and where they stand with respect to different timetables and roles. A 40-year-old woman, for example, may be "launching" her teenage children or embarking on first-time motherhood, "peaking" in her profession or reentering the labor force. Complexity and diversity are even more pronounced when we turn from individual lives to parent–child relationships. Not only do both generations bring different roles and experiences to the adult child–elderly parent relation, but over the course of their lifetimes, parents and children develop their own idiosyncratic strategies and understandings as well. By the time parents are elderly and children are in their middle years, both generations have acquired a repertoire of beliefs and practices that orient their behaviors toward one another and reflect how their lives have been organized and connected throughout the adult years. "With the passage of time," write Hess and Waring (1978), "so much diversity arises in family groups that possibly no two sets of parents and children in the society—or even in the same family—have traveled parallel paths" (p. 267, quoted in Hagestad, 1981, p. 21).

While complexity and diversity have been highlighted in theoretical and discursive accounts of parent–child relationships, they have not been emphasized in research reports on parent–child ties. To the contrary, researchers have tended to portray the interactions between daughters and their elderly parents in one-sidedly positive or negative terms. On the positive side, for example, survey after survey documents the persistence of social, emotional, and material exchanges between children and their elderly parents (e.g., Shanas, 1979a, 1979b, 1980; see Troll, Miller, and Atchley, 1979, for a review). Gerontologists have also highlighted the responsiveness of daughters in attending to parents' needs and serving as care-givers when necessary (Brody, 1981; Hill, Foote, Aldous, Carlson, and MacDonald, 1970). Indeed, much of the research over the past 30 years has been directed toward disproving the notion that family ties have withered with the advent of modern industrial society or that families—and, in particular, children—abandon the old. While there is recognition that the flow of goods and services may shift over the course of the family cycle and vary by social class, distance, and the like, the major thrust of this work emphasizes the persistence and reciprocal nature of intergenerational ties. Moreover, in drawing such a positive portrait, many researchers have discounted as simplistic or inaccurate such concepts as "role reversal," which implies that mothers and fathers become childlike in old age and children are pressed into assuming a parentlike stance.

In contrast to this fairly positive image of family relations, attention has more recently shifted to the difficulties adult children may encounter in maintaining good relations with their parents. In particular, social scientists and policy analysts have focused on issues of *parent-caring*, a term that refers to the unpaid work entailed in nurturing and meeting the needs of an elderly parent and implies some degree of dependency of the parent on the child (e.g., Cicirelli, 1981). A small but growing body of ethnographic, fictional, and autobiographic accounts (Archbold, 1978; Gordon, 1978; Isaacs *et al.*, 1972; Murphy, 1980) describes in detail the tensions that can be introduced into family life when children assume responsibility for chronically ill or disoriented parents: The work load increases, other family relations suffer, children's social activities are curtailed, and the relationship between offspring and their parents becomes strained. Current assessments of the state of the modern family also feed into this negative view of adult child–elderly parent relations as marked by dependency and difficulty. It has become almost commonplace for gerontologists to point to changes in the family that are likely to make it more difficult for children to act in a caring and responsible manner with respect to their aging parents. It is often noted that long-run declines in family size mean that while there are relatively more elderly parents today than in the past, there are relatively fewer children to share the burden of work and responsibility (Treas, 1977). Moreover, as parents survive to increasingly advanced ages, the children of elderly parents are more often approaching old age themselves (Brody, 1979). Perhaps most visible and talked about of all is the increased labor force participation of women. As opportunities and pressures for female employment increase, more and more women, it is conjectured, will be caught in the bind of weighing the needs and expectations of parents against employment aspirations and commitments of their own. While a number of studies are now under way to examine the ramifications of such changes—especially increases in women's employment (e.g., Brody, 1981)—it is too often taken for granted that such changes are limiting the capacity and willingness of family members to meet traditional responsibilities toward aging parents.

There are undoubtedly both positive and negative sides to the adult child–elderly parent relationship, yet to focus on one side to the exclusion of the other yields an incomplete and overly simplistic picture; it obscures the variety and complexity of the relationship. Children differ not only in the ways they experience the aging and death of a parent but also in how much they are called upon to help out when parents grow old. Following a description of the Adult Daughter Study, the remainder of the chapter addresses issues and variations that must be considered in order to develop more complex frameworks and models for understanding how the child–parent relationship develops in the latter half of the family cycle.

The Adult Daughter Study

The Adult Daughter Study consisted of interviews with 81 white women between the ages of 30 and 60, all of whom had at least one living parent 70 years of age or more.[1] The women were selected at random using annual town census listings from two communities in the

---

[1]These interviews were part of a larger study on families and care-giving strategies funded by the National Science Foundation (NSF DAR 7910358), Laura Lein, principal investigator.

Boston metropolitan area. One community housed a largely working- and lower-middle-class population; the second was more affluent, and its residents were more likely to be college-educated and working at professional and managerial jobs. Women were contacted during the spring and summer of 1980; among those who met the sample criteria, approximately 75% agreed to participate.

The daughters who were selected by this procedure are what we generally think of as middle Americans. All but one of the women had at least a high school education: 20% were high school graduates with no further schooling, 38% had received some technical training or completed some college, while 41% had finished 4 years of college or more. In addition, most (80%) were married and most (85%) were mothers, but, as reported later, they differed in where they stood in their family-cycle careers. The financial positions of these women and their families ranged from moderate to affluent. Sixteen percent reported annual family incomes of less than $20,000, 14% had incomes of over $60,000, while the incomes of most respondents were somewhere in between. Participants also differed in their ethnic heritages and religious affiliations and reflect the wide range of backgrounds commonly found in the Boston area. Forty-three percent of the women described themselves as Catholics, 23% were Protestants; 11% were Jewish, and the remaining 22% did not identify with an organized religion or church.

The parents of these women also varied considerably in terms of their ages, marital status, and early life experiences. Forty percent of the women interviewed reported that their older (or only) parent was between the ages of 70 and 74, while 30% had at least one living parent who was 80 years or more. Three-fifths of the respondents were daughters of widowed parents, with widowed mothers outnumbering widowed fathers four to one. Although virtually all of the daughters were born in this country, almost half (48%) reported that at least one of their parents was foreign-born. Not surprisingly, these older parents were generally less well educated than the daughter generation. Over one-third of the older mothers (35%) had completed less than 4 years of high school, and several had received little formal schooling at all; 29% of the mothers were high school graduates, 16% had received some technical training or college after high school, and 19% had completed the requirements for a B.A. degree. The financial status of parents was more difficult to assess than their other characteristics because most of the daughters reported being uninformed about this aspect of their parents' lives. Only 21% reported knowing their parents' incomes, while an additional 41% were willing to wager a guess. About half of those who knew or guessed at parents' incomes reported that mothers and fathers lived on less than $10,000 annually, but only 15% of the daughters reported that they were helping parents out with financial contributions, and half of these reported doing so only from time to time.

It is important to note that the women who participated in this study were not selected because of some special relationship they shared with their elderly parents. They were not picked because their parents were particularly healthy or particularly needy, or because their parents lived especially close by or far away. Nine percent of the daughters shared a home or lived in a two-family dwelling with parents, 34% lived either in the same community as parents or in a bordering town, and 30% lived more than an hour's drive away. Similarly, respondents were not selected because they were especially concerned about the aging of parents or because they were heavily involved in providing parents with help. While some of the women were, or expected to become, their parents' primary care-givers, others anticipated that a sibling would take on most of the responsibility and work. In addition, the participants do not solely represent daughters who get along well with elderly parents or daughters whose relationships are marked by conflict and strain. Rather, they are a diverse and random sample of white working- and middle-class daughters of elderly parents, and they provide a variety of situations and experiences to examine and compare.

The Interlocking of Generations

Perhaps the most basic question to address in identifying important variations in the adult child–elderly parent relation is: Who are the daughters of aging parents? Most often, we think of these daughters as a generation "caught in the middle," women in their 40s and early 50s who are responsible for meeting the needs of both their elderly parents and their adolescent children while often working at a paid job as well. If we look at this characterization more closely, however, we see that it understates the many different ways in which the life cycles and life commitments of adult children and elderly parents interlock. First, not all daughters of elderly parents are similar in age. Although the modal respondent in our study was in her late 40s, 25% of the women interviewed were less than 40 years old while nearly 13% were approaching 60, the upper age limit in this sample. Indeed, demographic trends indicate that an increasing number of men and women who are 65 years or older themselves still have a parent or parent-in-law alive (Harris and Associates, 1975; Brody, 1979). Second, not all daughters of aging parents are at similar points in their own family cycles. While the modal respondent was a mother of teenage children, 27% of our sample were currently raising preschool- or school-age children and a similar percentage had no child-care responsibilities, typically either because they had not yet had children or because their children had grown and left home. In addition, a few midlife women had decided to remain childless. Third, while clearly more daughters of elderly parents hold paid jobs than in previous generations, there is a wide variation in the extent of their labor force involvement and in how they strike balances between paid work and family roles. Although nearly 70% of the daughters we interviewed were in the labor force, half of these women worked only part-time hours. Thirty-one percent of the sample were full-time homemakers.

In large part, these variations reflect the family-timing decisions made sequentially by members of each of the two generations involved. How old you are when your parents turn 70 is obviously a function of how old your parents were when they started their families and your own place in the sibling hierarchy. How elderly parents fit into your family cycle then depends on the timing and spacing of your own children, which, in turn, affect how and when you become involved in other roles such as that of paid worker. The members of a multigenerational family are thus interlocked in ways that reflect the aggregation of family-timing patterns and decisions made by all of the nuclear families involved. As a result, it is not surprising that there is wide variation in the ways the life cycles of daughters and elderly parents intersect since normal variations in the family-timing patterns within any one generation, here the elderly parents, are then compounded by the different decisions made by members of the next generation, their children. To date, however, there has been little effort to examine how these different family configurations influence the relationships between children and elderly parents. In the next section, some of the implications of different timing patterns are discussed.

The Impact of Timing Patterns

Most of us carry a standard image of how the parent–child relationship progresses in adulthood, an image that is accurate in many cases. The relationship between young adults and their parents is most often characterized by issues of separation, with children establishing separate identities and households at a time when their midlife parents are still vigorous and healthy. As children settle into adult roles and have offspring of their own, a period of rapprochement and stability is likely to follow, with both parents and children remaining relatively independent; Baruch and Barnett (1983) describe this period as the "era of good feelings." Finally, as middle-aged children become established and prepare to launch their own offspring into the adult world, they begin to deal with the aging of their parents and the inevitability of their parents' death. This is an accurate description of how the life-courses of some daughters and their parents are interlocked, but, as the data presented above suggest, many daughters are off time with respect to this standard image and encounter the aging and death of parents at earlier or later points in their lives. Neugarten (1968), among others, suggests that being off time may make such transitions more difficult. A thematic reading of the interview protocols suggests that variations in family-timing patterns play an important role in shaping how daughters deal with some of the psychological issues and considerations that arise when parents grow old.

Several case studies illustrates how different family-timing patterns shape the ways daughters frame the issues of loss surrounding the possibility of a parent's death. Theresa Camilli, who is in her 30s, and Ethel Lindstrom, who is in her 50s, are both faced with the possibility that their parents may not have much longer to live.[2] Yet contrast the different ways they deal with their impending loss: Mrs. Camilli, when asked to describe her parents, responded in this way:

> They are very understanding. I'd be lost without them. They've helped me through many, many hard times. I really wouldn't know what to do [if they died]. I don't even want to talk about them leaving because I just want them around forever. I just kind of block that right out my mind. When my father had the heart attack, it scared me half to death. And when my mother had her operation, that made me very nervous. I made it on my own with my husband, but there's lots of times you just can't tell a friend something, and you need somebody. And then I go talk to my mother. I'm very close with my mother. . . . If I have a problem, I know that she'll give me good advice and so will my father. They do not beat around the bush. They just come straight out and tell you what they think.

Over the course of her interview, Mrs. Camilli emphasized the loss she would feel should her parents die at this point in her life, and her words expressed fear and apprehension about whether she could make it on her own. The older Mrs. Lindstrom described her concerns about her mother's death in a very different way:

> Well, the thing that concerns me most is that I hope my mother will go very quickly. I hope she will die and not be prodded and poked and all these things they have to do to you. And I hope that she won't be uncomfortable and not tell us about it, because she's apt to do that. And I hope that she will just go and not be frightened at the time. . . . If they told me that she would die tomorrow, I think I'd be very, very happy because I'd know that she had a happy life to the last moment. That's the thing that concerns me the most—not how soon she will go, but *how* she will go.

Mrs. Camilli was barely able to consider her parents "leaving" and clearly had not accepted the possibility of their loss, whereas Mrs.

---

[2]Names have been changed to assure the confidentiality of respondents.

Lindstrom appeared resolved to the inevitability of her mother's death and more concerned about her mother's suffering than her own. These differences can be linked in part to the life stages of both the daughters and their parents. Mrs. Camilli is still reliant on her parents, both psychologically and instrumentally. She counts on her mother and father both for advice and for practical support in raising her four young children. Mrs. Lindstrom, by contrast, is happily employed full time and busy establishing a second marriage. Although she used to confide in her mother at length when she was younger, she now finds that her life is fairly stable, and she has others with whom she can talk and who are often more helpful than her ailing mother. While the two women both maintain daily contact with their parents through phone calls and visits, Mrs. Camilli looks upon these encounters as at least as important for herself as for her parents, while Mrs. Lindstrom realizes how much her mother looks forward to such contacts and continues them primarily for this reason.

Mrs. Camilli and Mrs. Lindstrom illustrate how the impact of a parent's aging can differ depending upon the extent of one's psychic and emotional separation from parents. Psychologists point out that some women never effectively separate, particularly from their mothers, since the transition from a childlike and dependent status to equal footing as an adult can be difficult even under the best of circumstances (e.g., Cohler and Grunebaum, 1981). While much of the psychological work of separation occurs in the adolescent and young adult years, the issues often extend into later years as well. Women in their 30s in our sample were more likely than older women to still be preoccupied with establishing their own identities and disengaging from their parents. As the case of Mrs. Camilli suggests, when an adult child must simultaneously deal with issues of separation and with the reality of a parent's failing health and death, resolution can become more difficult and complex. When daughters are still emotionally dependent on their parents, they feel especially vulnerable and threatened by signs of their parents' old age. Under these circumstances separation can be difficult, and perhaps even prolonged, both for daughters who are close to and still reliant on parents and for daughters who have not resolved the ambivalence and conflict with parents often associated with establishing an adult identity.

Lauren Jarvis, who is approaching 40, expresses how much easier it is to accept parents' old age once children come to terms with their own adult identity. She recounted her experiences with her 88-year-old father in this way:

> I feel fairly comfortable with the way things are now . . . and I certainly hope that our relationship won't dissipate before my father dies. If he dies today, I would feel very comfortable with it—beyond the missing him—but I would

have no regrets. I've said what I wanted to say. I've expressed what I've wanted to, and so has he. It's not going to get any better. I hope it doesn't get worse. It's OK. Everything is comfortable. Now had he died, say, in my late twenties, ten or eleven years ago, I couldn't have said that. There was still a lot to be resolved.

Losing a parent when both you yourself are older and your parent is older seems more a part of the natural timing of events. In addition to their greater readiness to accept the aging and death of a parent, adult children in their 40s and beyond are more likely to have friends and acquaintances who have also experienced some of the difficulties surrounding a parent's aging and who can act as role models and confidants. As one woman explained: "I talk with my friends about my parents because so many of my friends are in the same boat. Practically all of my friends who are my age or older have gone through it."

While men and women have gained increasing control over decisions about whether, when, and how many children to have and often weigh a large number of factors in making these family-timing decisions, they rarely think ahead to how their decisions will shape the nature of their involvement in an adult child–elderly parent relationship. While many couples may look forward to the security of having a child to fall back on in old age, few consider the ramifications of their family-timing patterns on the availability and willingness of children to respond should the need arise. For example, how many people who marry young and have children immediately realize that the advantages of being relatively young when their children are young may turn into a disadvantage when they are old and find that their children are old as well? Similarly, a growing number of couples are postponing children until they are in their 30s and even early 40s so that they have time to establish careers and solidify marriages, but they rarely take the needs and expectations of elderly parents into account. For example, how many realize they may be trading off time for themselves at the beginning of the adult life course against time for themselves once children have left home and old parents are needy? As Daniels and Weingarten (1982) describe, there are long-term ramifications and trade-offs with all family-timing patterns. With issues of timing becoming more and more a matter over which couples have control, it is important to bring these ramifications and trade-offs to the attention of both generations.

Parents' Needs and Daughters' Responses

Just as variations in family-timing patterns shape the nature of the relationship between children and parents in later life, so do the vagaries of parental health and life circumstances. No one can predict when a parent's health will decline or when an elderly mother or father will be widowed. As a result, the characterization of daughters as being "caught in the middle," responsible for meeting the needs of both growing children and ailing parents, is inaccurate not only because of variations in ages and life stages but also because it rests on the assumption that elderly parents are typically needy and dependent. When we examine statistics on the physical and mental health status of the older generation and look at the ways daughters in our sample describe their parents, we see that many parents remain quite healthy and self-sufficient throughout most of the period we call old age and that patterns of interdependence between the generations that are evident in the latter part of the family cycle are often patterns that developed long before parents grew old.

While older people on the average certainly have more chronic diseases and disabilities than do young people, the majority are in good health. In 1975 interviews conducted by the National Center for Health Statistics found that almost 70% of the elderly questioned rated their health as excellent or good; only 9% described their health as poor (Kovar, 1977). Recent estimates also indicate that only about 4 to 6% of the population 65 years or older suffer from organic brain syndrome (Raskind and Storric, 1980) and only 10% show any signs of senility whatsoever (Fighting off old age, 1981). Even though these percentages are higher among the very old, our fears of senility and mental impairment are greatly exaggerated. When we turn from mental and physical health and look at the day-to-day functioning of older people—what gerontologists call the activities of daily living—the story is much the same. One needs-assessment survey conducted in Massachusetts found that over half of the elderly people interviewed were self-sufficient when it came to transportation, housekeeping, food shopping, and food preparation; over 80% were self-sufficient when it came to personal hygiene (Branch, 1977). Moreover, these figures are really underestimates since many of the older people who were not classified as self-sufficient actually relied on their spouses for help, and clearly, turning to one's spouse is not unique to the elderly.

These positive figures on the health and independence of the old coincide with the ways daughters in our sample described the health of their parents and how much support they have been called upon to provide. Not only do older people describe themselves as healthy and active, but their children do so as well. When asked, "How would you describe your parents' health?" 69 of the women interviewed answered with a label resembling the categories used in survey questionnaires. One-third of these daughters characterized their parents' health as excellent or very good; an additional 42% characterized it as good, while only one-quarter portrayed the health of either parent as only fair or poor. Even fewer described their parents as disoriented, confused, senile, or forgetful to the point of its hampering their daily functioning. Interestingly, although every respondent had at least one mother or father who was 70 years of age or older, the majority (61%) did not think of their parents as old. In response to the question "Do you think of your parents as young, middle-aged, old, or what?" most daughters spoke of them as "getting older," middle-aged, or in terms of some other more youthful-sounding category. Parents did not seem to fit the stereotypic image of befuddled and inactive old people. Even in those cases when daughters initially responded that they thought of their parents as old, several quickly qualified their answers, as illustrated by the following response:

> Well, I guess I'd have to think of her as old, but not very old. She's youthful for her age. I mean, she is old, she's seventy-three. But she is certainly younger in her appearance and her actions than some women I've seen in their fifties. She's very agile and gets out and does everything and doesn't depend on anyone for anything. [Interviewer: What makes you think of her as old?] Well, that's a good question. I guess the fact that I know she's old. I really don't think of her as old, but middle-aged seems more what I am—I'm fifty-three. So I really couldn't say that she was middle aged. . . . I guess I think of her as "getting older," perhaps that would be more correct.

It is possible to interpret the unwillingness of some daughters to label their parents as old as a defensive response, a denial of both their own and their parents' aging. However, given the descriptions of parental health and the national figures cited above, a more likely explanation is that in many cases their parents have, in fact, remained vigorous and active despite their advanced chronological ages.

It is therefore not surprising that the majority of daughters were only minimally involved in what could be termed "parent-caring" at the time of the interview. On the basis of a thorough reading of the interview protocols, we scored the respondents on the extent to which they were involved in providing instrumental support to their parents. More specifically, we rated respondents on whether they provided no, some, or substantial help (score = 0, 1, or 2, respectively) with the following seven tasks and activities: personal care and hygiene, household chores, errands, transportation, financial management, institutional interactions (e.g., dealing with Medicare forms), and actual financial contributions. Out of a possible score of 14, respondents received scores ranging from 0 to 12. Two out of every five daughters, however, received scores of 0, meaning that they provided no regular help with the activities of daily living, and only one out of every five received a score of 5 or higher.

For the most part, these relatively low scores reflect the fact that the parents of the women interviewed were free of major physical and mental impairments that would call for prolonged and intensive time investments on the part of children. Good health, however, is not the whole explanation. First, many of the illnesses associated with aging are chronic in nature. In living with a chronic illness such as arthritis or diabetes, older people learn to adapt and make do. Instead of major weekly shopping trips, parents go to the local store several times a week; instead of cleaning the entire house at once, they clean one room at a time; instead of mowing the law in one afternoon, they spread the chore out over several days. Putting a premium on their own independence, parents learn how to live within their limitations. Second, although the elderly are more likely than their children to have serious illnesses, more frequent hospitalizations and surgery, and longer recuperative periods, many do, in fact, recover. While daughters may be quite involved during intensive periods of need, parents often get back on their feet again. Paula Bird's situation is fairly typical.

> My father had pneumonia from Thanksgiving until after Christmas. He had it and we didn't know it. He was falling a lot. I was going over, doing his breakfast dishes, getting some type of lunch for him and seeing that something was cooked for dinner, because I knew he was falling and he was weak. I though, Gee, what are we going to do? Finally, since my sister had had pneumonia the month before we said, "Dad, I think you ought to go to the doctor." And sure enough, he had pneumonia.
>
> It was scary. It was before Christmas and we were very, very busy. I had to go over every day because I am the only one in my family who is "not working." . . . It was a drastic change, and he became very dependent on me. He was very weak. He was falling asleep all the time. But the pneumonia took care of itself, and now he's better.

While to this point we have emphasized how many parents remain in good health throughout most of their lives, it is undeniably true that many elderly people get seriously or terminally ill. In such circumstances, parents typically turn first to each other and then to their children for care (Cantor, 1980; Lewis, Bienenstock, Cantor, and Schneewind, 1980; Shanas, 1979b, 1980; see also case studies reported in self-help books, such as Silverstone and Hyman, 1976). The vast majority of children are at their parents' beck and call when catastrophic illness does arise, whether it means traveling to be on hand for a parent's serious operation and recuperation, being there when a parent is dying, or helping a parent make funeral arrangements and adjust to widowhood.

There is considerable variation, however, in how much and what types of care children are called upon to give to parents, both in cases of dire emergency and in borderline situations where parents are becoming more frail and needy. There is also variation in how graciously daughters accept the role of helping parents and adapt their lives to fit parental needs. First, daughters from working-class backgrounds are more likely to live with or near their parents and to have built up patterns of interdependence and helping out, which more easily slide into patterns of parent-caring when the need arises. By contrast, middle-class daughters, particularly women who have left home to attend college, are more likely to have drawn strict boundaries between their own nuclear families and those of their parents and to have constructed lives that are separate from those of their parents and siblings. Working-class daughters are therefore more likely to find themselves in circumstances that pull them into parent-caring, circumstances (such as living in the same neighborhood or town) that are in turn shaped by a value system that emphasizes interdependence and the responsibility of one nuclear unit of the extended family for another. For such daughters, taking care of a frail or ailing parent is virtually taken for granted, as illustrated by the following case study.

> Nora Dubchek lives two miles away from her widowed father. She works part time as a hairdresser, and her husband is a self-employed gardener. When she was first asked if her father had come to rely on her, she replied, "No. No. Only when he doesn't feel well. You know, I will sometimes take him to the post office, or drive him here, or go over and do a few things in the house." When asked how often she saw her father, however, she went on to say, "Oh, I see him every day. I was there this morning. This morning I did the dishes for him because he has a bad hand. And I just talked to him." Later in the conversation, it came out that Mrs. Dubchek did many other things for her father—she tends to home repairs, makes sure his house is properly cleaned, takes him places in bad weather, and nudges her brothers and children to make regular visits. She has thought about her father's advancing age and the possibility that at some point he may not be able to live alone. She anticipates becoming more involved in his life, even to the point of establishing a joint residence.

In the case of Mrs. Dubchek and other working-class women like her, parents are seen less as presenting problems and complicating their lives than as being a part of their immediate family; parents' needs are part of the fabric of daily life.

Middle-class daughters, by comparison, are less likely to integrate parents into their lives to this extent or to provide parents with the type of support Mrs. Dubchek takes for granted. They typically made fewer visits to parents, even when they lived in the same metropolitan area. When we compared working- and middle-class women in terms of the amount of instrumental aid they reported providing to parents, we found that a disproportionate number of working-class daughters were among the most heavily involved. More specifically, whereas one-fifth of the women with only high school or vocational training received the lowest possible instrumental score, almost half (45%) of the women with at least college educations did so; whereas half of the less educated women received instrumental scores of 4 or higher, only 15% of their better educated counterparts were this involved.

Even among the working class, however, it is not always daughters who are called upon for help. Just as elderly spouses turn to each other for assistance with routine chores, they also look to one another in times of illness and need (Johnson, 1980; Lewis et al., 1980; Stueve, 1982). Even in cases where parents call on children, one child is often singled out as primary care-giver rather than responsibility being equally shared among siblings. In our research, daughters typically reported providing more assistance than their brothers, proximate daughters tended to provide more help than respondents who lived farther away, and oldest and youngest daughters seemed to take more responsibility for elderly parents than women who held middle positions in the sibling line. Thus, while most studies (including this one) suggest that daughters are the major providers of instrumental support to needy parents, still many women do not expect to be called upon for more than occasional assistance because they know that a sister (or, less often, a brother) will step in instead. As one respondent with several brothers and sisters put it, "It's not that my oldest sister would *feel* most responsible but that the responsibility would fall on her because she would be the most accessible (should my parents need help)."

In addition, it is not uncommon, particularly in middle-class families, for parents to look to friends and neighbors for help rather than to family, especially if children live far away and a community of age-peers is available. Some older people, particularly those who are affluent enough to buy homes in retirement communities and who are accustomed to living apart from their children, prefer to hire services when necessary or to engage in reciprocal exchanges with friends rather than becoming dependent upon offspring. Carol Post, whose parents moved to a condominium limited to people 50 years and older, described some of the advantages of this living arrangement:

> My parents have a huge network of friends and people to bring them what they need. I mean if one of them is in the hospital, the other one gets invited out for every meal or people bring in things. People are just tremendously supportive. They'll drive you to the hospital to visit. My parents have a whole network there.

What differentiates this respondent from more interdependent working-class women is the notion that parents can be taken care of by people other than family members. This is a notion that appears to be shared by both daughters and parents. A middle-class daughter is more likely to assume that her parents would hire a housekeeper or, if necessary, a private-duty nurse than expect her to perform such tasks. Not only are parents seen as having the financial resources to purchase the services they need, but they are also perceived as having become accustomed to making arrangements without resorting to children. If both parents and children are used to maintaining boundaries between their respective households and leading separate and independent lives, they are less likely to look to one another for help if something goes wrong. Middle-class parents may hesitate to disrupt their children's lives and at times may actually prefer the less emotionally charged strategy of hiring help or relying on their informal networks. However, middle-class parents, like working-class mothers and fathers, expect their children to be available in serious situations, and their children acknowledge this claim.

One such serious situation that arises is the death of a parent, leaving a widowed mother or, less commonly, father alone. After an initial period of intense involvement, children may pick up some of the tasks previously performed by the deceased parent. Mothers may call upon their sons and sons-in-law, for example, for advice on financial matters and taxes; fathers may look to their daughters and daughters-in-law for help with housekeeping and the like. Children report making greater efforts to stay in touch, either by dropping in more often or by phoning, since widowed parents are often thought to be lonely. The different patterns of interaction characteristic of working- and middle-class families, however, persist. Working-class daughters continue to place a greater emphasis on integrating their widowed mothers and fathers into their lives, whereas middle-class daughters tend to do what they feel is necessary to help a widowed parent re-establish a life of his or her own.

In discussing the health and life circumstances of parents, it is difficult to strike a proper balance, to avoid presenting a picture that is either overly optimistic or too narrowly focused on the problems of old age. Our point is not that elderly parents never become dependent upon daughters. Some parents need a lot of help a lot of the time, especially those who are very old or who are seriously or terminally ill; some parents need a lot of help some of the time—for example, during spells of sickness or following the death of a spouse. However, when we consider the number of years adult children now have to relate to parents who are elderly, it is fair to say that the adult child–elderly parent bond is best thought of as an extension of the relationship that developed during early parts of the family cycle.

Women's Changing Roles

Thus far, we have argued that the image of daughters as being "caught in the middle" is inaccurate both because daughters differ in their own ages and family stages when they are faced with their parents' old age and because old age is an extended period of time during which most mothers and fathers remain active and healthy. In looking forward to how the adult child–elderly parent relationship will be shaped in the future, one additional question that must be addressed is: What is the effect of women's increasing labor force participation? To date, this remains a largely unanswered question. While a substantial amount of research has focused on the implications of women's employment on family interactions during the child-rearing years, less evidence has accumulated on the relationship between women's employment and interactions with older generations. Here again, it is easy to oversimplify the issue. It is often assumed either that employed women are pressed into relinquishing responsibilities to elderly parents or that the needs of elderly parents place undue constraints upon their daughters' workplace involvements. Our interviews with midlife women suggest that the relationships are more complex and that we must look at employment in light of what we have learned about the nature of the adult child–elderly parent tie.

First, there are many circumstances and situations in which women's employment is of negligible importance. Whether or not employment constrains the amount of care-giving daughters provide to parents is a moot point if parents are healthy and managing on their own. Similarly, employment makes little difference if daughters live several hundred miles away, since face-to-face contact is limited whether or not a woman is employed. Employment also makes little difference if parents and daughters have become accustomed to independent lives and daughters are not relied on as the first line of defense against the day-to-day problems of old age.

Second, there any many situations in which daughters have learned to maneuver around employment, especially if their schedules are flexible or they work part-time hours. Among daughters who lived within an hour's drive of parents, part-time employees actually visited parents more often than either full-time workers or full-time homemakers, and they provided more instrumental assistance when parents lived very close by. Clearly, many of the ways daughters assist parents can be accommodated into a part-time work routine. Reassuring phone calls can be made before or after work hours, errands can be run on weekends, and so on. In addition, in cases of necessity, women make efforts to accommodate paid work to the needs of parents. Approximately two-fifths of the employed women we interviewed had taken time off from work to aid parents, yet most often the time required was minimal—for example, an afternoon to take a mother to a doctor's appointment—and the women did not see it as interfering with their responsibilities on the job. For those women who had been employed for long periods of time, patterns of mutual assistance were often developed before parents grew old.

Third, women's decisions about whether and how much to work typically take into account a number of factors—financial considerations, the needs of children and spouse, volunteer work and other commitments, and, in some cases, the needs of parents. About 10% of the women in our sample mentioned that their parents' failing health and reliance upon them was one factor in their decisions to postpone or terminate employment or to limit their work hours. For example, one woman quit her full-time job in part so she would be more free to visit her recently widowed father, who lives several hours away. However, there were a number of other factors involved that reinforced this decision. She was also tired of the pressures her job entailed and was looking forward to starting a family and being a full-time mother. She quit her job as much in anticipation of pregnancy as she did because of her father. Another woman postponed going back to work because she was heavily involved in helping her widowed parent with day-to-day housekeeping, doctors' visits, and the like. Additional factors entering into her decision, however, were her satisfaction with being a full-time homemaker and her ambivalence about leaving a young teenage daughter at home alone. As these examples illustrate, it was usually a composite of factors, rather than the needs of aging parents alone, that influenced daughters' employment decisions, and even the women themselves had difficulty in ranking their relative importance.

In some cases, however, it does appear that employment—especially full-time employment—makes a difference. Among daughters who lived within an hour's drive of parents, full-time employees provided less instrumental assistance and visited parents less often than either part-time workers or full-time homemakers. Not surprisingly, full-time employment placed greater constraints on those forms of parent–child interaction that require more time and energy: Visits were more affected than contacts by phone. To what extent a decline in face-to-face contact is experienced as a loss either by daughters or by parents is unclear. For example, in returning to the labor force, daughters may be trading the social contact with parents for social contact with fellow workers. Parents, likewise, may offset the decline in daughters' visits by increasing contacts with neighbors and friends; alternatively, they may miss the more extensive contact with kin since they are at a time in their lives when other forms of social participation may be constrained. Among the women we interviewed, employment-related cutbacks never meant that daughters stopped seeing their parents but rather that they decreased their visits incrementally from daily to several times a week, from bimonthly to monthly, and so on. In addition, there is evidence that some employed daughters cut corners with parents in other ways as well. Special favors may be shaved; employed daughters may not be quite as available to listen to a mother's problems or talk on the phone several times a day; they may suggest taking a cab rather than offering to chauffeur; they may still be willing to run errands or take a parent to a doctor's appointment, but everyone is more constrained to a tight schedule. What difference this trimming makes in the lives of daughters and parents remains unclear and merits further investigation.

Employment can also serve as a legitimate excuse to pass on some of the work involved in keeping a parent comfortable to an unemployed sibling, although some unemployed siblings are less willing to accept this excuse than others. One woman, for example, complained that her brother and sisters expected her to fill in and be on call for her widowed mother since she was the only one "not working." As she herself was currently raising young children and involved in a number of community activities, she sometimes felt she was doing more than her share.

Finally, there is the matter of cohort differences. The present daughter generation is composed of members of several different cohorts, each of which has faced the impact of women's changing roles at a different point in the life cycle. What paid work means to a woman in her 30s today and what kind of balance she strikes between paid work and family roles may be quite different from how a woman in her 50s orders her priorities. With growing numbers of midlife women in the labor force, it will be important to pay attention to such cohort differences in our efforts to understand the ramifications of women's employment on family ties in the years to come. In light of these considerations, it becomes apparent that assessing the impact of employment on daughters' responses to aging parents is no simple matter. Just as we are beginning to develop more complex models for understanding how women strike balances between their work and family roles in the early part of the family cycle, we will need equally complex models in examining the work–family interface in the latter half of the family cycle as well.

Conclusion

In this chapter, we have examined the adult child–elderly parent relationship from the vantage point of daughters and discussed some of the ways daughters differ in how they respond when parents grow old. Our analysis suggests that while most women's lives are touched by the aging of parents, simplistic stereotypes, such as that of daughters being "caught in the middle," distort our understanding of parent–child relationships in later life.

In closing, there are three further considerations that warrant attention. First is the matter of women's involvements with other elderly kin.

Women may be pressed into a care-giving role not only by the needs of their own mothers and fathers but also by their parents-in-law and other elderly kin. For example, at the time of the interviews, among married respondents with at least one parent-in-law still living, three-quarters reported that at least one parent-in-law was 70 years or older. The question of how and when women become involved in the care of elderly mothers- and fathers-in-law merits its own discussion and cannot be adequately treated here. Suffice it to say that while some respondents were quite involved in helping out their husbands' elderly parents, most often this responsibility was assumed by a sister-in-law.

Second, there is the question of whether women with elderly kin *feel* caught in the middle, whether they find that being a daughter or daughter-in-law conflicts with their roles as wives and mothers or interferes with their efforts to pursue careers. This again is a difficult and complex matter, one that can only be touched upon here. A number of the women interviewed felt pulled by the competing demands of some combination of parents, children, spouses, employment, and other activities. These pulls were experienced not only by employed women but by busy homemakers as well. When parents do need help, it can be draining and time-consuming; even in the best of circumstances, it can be emotionally difficult to watch a parent grow old. Adult children do worry about their parents, and their worries range from concern over whether parents will have an accident while they are vacationing in Florida, to whether a widowed mother will be able and willing to make it on her own, to whether an elderly relative will take a turn for the worse and have to be placed in a nursing home. Elderly kin can and do complicate the lives of daughters, but so do husbands, children, grandchildren, and younger relatives. These complications are part of family life, a part that a growing number of midlife women are now experiencing and fitting into the rest of their lives.

Finally, while the current generation of daughters is accommodating to the needs of aging parents, it is less clear what will happen when these women are elderly mothers themselves. For example, will they want the same things from their daughters as their mothers now want from them? Can they reasonably expect the same kinds of help and attention from daughters that their mothers expect and receive from them? Given the decisions of more men and women to limit the size of their families, how many elderly mothers and fathers of the future will have daughters to call on and rely upon at all?

REFERENCES

Archbold, P. G. *Impact of caring for an ill elderly parent on the middle-aged or elderly offspring caregiver*. Paper presented at the 31st Annual Scientific Meeting of the Gerontological Society, Dallas, November 1978.

Baruch, G., and Barnett, R. C. Adult daughters' relationships with their mothers: The era of good feelings. *Journal of Marriage and the Family,* 1983, 45, 601–606.

Branch, L. G. *Understanding the health and social service needs of people over age 65.* Center for Survey Research, University of Massachusetts and the Joint Center for Urban Studies of M.I.T. and Harvard University, 1977.

Brody, E. M. Aged parents and aging children. In P. K. Ragan (Ed.), *Aging parents.* Los Angeles: The Ethel Percy Andrus Gerontology Center, 1979.

Brody, E. M. "Women in the middle" and family help to old people. *Gerontologist,* 1981, 21, 471–480.

Cantor, M. H. The informal support system of New York's inner city elderly: Is ethnicity a factor? In D. E. Gelfand and A. J. Kutzik (Eds.), *Ethnicity and aging.* New York: Springer, 1979.

Cantor, M. H. *Caring for the frail elderly: Impact on family, friends, and neighbors.* Paper presented at the 33rd Annual Scientific Meeting of the Gerontological Society of America, San Diego, November 1980.

Cicirelli, V. G. *Helping elderly parents.* Boston: Auburn, 1981.

Cohler, B. J., and Grunebaum, H. U. *Mothers, grandmothers, and daughters.* New York: Wiley, 1981.

Daniels, P., and Weingarten, K. *Sooner or later: The timing of parenthood in adult lives.* New York: Norton, 1982.

Fighting off old age. *Time,* February 16, 1981, p. 54.

Gordon, M. *Final payments.* New York: Ballantine, 1978.

Hagestad, G. O. Problems and promises in the social psychology of intergenerational relations. In R. W. Fogel, E. Hatfield, S. B. Kiesler, and E. Shanas (Eds.), *Aging: Stability and change in the family.* New York: Academic Press, 1981.

Harris, L., and Associates. *The myth and reality of aging in America.* Washington, D.C.: National Council on Aging, 1975.

Hess, B. B., and Waring, J. M. Parent and child in later life: Rethinking the relationship. In R. M. Lerner and G. B. Spanier (Eds.), *Child influences on marital and family interaction.* New York: Academic Press, 1978.

Hill, R., Foote, N., Aldous, J., Carlson, R., and MacDonald, R. *Family development in three generations.* Cambridge, Mass.: Schenkman, 1970.

Isaacs, B., Livingstone, M., and Neville, Y. *Survival of the unfittest.* London: Routledge and Kegan Paul, 1972.

Johnson, C. L. *Obligation and reciprocity in caregiving during illness: A comparison of spouses and offspring as family supports.* Paper presented at the 33rd Annual Scientific Meeting of the Gerontological Society of America, San Diego, November 1980.

Kovar, M. G. Elderly people: The population 65 years and over. In National Center for Health Statistics, *Health, United States: 1976–1977.* Washington, D.C.: United States Government Printing Office, 1977.

Lewis, M. A., Bienenstock, R., Cantor, M., and Schneewind, E. *The extent to which informal and formal supports interact to maintain the older people in the community.* Paper presented at the 33rd Annual Scientific Meeting of the Gerontological Society of America, San Diego, November 1980.

Lopata, H. Z. *Women as widows: Support systems.* New York: Elsevier-North Holland, 1979.

Lowenthal, M. F. *Lives in distress: The paths of the elderly to the psychiatric ward.* New York: Basic Books, 1964.

Murphy, D. *Wheels within wheels.* New York: Ticknor and Fields, 1980.

Neugarten, B. L. The awareness of middle age. In B. L. Neugarten (Ed.), *Middle age and aging.* Chicago: University of Chicago Press, 1968.

Raskind, M. A., and Storric, M. G. The organic mental disorders. In E. W. Busse and D. G. Blazer (Eds.), *Handbook of geriatric psychiatry*. New York: Van Nostrand Reinhold, 1980.

Shanas, E. Social myth as hypothesis: The case of the family relations of old people. *Gerontologist*, 1979, *19*, 3–9. (a)

Shanas, E. The family as a social support system in old age. *Gerontologist*, 1979, *19*, 169–174. (b)

Shanas, E. Older people and their families: The new pioneers. *Journal of Marriage and the Family*, 1980, *42*, 9–15.

Silverstone, B., and Hyman, H. K. *You and your aging parent*. New York: Pantheon, 1976.

Soldo, B. J. America's elderly in the 1980s. *Population Bulletin*, 1980, *35*, whole volume.

Stueve, A. The elderly as network members. *Marriage and Family Review*, 1982, *5*, 59–87.

Treas, J. Family support systems for the aged: Some social and demographic considerations. *Gerontologist*, 1977, *17*, 486–491.

Troll, L. E., Miller, S. J., and Atchley, R. C. *Families in later life*. Belmont, Calif.: Wadsworth, 1979.

Chapter 9

Motherhood in the Middle Years
Women and Their Adult Children

VIVIAN WOOD, JANE TRAUPMANN, AND JULIA HAY

The mother–child relationship may well be the most salient and enduring relationship in human experience, and its importance does not stop when the child reaches adulthood. When Troll (1972) asked adult women and men of a wide age range to describe a person they knew, mothers and fathers were spontaneously referred to more frequently than any other persons. Baruch and Barnett (1983) found in a recent study that midlife women generally have very positive feelings about their mothers, and indeed their sense of well-being was tied to the quality of that relationship. Further, mothers relate to their offspring as adults for a much longer period than they relate to them as children (Goldberg and Deutsch, 1977, p. 317), and the time period during which mother and child relate to each other as adults is increasing. As Hagestad (1981) has pointed out, increased life expectancy is producing longer-term intergenerational bonds and, increasingly, the possibility that parents and children will grow old together. And because women generally outlive their husbands, it is mostly mothers and daughters who grow old together, often one or both having been widowed or divorced.

In this chapter[1] the focus will be upon the relationship between

[1]Support for the development of this chapter and for carrying out the reported research was received from several sources: Administration on Aging Grant No. 90-A-1230 to the Faye McBeath Institute on Aging, University of Wisconsin-Madison; a project assistantship funded by a Ford Foundation grant to the Women's Studies Research Center, University of Wisconsin-Madison; and funds from the The Andrew W. Mellon Foundation grant given by Radcliffe College for research by Dr. Traupmann at the Henry A. Murray Research Center of Radcliffe College.

VIVIAN WOOD • School of Social Work, University of Wisconsin, Madison, Wisconsin 53706. JANE TRAUPMANN • Family Development Center, Cambridge, Massachusetts, and 39 Pond Street, Natick, Massachusetts 01760. JULIA HAY • Wisconsin Family Studies Institute, 1906 Monroe Street, Madison, Wisconsin 53711.

women and their adult children from the mother's perspective. The concern is with the relationship but the emphasis is on its meaning and consequence for the mother. For professionals concerned about the well-being of older people, it is of more than academic interest to understand what leads to the maintenance of good relationships between mother and child. Women, because they usually outlive their husbands, often find themselves in need of help in the later years of their lives. Studies indicate that the most likely source of help is their children, particularly their daughters (Shanas, 1979).

Because of the salience of relationships to older parents, gerontologists have given some attention to this area in their studies of old age. Much of the existing research, however, has not been systematic or explicit with regard to many dimensions. Studies often do not differentiate between sons and daughters or between fathers and mothers, and the ages of either the parents or the children are often not given. Furthermore, gerontologists' studies have focused primarily on proximity, social support, and help patterns, rather than on the quality of the relationships between elderly parents and their adult children (Rosow, 1965; Gibson, 1972). These studies generally have emphasized the positive aspects of the relationship—namely, that one or more of the older parents' children live nearby, and that they interact regularly and help each other in times of need.

The problem aspects of the relationship at this stage of the older generation's lives have for the most part been neglected. Incidents of elderly parents abused by their adult children, which have recently appeared in the media, suggest that this relationship can be fraught with problems and can lead to tragic results. Exploratory research in this area suggests there is parent abuse, but its prevalence and severity are still unknown (U.S. House of Representatives, 1980).

Because of the scientific neglect of what McCall and Simmons (1966, p. 202) have referred to as the "career of a relationship," the existing literature provides little understanding of the factors that influence the development and maintenance of the mother–child relationship as the child moves into and through adulthood. With the focus largely on infancy and childhood, the developing relationship of the mother with the child once he or she becomes an adult is little understood. There is some research on early-middle-aged parents launching their children into young adult roles; a hiatus in the research exists, however, between this stage and the point when parents are elderly and the children are middle-aged (Troll, Miller, and Atchley, 1979). What happens in the intervening 20 or more years? It seems highly unlikely that the relationship remains static, but we have very little knowledge of how changes in the lives of the mother and of the adult child affect the relationship. The offspring's becoming a parent automatically makes the mother a grandmother. How do the mother's and the child's new roles affect the relationship? Does the fact that both the mother and the offspring are now parents change the relationship? Is the impact different for mother–daughter and mother–son relationships? In these days when multiple generations are alive at the same time, often the mother will also be the daughter of elderly parents; thus, the mother and her offspring will share the fact that each of them is fulfilling both the parent and child roles at the same time. Does the mother's relationship with her offspring change when her parents die, she loses her daughter role, and becomes the oldest generation in her family?

In sum, research on the mother–child relationship, with a few important exceptions, has focused on the early years and has neglected critical issues concerning the relationship after the child becomes an adult. When mothers and offspring first relate to each other as adults, the former are usually in their early middle years. This is apt to be an important period developmentally for the mother as well as for the child. Not only must mothers learn to relate to offspring as adults, these "women in the middle" (Brody, 1981) are adjusting to the empty nest and perhaps becoming mothers-in-law and grandmothers. Moreover, mothers of this age may be dealing with developmental changes as profound and diverse as going back to school (Traupmann, 1981), reentering the labor force, working out different relationships with their husbands, and helping their elderly parents deal with the problems of old age. Finally, there is the added dimension of integrating with these activities the new realization that their own lives are finite, that they too may find themselves old, feeble, and in need of care one day.

FRAMEWORKS FOR STUDYING ADULT FAMILIES

Models of socialization that imply a one-way flow of influence have not been found to be very useful as a framework for examining the mother–adult child relationship. Early students of adult intergenerational relations were generally concerned with values and behaviors transmitted from older to younger generations, usually from parent to child (see Troll and Bengtson, 1979, for a discussion of transmission research). These studies showed that there is substantial but selective intergenerational continuity within the family. Parent–child similarity (which is considered evidence for transmission) is most noticeable in religious and political areas, least in sex roles and life-style characteristics. Yet, as Troll and Bengtson (1979) point out, systematic theory in this area remains undeveloped and generalizations remain tentative. Formulations of socialization as a process of bilateral negotiation seem to offer a more fruitful perspective for looking at such transmission phenomena. According to this approach, "relations between generations are seen as a continuous bilateral negotiation in which the young and the old exchange information and influence from their respective positions in developmental and historical time" (Bengtson and Black, 1973, p. 207).

Findings from Fischer's (1981) research support the notion of continuous negotiation. She found that a daughter's marriage and becoming a mother led to a reordering of the mother–daughter relationship, on both symbolic and interactional dimensions: Mothers and daughters reevaluated each other at the same time that they became more involved in each other's lives. For daughters, marriage was a way of demonstrating to their mothers a new adult status; becoming mothers themselves gave the daughters a new appreciation of their mothers' parenting role. With regard to interaction, married daughters with children had significantly more frequent contact with mothers than did married daughters without children.

Hagestad (1981) expands the notion of "continuous negotiation" with her discussion of historical changes in the family cycle, which have been brought about in part by increased life expectancy. Adults in the family, she points out, "now confront each other in relationships for which there is no historical precedence and minimal cultural guidance, while they individually find themselves in life stages that also have few culturally shared expectations attached to them" (p. 25). Examples of these uncharted relations are a mother and a daughter who are both old and widowed at the same time; or the woman who becomes a stepgrandmother when her daughter marries a divorcee with children from an earlier marriage. Hess and Waring (1978, p. 242), in a similar discussion of intergenerational relations among adults, conclude, "Clear normative prescriptions are lacking at the same time that choices of what to do are expanding." As Hagestad (1981, p. 25) has pointed out, adults in these ambiguous new relationships to a large extent have to negotiate and "create the structure and meaning of their bonds."

While the idea of continuous negotiation as "a process through which shared expectations are created" makes good sense, research for studying ongoing relationships faces tough methodological problems. The methodological issues of studying the development of an *individual* over time have been pointed out by developmental psychologists, with partial resolution of some issues through the use of cross-sequential methods (Schaie, 1970). Studying a *relationship* over time undoubtedly introduces new complexities that are yet to be dealt with. Not only does the relationship itself change with the passage of time, but also the two parties to the relationship dyad are changing; furthermore, these changes occur within a changing social milieu. (See Troll and Bengtson, 1979, for a discussion of these issues.)

Dimensions of Relationships in Adult Families

The study of an ongoing relationship at any stage in the life cycle requires a determination of the salient issues or dimensions of the relationship. This is complicated because some issues may be relevant to only one stage while others are pertinent to all or several stages, as Neugarten (1968) has pointed out in her essay on *individual* adult development. Bengtson (1982) has outlined four problem areas that family members often mention in regard to interaction between adult generations: (1) the challenges presented by changing roles and expectations accompanying growing up and growing old; (2) issues of autonomy and dependency—issues that seem to predominate when the child is young and again when the parent is old; (3) a just balance of giving and receiving between generations or, put another way, the issue of maintaining equity; and (4) the maintenance of continuity in the family and the avoidance of, or dealing with, disruptions such as those caused by divorce or death.

There has been research about each of these problem areas but its usefulness for understanding the mother–adult child relationship is limited. For example, many studies, such as Lowenthal and Chiriboga's (1972) study of the "empty nest," focus on one or the other member of the dyad—either the mother or the child—rather than on their relationship. Research on interaction and exchange of help between generations (Hill, Foote, Adlous, Carlson, and MacDonald, 1970; Shanas, Townsend, Wedderburn, Friis, Milhoj, and Stehouver, 1968; Sussman and Burchinal, 1962) has been largely descriptive and has been only peripherally concerned with the effect of such exchanges on the relationship between parent and child. Such research indicates that most older persons have at least one adult child living nearby with whom they interact regularly and exchange help when needed (see, for example, Shanas, 1979). The parents do most of the visiting and helping when the children are young adults, but the pattern is often reversed when parents move into advanced old age, particularly if they become ill and disabled. This research has emphasized that children do keep in touch and aid their older parents if needed. But researchers generally have not asked about children who fail to keep in touch and their reasons for lack of contact, leading Hagestad (1981) to suggest that it is time for such studies.

Schorr (1960) points out a gender difference in the mother–adult child relationship. He suggests that the widowed mother–daughter relationship is smoother and closer than the mother–son relationship. Because females in families have been primarily responsible for care-giving and household tasks, mothers and daughters can reciprocate these services, but mothers and sons often cannot. Sons are more likely to provide instrumental help such as financial assistance and advice—services mothers usually cannot return. The reciprocity of the mother–daughter relationship produces a more balanced relationship, while the one-way flow of the mother–son relationship tends to cause imbalance and often dependency. Data from our own study on differentiation in the relationship of mothers to their daughters and to their sons will be presented later in this chapter.

We turn now to a closer examination of two of the issues—dependency and equity—which Bengtson (1982) has designated problem areas.

Dependency

The mother–child relationship is unique in that dependency *is* so central—dependency of the infant and young child on the mother in the early years, a renegotiation of that dependency in the child's adolescence, typically a trading back and forth of the dependent role during the mother–adult child "middle period," then the possibility of increased dependency of the mother on the adult child in her old age.

Dependency, as a dimension of the mother–adult child relationship, is undoubtedly different from dependency in the mother–young child relationship, but the distinction has not been considered in much depth in the literature. Dependency is a major issue in old age; in literature on this period, however, the concept of dependency is used in many ways. In a monograph on dependency in old age, for example, the editor (Kalish, 1969) points out that the term *dependency* is used to refer to an interpersonal relationship, a condition, a personality characteristic, and a particular example of behavior. In this chapter, of course, we are concerned with dependency in the mother–adult child relationship. If we say that the mother is dependent on her daughter, for example, we imply that the daughter gives more than she receives in the relationship. Interrelated elements such as the sense of obligation, duty, and the norm of reciprocity muddy the picture and make clear distinctions difficult. The fact that dependency in old age is a sensitive topic further complicates the tasks of examination; while the dependency of the young child on the parent is normative, there is ambiguity concerning the dependency of the parent on the adult child. In addition, there are sensitive potitical implications embedded in the issues of dependency for women. Power, and thus powerlessness, are always factors in relationships in which one person necessarily depends on another. Most research has ignored these touchy issues when looking at family relationships. However, as women, often both daughters and mothers themselves, strive to understand their relationships better, this area is no longer being ignored (Dinnerstein, 1976; Matthews, 1979; Rubin, 1979).

What have life-span scholars to say about dependency in adulthood? Rosow (1965) claims that the fact that children see and help their older parents has been seen by many researchers as evidence of good relationships based on affection and positive sentiments. He argues that this should not be assumed but should be a question for investigation, pointing out that children may maintain these ties out of a sense of obligation that may strain rather than strengthen affectional bonds. Blenkner (1965), in contrast, claims that a sense of duty enhances relationships between adult children and older parents, and Cicirelli's (1980) research tends to support this idea.

Another body of research suggests an intriguing picture of the effects that feelings of obligation may have on mother–adult child relationships. On the one hand, research by Adams (1968b) and Lopata (1973) shows that widowhood, which often creates a state of increased need for the mother with resultant feelings of obligation on the part of her children, may strain the relationship. On the other hand, divorce of adult children, which may involve increased dependence of the younger member of the dyad, may actually lead to an improved relationship between the mother and her divorced child (Hagestad, Smyer, and Stierman, 1983). A shift or an imbalance in dependency may be detrimental to the relationship. The importance of both parent and adult child maintaining independence has been stated by anthropologists Clark and Anderson (1967):

> A good relationship with children in old age depends, to a large extent, on the graces and autonomy of the aged parent—in short, on his ability to manage gracefully by himself. It would appear that, in our culture, there simply cannot be any happy role reversals between the generations, neither an increasing dependency of parent upon child nor a continuing reliance of child upon parent. The mores do not sanction it and children and parents resent it. The parent must remain strong and independent. If his personal resources fail, the conflicts arise. The child, on the other hand, must not threaten the security of the parent with requests for monetary aid or other care when parental income has shrunk through retirement. The ideal situation is when both parent and child are functioning well.

Bengtson (1982, p. 92) agrees, arguing that "much of the drama of intergenerational relations concerns issues of autonomy on the one hand and dependency on the other." Kerckoff (1966), in a study of 135 couples, found that those who had the lower levels of mutual support activities with their children had higher morale, noting that both dependency on children for living arrangements and propinquity of offspring appeared to contribute to unhappiness in later life. In other words, high morale was associated with relative independence of the two generations. But, as Kerckoff suggests, there is no way to identify the direction of causality in these findings since an elderly parent's low morale may require the offspring to provide assistance, rather than the assistance fostering low morale. Johnson and Bursk (1977) found that poor health and poverty contribute to dependency, and the greater the dependency, the more likely parents and children are to have negative feelings toward themselves and toward each other. It is important to note that mothers much more often than fathers are at risk of being dependent on children. While 52% of women 65 and over are widowed, only 14% of older men are. And women are more highly represented among the aged poor than are men.[2] Thus, men more often than women have a spouse to depend on in later life; women, on the other hand, usually must turn to their children for care and assistance. So it is more often a mother's dependency than a father's that strains the relationship between parent and adult child.

Matthews (1979), in looking at dependency and the balance of exchange in elderly mother–adult child relationships, focuses on the idea of power. Matthews argues that the current structure of the "modified extended family" does not give the old widowed mother a viable position in this group. The old mother, she suggests, is in a subordinate position in her family because she is very likely to have only her offspring as a source of support and needed services, and at the same time may have very little to offer in return. From the exchange theory perspective that Matthews uses, the old mother with few resources has little power in relation to her offspring, creating an imbalanced relationship. While the likelihood is high that the old widow's offspring have other sources of rewards and help, she may depend only on the relationship with her children for rewards, particularly if she has always been family-centered. The importance of maintaining good relationships with her children is great and explains the necessity for complying with her offspring's definition of her position in the family. Matthews gives examples of how the children's treatment of their mother—unconsciously, perhaps—emphasizes her subordinate position. They drop in to see her, at their convenience, for example, but she is never made to feel free to visit the children unannounced. Old mothers of the future, with more education and more advantageous economic positions, are less likely to be dependent on children in later life. Indeed, one can imagine children

---

[2]In 1978 36% of nonmarried older women had incomes below the poverty level, as compared with 27% of nonmarried older men; only 8% of older men and women in couples had incomes below the poverty level (U.S. Department of Health and Human Services, 1981).

and grandchildren vying for invitations to the elderly widow's retirement condominium complete with swimming pool and other amenities.

In summary, many investigators consider dependency a key dimension in the "career" of the mother–adult child relationship. Dependency is particularly salient when the child is an adolescent and is striving for autonomy, and again when the mother is old and is attempting to maintain her independence. The mother–child relationship seems to be at its best during the mother's middle years, when both parent's and child's autonomy is unthreatened and both are capable of reciprocating care and assistance.

Maintenance of Equity

The second key issue to be discussed here is related to what Bengtson (1982) called "a just balance of giving and receiving between generations." Family theorists have suggested that the norm of reciprocity (Gouldner, 1960) is one of the most powerful of social forces sustaining intergenerational ties for the middle-aged and their elderly parents. Sussman (1976) describes this as an implicit bargain struck between the generations such that the daily maintenance, provisions for education, and general caring during the child's infancy and early years will be reciprocated with similar services and caring in the parents' later years. In the words of a mother of three boys now in their 30s, "My sons are my old-age insurance."

There is disagreement among theorists, however, as to the effectiveness of the reciprocity norm for ensuring intergenerational care for the elderly. Clark (1969) points out that social reciprocity is temporal in nature. Because our culture is strongly oriented to present and future, past services rendered or aid given does not bind the recipient for very long to a request for reciprocity. Is a sense of fairness or equity apparent between mothers and their adult children? Or is the current generation of older mothers feeling a distinct lack of reciprocity for their long labors of child-rearing?

A recent study of middle-aged and older women (Wood and Traupmann, 1980) sheds some light on these questions. A total of 187 mothers were interviewed about their feelings as mothers and as daughters. The interview was part of a large multidisciplinary study of women aged 50 to 93 conducted by the Faye McBeath Institute on Aging of the University of Wisconsin-Madison. The sample for the larger study was composed of 240 randomly selected women living in five different areas of a small midwestern city. The theoretical framework for this research was equity theory (Walster, Walster, and Berscheid, 1978), a social psychological theory concerned with fairness in interpersonal relations. Equity theory states that individuals in equitable rather than inequitable relationships are happier and less distressed and are more likely to remain in the relationship. Inequities in either an overbenefited or an underbenefited direction can be distressing, though the degree of distress for those feeling they are getting more than they deserve (overbenefit) is less severe than for those who feel they are getting less than they deserve (underbenefit).

There has been criticism of equity theory when applied to intimate relationships, largely because it offends people's ideas of what such relationships should be like. Many people believe that in relationships based on love and family ties, people are not aware of what they give and get but, rather, love unconditionally (e.g., Fromm, 1956), and that an awareness of the patterns of give and take would surely spell the relationship's demise (e.g., Murstein, Cerreto, and MacDonald, 1977).

Other theorists take the opposite view, that it is only through a relationship based on the equality of contributions and of rewards that intimacy flourishes (e.g., Scanzoni, 1972; Lederer and Jackson, 1968). It may be that an awareness of the implicit bargain surfaces *only* when an imbalance becomes acutely apparent—as when, for example, the wife who has put her husband through medical school later finds him uninterested in her, or the mother who has struggled to raise four children finds that they all settle thousands of miles away and only send birthday cards once a year.

Miller (1976) suggests another twist to the issue of fairness in family relations. She hypothesizes that women are socialized to accept less than "a fair shake" from life. These expectations lead women to feel distinctly guilty when they are the recipients of nurturance or special kindnesses because they feel they do not deserve such benefits. Mothers, they believe, should be givers but not receivers.

The questions investigated in the Wisconsin study were whether women would report an awareness of the fairness of exchanges that go on in their family relationships and, if so, whether fairness or equity in these family relationships was important to them. If the reciprocity norm is operating with mothers and their adult children, it was expected that women who feel content and happy with their sons and daughters would report a sense of fairness about the relationship overall. Those who feel distressed—angry, resentful, or guilty about their relationships with their adult children—would report a distinct lack of fairness.

Most crucial to a test of the reciprocity norm, however, is a comparison of the perceived fairness in the childhood *and* in the parenthood of the same individuals. Do men and women who have been generously overbenefited in childhood then raise their own children in a similar manner by giving so much that they then place themselves in an underbenefited position? And conversely, do underbenefited children go on to underbenefit their own offspring 20 years hence, thus putting themselves in an overbenefited position when their children show kindness and concern? In other words, is a repetition of the equity/inequity conditions across generations the pattern we would be most likely to encounter in a study of today's older generation?

An equally plausible prediction, elaborated by family theorists, takes just the opposite position (see Boszormenyi-Nagy and Spark, 1973). Men and women who were underbenefited in childhood attempt to undo the inequity by overbenefiting their own children, thereby putting themselves in an underbenefited position in adulthood with respect to their children. Examples of this cross-generational undoing abound in popular folklore—the poor uneducated cleaning woman who works at three jobs to put her son through college, or the immigrant father who sacrifices in order to set his son up in business.

Since most of the respondents in the Wisconsin study were both daughters and mothers, it was possible to examine equity/inequity effects across two generations. Respondents were asked to reflect on their relationships with their adult children and with their parents. The questions asked were modified versions of standard equity questions used in previous equity/intimacy research. (See Traupmann, Petersen, Utne, and Hatfield, 1981, for a description of the development of these measures.)

First, after a series of questions about children and a brief introduction to conceptualizing the complexities of family life in terms of "give and take," respondents were asked the following question:

> When you think about all you did and do for your children and the joys and frustrations of raising them . . . and . . . all that they did and do for you and their joys and frustrations from their life with you, how do things "stack up"?
> 1. They got a much better deal.
> 2. They got a somewhat better deal.
> 3. They got a slightly better deal.
> 4. We got an equal deal.
> 5. I got a slightly better deal.
> 6. I got a somewhat better deal.
> 7. I got a much better deal.

Much later in the interview, after a series of questions about parents, the following question was asked:

> When you think about what you did for your parents and what you got from them and . . . what they did for you and got from you, how do things "stack up"? [The same 7-point scale for responses was used.]

The respondents were first placed in one of three groups on the basis of relationships with children: (1) women who felt their children got a better deal—or who felt *underbenefited,* (2) women who felt the deal was *equitable*, and (3) women who felt they got a better deal than their children or who felt *overbenefited*. A similar grouping was done in regard to their relationships with their parents.

The results were as follows: Most women felt a sense of fairness in both their relations with children and their relations with parents. Over two-thirds of the women reported that the relationship with their children was equitable, and nearly two-thirds reported the same about their relationship with their parents.

Second, most of those who felt relations were inequitable, whether they reported from the perspective of daughter or from that of mother, thought children generally got the better deal in relation to their parents. Of the daughters who perceived themselves inequitably treated, almost twice as many (64% compared to 36%) felt they, not their parents, had gotten a better deal. When the respondents changed their perspective to that of mother, the pattern of inequities remained in favor of children. Over twice as many mothers (68% vs. 32%) felt their children had received a better deal in the relationship than they had.

Turning to the cross-generational question either of repetition of inequities experienced in childhood or of the undoing of childhood inequities, an interesting pattern emerges. Those overbenefited as children tend to *repeat* that pattern with their own children (62% vs. 38%). Those underbenefited as children tend to report *undoing* that pattern with their own children (73% vs. 27%).

THE CONSEQUENCES OF INEQUITIES WITH PARENTS

If a sense of fairness or unfairness exists between mothers and adult children, how does it affect what they are willing to do for each other? One would expect that the underbenefited would have concluded in their own adulthood that their parents deserved little if anything from them now, since the balance had been tipped in the other direction for so long. Conversely, the overbenefited might feel a strong sense of obligation to repay the generous favors they received in childhood. In order to explore the consequences of inequities, women were asked to reflect on how the responsibility for care of their aging parents had been divided between them and their siblings, using the following question:

> In some families one son or daughter is primarily "in charge" of caring for aging parents. In other families these responsibilities are shared among the sons and daughters. How was it in your family?
> 1. Others (brothers, sisters, etc.) were solely in charge. I gave them no help or almost no help.
> 2. Others (brothers, sisters, etc.) were primarily responsible but I helped some.
> 3. We shared the responsibilities more or less equally.

4. I was primarily responsible but got some help from others.
5. I was solely in charge, I got no help or almost no help from others.

The results were surprisingly inconsistent with expectations. Of the women who felt underbenefited with respect to their parents—those expected to take little responsibility for parents in old age—a much greater percentage (57% vs. 26%) were taking primary responsibility for them than those in the overbenefited group were doing. Those in the overbenefited group either let others take responsibility (39%) or shared the responsibility with siblings (35%).

A word of caution: The data are complicated by the fact that some women had two living parents, some had only one living parent, and for the majority both parents were dead. Thus, some respondents, in answering the questions about their parents, were talking about ongoing relationships while others were speaking retrospectively of past relationships.

Given that qualification, the inconsistency between the reported inequities in older women's relationships with their parents and the parent care-giving they are subsequently prepared to do poses further interesting questions. Are parent–child relationships different from most relationships? Are the norms of expected behavior in the parent–child relationship so strong that what one *should* do overrides what one feels like doing? Are the patterns of the relationship so set when the children are young that they are not easily changed?

The reasons our respondents gave for keeping in contact with their parents had some relevance to these questions. Using scales developed by Adams (1968a), we asked women to assess the importance for them of different reasons for keeping in close contact with aging parents. The list of reasons included "feelings of obligation," "I need their help," "they need my help," and "enjoyment." Underbenefited women, we found, were most likely to place emphasis on a sense of obligation or on the fact that their parents needed them as the reasons for keeping in touch. The overbenefited women—those who thought they'd gotten the best of the deal in the relationship with their parents—were most apt to say they kept in touch with their parents because *they* needed their parents. These results suggest that early relationship patterns tend to persist, and that in some cases the norms of expected behavior override more immediate feelings.

The Consequences of Inequities with Adult Daughters and Sons

We have seen that feelings of inequity with parents in adulthood may affect one's sense of responsibility for care-giving and even one's feelings about simply keeping in touch with parents. What is known about the consequences of inequity with sons and daughters in adulthood? First, we found evidence that contradicts Miller's (1976) prediction that women prefer inequitable (underbenefited) rather than equitable relationships with their adult offspring. The happiest and least distressful relationships were the equitable relationships, followed first by the overbenefited and then by the underbenefited relationships. Also noteworthy is the fact that the curve for daughters diverges at the two inequity points from that for sons, suggesting that there may be more distress associated with inequities with daughters than with inequities with sons, though the interaction was not statistically significant. This differential distress between daughters and sons emerges clearly (and is statistically significant) in the women's pattern of resentment about inequity. Women express virtually no resentment toward sons, regardless of whether their sons have treated them fairly or unfairly. However, resentment is expressed toward daughters who have given their mothers less than the mothers feel they deserve. This supports Gunhild Hagestad's observation (cited in Troll *et al.*, 1979, p. 97) that middle-aged mothers expect more interaction and help from their daughters and are upset when they do not get them. On the other hand, they expect much less from their sons and are delighted with anything they get.

In sum, there does not seem to be a simple relationship between feelings of equity in cross-generational relations and the way these relationships are subsequently maintained. Equitable relationships seem to be the predominant type and can be comfortably maintained in later adult life. However, when feelings of inequity arise early on, a more complicated set of consequences seems to ensue that is not so readily predictable from a simple equity theory framework. Inequities in the overbenefited direction are more often attributed to children and are more likely to be replicated in the next generation than are inequities in the underbenefited direction. However, overbenefited feelings do not seem to motivate subsequent care-giving behavior. Remarkably, it was those who felt underbenefited who more often took responsibility for care of parents in old age.

OTHER ISSUES

Dependency and equity were considered as independent concepts in this discussion. It should be apparent, however, that the two concepts are related. Dependency refers to a situation in which one member of a dyad receives more from the other member than he or she gives in return. Equity, on the other hand, refers to the reaction of either member of the dyad in terms of whether he or she thinks the particular balance of give and take is fair. These two concepts and related ones such as obligation, duty, and reciprocity need further conceptual clarification and deserve further study.

An important issue with regard to the mother's old age is whether the offspring's dependency on the mother in childhood has allowed the mother to build up "credit," which is repaid in old age with care from her child when needed. Johnson (1978), in an analysis of what contributes to a good relationship between older mothers and their daughters, found that the relationship the pair developed over many years and through many crises appeared, from the perspective of both the mothers and the daughters, to have great relevance for the current quality of that relationship. One research question to be resolved regarding the quality of the mother–child relationship when the mother is old is whether the past long-term relationship or the current situation of the older mother has greater effect.

One might also conjecture that the *objective* balance between dependence and autonomy in the relationship is often less important than the *subjective* reaction—whether both the mother and the child feel there has been a fair and equitable give and take in the relationship. A relationship that seems imbalanced and unfair to an outsider may be seen as perfectly fair and satisfactory to the parties involved. Relationships that may be most problematic are those in which one member of the dyad views the relationship as equitable and the other does not—for example, the son who takes for granted the scrimping and saving of his widowed mother to put him through medical school and who then, as a successful physician, is ashamed of and avoids his mother.

Summary

We have pointed out the neglect by researchers of the mother–child relationship after the child becomes an adult. We referred to the increasing duration of this relationship as life expectancy has increased. We pointed to the importance of understanding the development of this relationship over time and to the special significance of the relationship to mothers in their advanced old age. Failure to study this relationship stems in part from the lack of adequate frameworks for doing so, a situation that appears to be improving as students of intergenerational relationships turn their attention to the quality of relationships between parents and their adult children.

We examined in detail two dimensions of the relationship that the literature suggests are salient to our understanding of this bond: dependency and equity. Data from our own study of older women and their relationships to their parents and to their adult children were included in order to shed light on equity in mother–adult child relationships.

Attention was directed to the relationship between dependency and equity and to the need for conceptual clarification.

REFERENCES

Adams, B. N. *Kinship in an urban setting*. Chicago: Markham, 1968. (a)
Adams, B. N. The middle-class adult and his widowed or still-married mother. *Social Problems*, 1968, *16*, 51–59. (b)
Baruch, G., and Barnett, R. Adult daughters' relationships with their mothers: The era of good feelings. *Journal of Marriage and the Family*, 1983, *45*, 601–606.
Bengtson, V. L. A generation gap? Research perspective on ways that generations interact. In J. P. Rosenfeld (Ed.), *Relationships: Marriage and family reader*. Chicago: Scott Foresman, 1982.
Bengtson, V. L., and Black, O. Intergenerational relations: Continuities in socialization. In P. Baltes and W. Schaie (Eds.), *Life-span developmental psychology: Personality and socialization*. New York: Academic Press, 1973.
Blenkner, M. Social work and family relationships in later life with some thoughts on filial maturity. In E. Shanas and G. Streib (Eds.), *Social structure and the family: Generational relations*. Englewood Cliffs, N.J.: Prentice-Hall, 1965.
Boszormenyi-Nagy, I., and Spark, G. M. *Invisible loyalties*. Hagerstown, Md.: Harper & Row, 1973.
Brody, E. "Women in the middle" and family help to older people. *Gerontologist*, 1981, *21*, 471–482.
Cicirelli, V. *Age differences in adult children's feelings of closeness toward parents: Effects of filial obligation and partial dependency*. Paper presented at the annual meeting of the American Psychological Association, Montreal, 1980.
Clark, M. Cultural values and dependency in later life. In R. Kalish (Ed.), *The dependencies of old people*. Ann Arbor: University of Michigan, Institute of Gerontology, 1969.
Clark, M., and Anderson, B. *Culture and aging*. Springfield, Ill.: Charles C Thomas, 1967.
Dinnerstein, D. *The mermaid and the minotaur*. New York: Harper & Row, 1976.
Fischer, L. R. Transitions in the mother–daughter relationship. *Journal of Marriage and the Family*, 1981, *43*, 613–622.
Fromm, E. *The art of loving*. New York: Harper & Row, 1956.
Gibson, G. Kin family network: Overheralded structure in past conceptualizations of family functioning. *Journal of Marriage and the Family*, 1972, *34*, 13–23.
Goldberg, S., and Deutsch, F. *Life-span individual and family development*. Monterey, Calif.: Brooks/Cole, 1977.
Gouldner, A. The norm of reciprocity: A preliminary statement. *American Sociological Review*, 1960, *25*, 161–179.
Hagestad, G. O. Problems and promises in the social psychology of intergenerational relations. In R. Fogel, E. Hatfield, S. Kiesler, and E. Shanas (Eds.), *Aging: Stability and change in the family*. New York: Academic Press, 1981.
Hagestad, G. O., Smyer, M. A., and Stierman, K. Parent–child relations in adulthood: The impact of divorce in middle age. In R. Cohen, B. Cohler, and S. Weissman (Eds.), *Parenthood as an adult experience*. New York: Guilford Press, 1983.
Hess, B., and Waring, J. M. Parent and child in later life: Rethinking the relationship. In R. M. Lerner and G. B. Spanier (Eds.), *Child influences on marital and family interactions*. New York: Academic Press, 1978.
Hill, R., Foote, N., Aldous, J., Carlson, R., and MacDonald, R. *Family development in three generations*. Cambridge, Mass.: Schenkman, 1970.

Johnson, E. S. "Good" relationships between older mothers and their daughters: A causal model. *Gerontologist*, 1978, *18*, 301–306.
Johnson, E. S., and Bursk, B. Relationships between the elderly and their adult children. *Gerontologist*, 1977, *17*, 90–96.
Kalish, R. Introduction. In R. Kalish (Ed.), *The dependencies of old people*. Ann Arbor: University of Michigan, Institute of Gerontology, 1969.
Kerckoff, A. C. Family patterns and morale in retirement. In I. H. Harper and J. C. McKinney (Eds.), *Social aspects of aging*. Durham, N.C.: Duke University Press, 1966.
Lederer, W. J., and Jackson, D. D. *The mirages of marriage*. New York: Norton, 1968.
Lopata, H. Z. *Widowhood in an American city*. Cambridge, Mass.: Schenkman, 1973.
Lowenthal, M. F., and Chiriboga, D. Transition to the empty nest: Crisis, challenge or relief? *Archives of General Psychiatry*, 1972, *26*, 8–14.
Matthews, S. H. *The social world of old women*. Beverly Hills: Sage, 1979.
McCall, G., and Simmons, J. L. *Identities and interaction*. New York: Free Press, 1966.
Miller, J. B. *Toward a new psychology of women*. Boston: Beacon Press, 1976.
Murstein, B. L., Cerreto, M., and MacDonald, M. G. A theory and investigation of the effect of exchange orientation on marriage and friendship. *Journal of Marriage and the Family*, 1977, *39*, 543–548.
Neugarten, B. Adult personality: Toward a psychology of the life cycle. In B. Neugarten (Ed.), *Middle age and aging*. Chicago: University of Chicago Press, 1968.
Rosow, I. Intergenerational relationships: Problems and proposals. In E. Shanas and G. Streib (Eds.), *Social structure and the family: Generational relations*. Englewood Cliffs, N.J.: Prentice-Hall, 1965.
Rubin, L. *Women of a certain age*. New York: Harper & Row, 1979.
Scanzoni, J. *Sexual bargaining: Power politics in the American marriage*. Englewood Cliffs, N.J.: Prentice-Hall, 1972.
Schaie, W. A reinterpretation of age-related change in cognitive structure and functioning. In L. R. Goulet and P. B. Baltes (Eds.), *Life-span developmental psychology: Research and theory*. New York: Academic Press, 1970.
Schorr, A. L. *Filial responsibility in the modern American family*. Washington, D.C.: Social Security Administration, 1960.
Shanas, E. Social myth as hypothesis: The case of the family relations of old people. *Gerontologist*, 1979, *19*, 3–9.
Shanas, E., Townsend, P., Wedderburn, D., Friis, H., Milhoj, P., and Stehouver, J. *Old people in three industrial societies*. New York: Atherton Press, 1968.
Sussman, M. The family life of old people. In R. Binstock and E. Shanas (Eds.), *Handbook of aging and the social sciences*. New York: Van Nostrand Reinhold, 1976.
Sussman, M., and Burchinal, L. Kin family network: Unheralded structure in current conceptualizations of family functioning. *Marriage and Family Living*, 1962, *24*, 231–40.
Traupmann, J. *Women in midlife: The choice of continuing education*. Paper presented in the symposium Middle-Aged and Older Women and Achievement: Process and Implications, at the meeting of the American Psychological Association, Los Angeles, September 1981.
Traupmann, J., Petersen, R., Utne, M., and Hatfield, E. Measuring equity in intimate relations. *Applied Psychological Measurement*, 1981, *5*, 467–480.
Troll, L. *Salience of family members in three generations*. Paper presented at the meeting of the American Psychological Association, Honolulu, 1972.
Troll, L., and Bengtson, V. L. Generations in the family. In W. Burr, R. Hill, F. Ivan Nye, and I. Reiss (Eds.), *Contemporary theories about the family* (Vol. 1): *Research-based theories*. New York: Free Press, 1979.
Troll, L., Miller, S., and Atchley, R. *Families in later life*. Belmont, Calif.: Wadsworth, 1979.

U.S. Department of Health and Human Services, Social Security Administration, Office of Research and Statistics. *Income and resources of the aged, 1978* (SSA Publication O. 13–11727). Washington, D.C.: U.S. Government Printing Office, October 1981.

U.S. House of Representatives, Select Committee on Aging (96th Congress, First Session). *Elder abuse: The hidden problem* (Comm. Pub. No. 96–220). Washington, D.C.: U.S. Government Printing Office, 1980.

Walster, E., Walster, G. W., and Berscheid, E. *Equity: Theory and research.* Boston: Allyn and Bacon, 1978.

Wood, V., and Traupmann, J. *The aging women project: Final report.* Unpublished manuscript, University of Wisconsin, 1980.

Chapter 10

Black Women in the Middle Years

JEANNE SPURLOCK

WHO ARE WE?

According to the U.S. Bureau of Census (1980), Afro-American women in the 35–54 age range represented 1.23% of the total population in 1979. Black women between the ages of 55 and 60 represented less than .5% of the population.

Like all groups of people, there is diversity among us. Because a greater percentage of us are from poverty backgrounds, we are likely to age quickly and are vulnerable to disorders that are related to poverty. For example, we are likely to have had poor or limited access to adequate health care services, and to face middle age with concern about our physical health. If we have had limited formal education, we are still likely to be working at lower level, low-paying jobs, or, burdened with physical and mental health problems, we survive with welfare assistance and/or Social Security disability payments. Not all of us, though; some of us struggle out to work daily even though feeling poorly.

Those of us who were born into families that were relatively free of economic crises are more likely to have had reasonably adequate health care. Even so, we may be experiencing concern about current physical health problems. Many are likely to be taking medication for hypertension, a common disorder among the Afro-American people. We may be troubled about the flare-up of arthritis or complications of diabetes, or other chronic physical disorders. Some of us are bothered with the physical signs of menopause; others experience no untoward physical reactions and have a sense of freedom.

JEANNE SPURLOCK • American Psychiatric Association, 1700 18th Street, N. W., Washington, D.C. 20009.

Having been motivated to pursue formal education, some of us have become reasonably financially secure in our chosen careers. In some professions, we find ourselves stuck at the lower levels of pay scales even though our responsibilities have expanded during the course of employment.

We are represented in politics, in both elected and appointed positions. Some of us have become nationally known in various fields; for others, the fame of yesteryear has faded, and some are yet struggling for recognition in their middle years. So it is in academe, journalism, and any number of other professions. Perhaps a greater number of us are invisible to the broader community.

We are never-married, married, separated and/or divorced, and widowed. Our coloring is black, brown, "high yellow," and even lighter. Some of us may be more preoccupied about our weight, age spots, and dry skin than we were about color in our adolescence. At middle age, many of us are more concerned about the thinning of our hair than about its texture. Others are taking the physical signs of middle age in stride, and fret little, if any, about the natural youthfulness of some of our sisters. We are represented in the statistics of the depressed and the well-adjusted. Some of us are involved in midcareer changes; others are adjusting to early retirement. We are represented among blue- and white-collar workers, as well as among the self-employed in both stable and unstable businesses.

Our sources of entertainment are varied. For some of us weekly bowling is a must; others struggle to play a decent game of tennis. Some of us are not so physically active and seek entertainment in sedentary activities. Because of financial restrictions and/or fear of night travel, television is the primary source of entertainment for many.

As most of the foregoing examples show, we respond to middle age no differently than women of the majority group in the United States. These examples also show the need to counteract concepts stereotyping Afro-American women. However, our position of double jeopardy—our race and our gender—often accounts for differences when we are compared to white women. Some of us bring to middle age the painful memories of overt racial discrimination and continue to maintain a stance of assertiveness, if not militancy. Others of us appear to have become masters at denial.

The range of differences has been observed in both personal and professional contacts, and within the author's family structure. These differences were also reflected in the answers to a questionnaire that was circulated informally to a small sample of black women (50 in number).

The differences and similarities among us are outlined in more detail in the sections to follow. Sketches from the professional literature and a view from the popular press precede a series of vignettes from the pens of Afro-American women poets and writers. Descriptions of various intrafamilial relationships are extracted from personal and professional experiences. Subsequent sections focus on the men (or absence of men) in our lives, the range of our economic status, our involvement (or lack of involvement) in the women's movement, and patterns of adaptation or maladaptation.

BEHAVIORAL SCIENCE AND BLACK WOMEN

The absence of specific references to black women of middle age in a number of widely read publications of black behavioral scientists is striking. Aging, middle age or midlife, and menopause are topics not to be found in the index of Staples's (1973) *The Black Woman in America*. Although the entries that focus on other topics such as "marriage," "matriarchal structure," "role, female" can relate to the period of middle age, this particular phase of life is not specifically referred to in the text. Jackson's (1973) excellent review of the role of Afro-American women does not specifically address life phase differences. However, a number of class and educational differences addressed by Jackson are of significance in the middle years. She challenges the premise that black women have had greater opportunities for varied occupations than white women and suggests that only two kinds have been available for the most part—(1) the traditional female profession of teaching, and (2) domestic employment, the latter "almost solely reserved for Black females in the South."

Ladner (1972) discusses the black female-headed household, vis-à-vis the roles necessary for the black women to play: "Today Black women play highly functional and sometimes autonomous roles within the family and society because the same economic and social conditions which allowed for the emergence of a female dominated society during slavery still perpetuate this type of family structure." According to Ladner, black women are perceived dualistically—the pillar of strength versus the symbol of immorality. This duality renders the black woman unable to compete with white women, a condition which has until recently accounted for many of the problems and conflicts of black women. It should be emphasized that Ladner sees this problem primarily as a thing of the past: "the new thrust toward Black consciousness and Black identity have allowed for the development of an internal set of standards by which many Black women have begun to judge themselves. Therefore, the conflict which was caused because of the incongruity between white versus Black identification models has lessened, and white conceptions of womanhood have ceased to have the same relevance they once had" (p. 42).

Illustrations of Ladner's premise can be found in a number of areas—from the selection of campus queens to the latest fashions in various fields of advertising. Those of us with broad facial features, dark complexions, or short hair can see similar images in fashion magazines, in campus publications, and/or on the television screen. This is not to suggest that a positive sense of self is dependent upon the external environment, but it serves to underscore the importance of cultural beliefs and mores.

In their 1968 publication, *Black Rage*, Grier and Cobbs describe in narrow, if not biased, language the black woman's effort to cope with her negative image, as defined by the broader society: "Letting youth go, beauty go, and sex go, they narrowed their vision to the most essential feminine function—mothering, nurturing, and protecting their children" (pp. 53–54). The Grier-Cobbs premise does not stand up if one carefully surveys the various groupings within the black female population, or even within a single group. This author thinks it unlikely that "beauty products" are important only to nonblack women. The departure of a woman's mate is not necessarily accompanied by her "letting . . . sex go" and restricting herself to the mothering role. In advancing their premise, Grier and Cobbs overlooked the scores of black middle-aged women, of matronly and striking appearance, who are involved in an ongoing relationship with a male companion, or those who are actively involved in church and/or other community projects. This author suggests that the narrowness of vision is more that of Grier and Cobbs rather than that of the women they describe.

The rearing of her children's children, whether as her own or as her grandchildren, is commonly experienced by black women. As with women in other groups, these experiences may or may not be studded with conflict. Lawrence (1975) provided several vivid illustrations of generational relationships that are conflicted in her account of the nurturing figures and noxious elements of an inner-city community. The child is often caught up in the mother–grandmother antagonisms.

> When separation and loss are devastating, anger is severe. The nurse has brought a 20 year old mother, Ms. Jones, into the well-baby station for consultation with the psychiatrist. The woman was accompanied by two-year-old twins, a boy and a girl. The twins would talk to everyone in the house but the mother. The mother had been accused of "battering" her seven-year-old daughter, Patsy, who had then been removed to a small state school. During the consultation, the twins rarely made physical contact with the mother. As the mother talked . . . the girl twin began to cry. . . . One of the conference participants said to the mother, impatiently, "Pick her up." "What do you want me to do, pet her?" retorted the mother. "That's what

ruined my Patsy. My mother pet her." "You mean that your mother petted her more than she pet you," the psychiatrist proposed. "My mother didn't raise me. She sent me to my grandmother's when I was a baby." This mother had little insight into her own feelings of abandonment at this time; nor of their significance in her relations with her children. (Lawrence, 1975, pp. 72–73)

However, as Lawrence points out, grandmothers often comfortably share in the nurturing process and reinforce that which is provided by the parents. In their longitudinal study of the impact of family structure and functioning on the mental health of children, Kellam *et al.* (1978) also illustrate the positive role played by grandmothers in one-parent families. In addition, Furstenberg (1976) has found that the preschool children of black adolescent mothers whose relatives (particularly the maternal grandmothers) participated in child-rearing functioned at a more advanced level than those preschoolers who were not cared for part-time by relatives.

That so many black female-headed households exist is related to the increase in the divorce rate in the black population and to the apparent limited opportunity that black women have for remarriage (Staples, 1978). Barriers to remarriage, especially the diminishing number of available black men, are related to the existence of such households.

FROM THE PENS OF BLACK WRITERS

Black women in their middle years are portrayed both stereotypically and as diverse in contemporary writings. Guy-Sheftall (1979) notes the diversity and complexity of black women in the poetry created by Gwendolyn Brooks. Brooks's poem "Sadie and Maude" (1962) vividly illustrates the breadth of the diversity.

> Maude went to college.
> Sadie stayed at home.
> Sadie scraped life
> With a fine-tooth comb.
>
> She didn't leave a tangle in.
> Her comb found every strand.
> Sadie was one of the livingest chit
> In all the land.
>
> Sadie bore two babies.
> Under her maiden name.
> Maude and Ma and Papa
> Nearly died of the shame.
>
> When Sadie said her last so-long
> Her girls struck out from home.

> (Sadie had left as heritage
> Her fine-tooth comb.)
>
> Maude, who went to college,
> Is a thin brown mouse.
> She is living all alone
> In this old house.

The tone of loneliness that is experienced by Maude is again suggested in another Brooks poem, "A Sunset in the City" (1962).

> Already I am no longer looked at with lechery or love.
> My daughters and sons have put me away with marbles
>   and dolls,
> Are gone from the house.
> My husband and lovers are pleasant or somewhat polite
> And night is night.
> It is a real chill out,
> The genuine thing.
> I am not deceived, I do not think it is still summer
> Because sun stays and birds continue to sing.
> It is summer-gone that I see, it is summer gone
> The sweet flowers in drying and dying down,
> The grasses forgetting their blaze and consenting to
>   brown.

A mechanism for dispelling loneliness or an expression of a driving ambition for leadership, possibly arising from an unsatisfactory marriage—these are themes that Mary Carter Smith (1970) satirically presents in "Clubwoman."

> Chairman of many committees
> At club meetings she's a must—
> But her spouse scrambles eggs for his supper
> And her furniture's covered with dust.

For some black women, middle age, as portrayed by black writers, reflects the psychology of oppression. The need for and the protectiveness of silence is penned by Barbara Chase-Riboud (1979) in her novel, *Sally Hemming*. The author sets the stage in which Sally, at age 56, views the census taker at a distance and reflects on the past: "Her silence was what had kept her alive and sane in this world where everything had been taken from her except these last two sons. And even they knew little about her life. Slaves revealed as little as possible about their origin and background to their children. It was an old trick. Not to speak was not to put into words the hopelessness of having no future and no past" (p. 14).

The continuing pattern of "holding back" is described in a lighter vein by Mari Evans (1971) in "When in Rome." The experiences described in the poem are commonplace among the scores of domestic workers, who, in their middle years, continue in the only kind of work they know.

> Mattie dear
>   the box is full
> take
>   whatever you like
> to eat . . .
>   (an egg
>   or soup
>   . . . there ain't no meat).
> there's endive there
>   and cottage cheese. . .
>   (whew if I had some
>   black-eyed peas . . .)
> there's sardines
>   on the shelves
>   and such
>   but
>   don't get my anchovies . . .
>   they cost
>   too much!
>   (me get the
>   anchovies indeed!
>   what she tink she got—
>   a bird to feed?)
> there's plenty in there
> to fill you up . . .
>   (yes'm. just the
>   sight's
>   enough!)
> (. . . Hope I lives till I get home
>   I'm tired of eatin'
>   what they eats
>   in Rome . . .)

And a return to a somber tone in Gloria Gayles's (1979) "Sometimes as Women Only." In the last stanza, she writes:

> sometimes
> as women only
> do we weep
> we are taught to whisper
> when we wish to scream
> assent
> when we wish to defy
> dance pretty
>   (on tiptoe)
> when we would raise circles of dust
> before the charge

Intrafamilial Relationships

Information obtained from the returns of the questionnaire previously referred to, although only suggestive, parallels that reported by other investigators (Ladner, 1972; Staples, 1973, 1978) and observed in professional and personal life experiences of the author.

In response to a question about support networks, respondents listed family members as central figures. Significantly, this response characterized the unmarried as well as the married women. For example, a 35-year-old divorcee lives alone but is very much a part of her brother's family of five; a 50-year-old never-married educator holds a similar position in her married sister's family. It has been the experience of the author that many single adults who live alone are integral members of a family system, as are single adults who share a household with a family unit. The importance of the extended family was pinpointed in the frequent identification of the grandparents as the primary caregivers during the respondents' childhood years.

It is of some significance that the church was often identified as an important unit in the current support system. Fellow church members were viewed as the extended family by some. This view of the church was held both by women who had continued an affiliation with the denomination with which they were identified as children and by the converts to another denomination.

Stack (1974) has written of the successful development and utilization of kin networks among lower-class black women in urban communities. There is no question that such systems have reinforced strengths and permitted survival for many in the networks. Indeed, in the experience of this author, this pattern is not confined to the working poor but is commonly utilized throughout each socioeconomic class. The value of networking has been addressed and utilized by a number of black women's civic and social groups.

For most people, middle age brings about changes in intrafamilial relationships. It is no different for black women. Some relationships have improved; others have been terminated. One 50-year-old mother of three daughters reported that she now has a positive mother–daughter/friend relationship with each of her young adult children. The earlier relationships were studded with conflict, especially during the stormy adolescence of the middle child. Of significance, too, was the change in the nature of her relationship with her husband. After years of episodic philandering, he was now, at 58, continuously emotionally committed to his family.

For some women, middle age is equated with loss and with disruption of some family relationships. When marriages break up and the ex-husband becomes involved with a much younger woman, middle age can be a painful period. The pain is often compounded by financial difficulties, reinforced by the ex-husband's inability or unwillingness to assume responsibilities for child support. This kind of situation often lays the groundwork for difficulties in the divorcee's relationship with her children, whatever their age. On the other hand, for those women who feel secure about themselves as a person, the middle years are viewed as a new beginning; the divorce is a relief and paves the way for improvement of some intrafamilial relations.

Middle age has been a time of remarriage for some women, and for a first marriage for a smaller number. Such marriages mean the beginning of many new relationships with the spouse's family. New relationships and the modification of the old also develop as children marry and grandchildren are born. A number of factors will determine the nature of the changes. Some mothers (and fathers) like their children-in-law and easily establish rapport. In contrast, if marriage of one's child is viewed as a loss, the relationship is likely to be in some jeopardy.

Because of the greater vulnerability of black men to poor health, a black women is likely to face middle age as a widow or to face the added responsibilities of a chronically ill spouse. Again, the nature of the changes, if any, in the intrafamilial relationships is dependent upon a number of variables. The stability/instability of the family's economic status is not the least important.

For many black women, middle age is another period of mothering—now, the mothering of her grandchildren or children of her siblings or members of the extended family. Women in the lower socioeconomic bracket are more likely to bear the responsibility for the care of the children of their adolescent daughters. Women at every socioeconomic level are likely to assume at least partial responsibility for a grandchild as the young mother struggles alone or with her husband to "make it." Again, the nature of the relationships varies and sometimes parallels the character of the earlier mother–child ties.

The Absence and Presence of the Men in Our Lives

Staples (1978) notes that the "black underclass is prevented by internal colonialism from achieving success in marriage" (p. 82) and that black women have fewer opportunities than their white counterparts for remarriage. A sizable percentage of middle-aged black women, who are also a part of the underclass, are without husbands (although there may be men in their lives). This pattern may also be characteristic of middle-class women in their middle years. The diminishing number of available black men who are viewed as potential mates by the divorced, widowed, or never-married black woman has been attributed to a number of factors. Staples (1978) writes: "With 25 percent of Black males unemployed, it is not surprising to find a disproportionate number of them in prisons and the military or narcotized by drugs. But the most significant social trend is the spiraling mortality rate of Black males" (p. 86). According to 1980 Bureau of Census data, 125,000 deaths of black men took place in 1978, as compared to 124,000 in each of the previous 3 years, and as compared to 108,000 in 1960.

For some married women in their middle years the marriage is a union in name only. Staples suggests that "high status Black males often view women as property and impose rigid rules of sexual fidelity for their wives, while participating themselves in a number of extramarital affairs" (p. 84). The middle-class woman may be more likely to tolerate this behavior and seek to maintain the marriage because a divorce might well result in the modification of her middle-class status. She might elect to become involved in an affair herself, or to be celibate.

For other married women, their middle years have brought a closer union with their husbands of some 20–30 years. Some, after years of discord, and even after periods of separation, become friends again and enjoy doing things together.

Within each socioeconomic grouping there are men who are abusive and others who are considerate and supportive. The woman in the life of the abusive man is likely to be the victim of his anger and frustration, generated by his own victimization in the broader society. Some of the men in the lives of middle-aged women are younger; some are in the same age range; others are much older. There appears to be a lessening of criticism directed toward the woman who elects to form a relationship with a younger man, and clearly this kind of relationship occurs within all socioeconomic groups. Men from other racial groups play an integral role in the lives of some black women. No longer are "acceptable" interracial unions confined to individuals in the entertainment fields (if they ever were), as illustrated by Lewis (1978).

Economic Status

In our excellent historical review of the employment of black women from 1910 to the early 1970s, Jackson (1973) points out that "Black women have traditionally occupied positions of lower status than is true of Black men, assertions to the contrary notwithstanding" (page 255). Staples (1978) cites significant statistics from the United States Women's Bureau: "1,500,000 people were employed in private household work in 1970. Almost two-thirds of them were Black. The medial income for full-time, year-round household workers was approximately $1,800 per year. . . . Two out of three are at least partly self-supporting and one out of eight is head of a family." Ladner (1975), too, provides supportive evidence for Jackson's view in her citation of 1973 data for the year-round civilian labor force. The annual income of the black female worker was at the bottom of the heap when compared to her white counterparts, and to black as well as white men.

Black women have shared the benefits of the affirmative action and equal opportunity programs with black men, white women, and members of other minorities. It is often suggested that the gains made by black women have been greater than those experienced by black men. An argument sometimes used to support this notion is that hiring agents seize the opportunity to meet two goals of affirmative action policy by hiring a black woman, who is a "double minority." However, the tenacity of discriminatory patterns has prevented such a practice in many settings. Jackson (1973) cites an example:

> I, myself, have experienced several Southern situations where my educational attainment surpassed that of White female employees. Usually the racial undertones were onerous. In one specific local community mental health center, several educated Black females were categorically rejected for positions as nurses and social workers by the director (a psychiatrist of foreign birth), despite their over-qualifications. . . . The inexperienced and racially-prejudiced director catered to [the] White female prejudices . . . [that] it was too difficult for them to view any Black female in any working relationship exclusive of domestic service. The director assumed that the Blacks ought to understand that and wait until the attitudes of the Whites had changed. (p. 234)

Even with ongoing discriminatory practices, black women have become more visible in various professions, businesses, and other male-dominated careers and vocations. Ladner (1975) cautions that this new visibility is open to misinterpretation. The small number of black women who hold positions of status, or who have made considerable advancement in the world of work, "have had little effect on the status of the average black woman" (page 76). According to a report of the U.S. Department of Commerce, Bureau of Census (*The Social and Economic Status of the Black Population in the U.S.: An Historical View, 1970–78*), "The occupational changes for Black women from 1949 to 1970 . . . were mainly in the white collar and service groups."

The overwhelming majority of black women arrive at and live through the middle years burdened by economic problems. For them, the message penned by Langston Hughes (1970) in his poem "Mother to Son" conveys their feelings. For them, life "ain't been no crystal stair," nor do they expect it to be in their middle years, but they will keep on "climbin'."

The Women's Movement: Involvement versus Nonparticipation

The history of Afro-Americans is studded with references to the efforts of women in activities directed toward liberation of black people—both women and men—as well as of all women. Walker (1976) notes the activities of Sojourner Truth at women's rights meetings, and the active campaigning of others, directed toward full emancipation for black women. The encounters that black women have had with sexism have not been infrequent and are as much a part of contemporary times as they were during the height of the abolitionist movement. However, black women in general have not been active in the contemporary women's movement, nor have they shown much enthusiasm for the movement.

A question regarding support of the women's movement was included in the survey questionnaire. Responses were mixed. One respondent wrote, "The racist history of the Women's Movement and the plight of Blacks negates my being a member." Some noted only partial support; others responded affirmatively and with no words of exception. Some black women have expressed the feeling that efforts directed toward the women's movement would dilute those that are still needed in the arena of the civil rights struggle. Others, stunned at the accusations that the advancement of black women has stunted that of black men, have hotly refuted these charges, and have encouraged support of the women's movement and the ratification of the Equal Rights Amendment as furthering the liberation of men as well as women. Jackson's (1973) call has a tone of urgency:

> Black women must increase their participation in the racial and feminist liberation movements, and they can find no better role models than Sojourner Truth and March Church Terrell. Their direct participation in the women's liberation movement is very critical, so that there will be no question of Black women being left out in the kitchen or the nursery. The "heat" should be placed upon those White Women who persist in believing that Black women do not wish to be liberated! (p. 255)

The labeling of the women's movement as white, middle-class (and possibly middle-aged, in view of the limited attention given to the needs of elderly women) has limited the interest that black women have shown. Beal (1970) is as discouraging of black women's involvement as Jackson has been encouraging. It has also been suggested (Hare and Hare, 1972) that black women's inactivity in the movement is not necessarily related to lack of interest and/or objections to the stated goals, but is due to their having been denied policy-making roles—"white women always dominate in coalitions and are always in charge" (p. 180). They also note that "it appears to some that white and black women are in a race to change places. The white woman is trying to escape the drudgery of the home for rewarding employment outside, while the black woman still longs to escape the labor force and to get into the home."

Walker (1976) cites words of wisdom in an address given by Fannie Jackson Coppin, a black teacher, social worker, and lecturer. The date of the address is significant; it was given at the Woman's Congress of 1894:

> Not till race, color, sex, and condition are seen as the accidents and not the substance of life; not till the universal title of humanity to life, liberty and the pursuit of happiness is conceded to be inalienable to all; not till then is woman's lesson taught and woman's cause won—not the white woman's nor the black woman's nor the red woman's but the cause of every man and every woman who has writhed silently under a mighty wrong. (p. 361)

COPING PATTERNS AND BREAKDOWNS

Not unlike women of other groups, scores of black women face and live through middle age free of major conflicts. They just "keep on keeping on" For some, development continues; witness the growing number who are returning to school as reentry students, to begin or complete college or postgraduate education. The experiences of a friend of the author provide a vivid illustration.

> E.J., who had returned to college as a part-time student when her youngest was in upper elementary school, graduated at age 45. She states that reentry was not the easiest experience in her life. The encouragement and support she received from her family (husband and two children still at home) helped in the binding of her anxiety. She went on to graduate school and now holds a responsible administrative position.
>
> At first glance, one would assume that E.J. is an exceptional person. So she is, but she is not alone. A survey of black women students—all reentry students—at a state university in a midwestern city, reveals many similar situations. (Jones, in press)

Those of us who have experienced conflicts of significance have, in many instances, developed successful behavioral patterns to stem the tides of discomfort and unrest. For many (maybe more at the lower socioeconomic levels), a flight into religion and strict morality have been the routes taken. Novelist Toni Morrison's (1970) description of Pauline Breedlove (in *The Bluest Eye*), a mother of two, who had been verbally and physically abused by her husband, is a graphic example: "All the meaningfulness of her life was in her work. For her virtues were intact. She was an active church woman, did not drink, smoke or carouse, defended herself mightily against Cholly (her husband) . . ." For a multitude of black people, church services have been "a place to discharge frustration and hostility so that one could face injustice and hardship the rest of the week" (Comer, 1972, p. 16). Of equal importance is the feeling of belonging that is fostered in the black-oriented religious services.

Some of us have utilized defenses that have been maladaptive. Many of us have continued a lifelong tendency to be passive-aggressive; others have been given to hypochondriasis or somatization. A sizable number of us have continued to direct considerable energies to efforts to control others in our immediate environments. It is as if these maneuvers help to bind our anxiety generated by our powerlessness. A 53-year-old widowed mother of eight tended to accentuate her efforts to inject her comments and guidance in every contact (most of which she initiated) with her adult children. She recalled that the broadening of this pattern coincided with her perception of her entry into middle age, a period that she equated with losses.

Depression of incapacitating intensity has either become more commonplace in black women or is more frequently diagnosed. In the author's experience as a clinician, there has been more than a hint that many of these women, some of whom are driven to overeat and/or to drink too much, seek initial help from a primary care physician and are treated symptomatically. Thus, the core problem is not addressed.

It has been reported that involutional melancholia is higher in women from low-income groups and those in low-prestige occupations (Ford, 1975). Since the majority of black women are in such groupings, it might be assumed that this disorder is commonly experienced by them. However, it is also noted by Ford that "minority ethnic groups are relatively less evident in the psychiatric population during the involutional years" (p. 1027). It is possible that black women are not properly diagnosed and/or not treated, or are treated by physicians other than psychiatrists.

As previously pointed out, black women are likely to be more susceptible to specific physical disorders because of poor and limited health care services. Findings relevant to this point were described at a Mini-consultation on the Mental and Physical Health Problems of Black Women (1975). For example:

> The effects of hypertension are particularly significant for Black women: while it occurs less frequently among Black women than among Black men, it attacks Black women with greater severity. Heart failure is very common. . . . Physicians' figures indicate that hypertension is probably the primary cause of death for Black women between the ages of 40 and 45. (p. 1)
>
> Invasive cancer . . . has two times greater incidence than that occurring in the white population. . . . (p. 11)
>
> Poverty works to deny adequate medical attention for the Black victim of breast cancer. (p. 11)

Summary

In the preceding pages, emphasis has been placed on the diversity among us, as well as on the differences and commonalities when we are compared to white women. For the most part, what we bring to middle age depends upon how life has dealt with us before and how we have dealt with life.

Most of us are a part of a family unit, even if we live alone and the family members are our adoptive kin. Our relationships with the men in our lives are varied. We may be lonely at times, or a great deal of the time, but some of us are vibrant most of the time.

We are dirt-poor, and we are affluent. We work at blue-collar and white-collar jobs; we are represented in most of the professions. We are on welfare, and we are independently well off. We are Democrats, Independents, and Republicans (in alphabetical order); some of us have never voted. A few of us have been publicly rewarded for our achievements and our contributions to the betterment of black people and the society at large; some of us are unknown and unsung heroines. Some of us are sick, so very tired, and defeated at middle age. The more fortunate among us have successfully overcome obstacles or had few to circumvent, and are content in our middle years.

References

Beal, F. M. Double jeopardy: To be black and female. In R. Morgan (Ed.), *Sisterhood is powerful*. New York: Random House, 1970.

Brooks, G. A sunset in the city. In *Selected poems*. New York: Harper & Row, 1963.

Cannon, M. S., and Locke, B. Z. Being black is detrimental to one's health: Myth or reality? *Phylon*, 1977, 38(4): 408–442.

Chase-Ribaud, B. *Sally Hemmings*. New York: Viking Press, 1979.

Comer, J. P. *Beyond black and white*. New York: Quadrangle Books, 1972.

Evans, M. When in Rome. In J. David and M. Watkins (Eds.), *To be a black woman: Portrait in fact and fiction*. New York: William Morrow, 1971.

Ford, H. Involutional melancholia. In A. M. Feldman, H. I. Kaplan, and B. J. Sadock (Eds.), *Comprehensive textbook of psychiatry/II*. Baltimore: Williams and Wilkins, 1975.

Furstenberg, F. F. *Unplanned parenthood: The social consequences of teenage child bearing*. New York: Free Press, 1976.

Gayles, G. Parade. In R. P. Bell, B. Guy-Sheftall, and B. J. Parker (Eds.), *Study black bridges: Visions of black women in literature*. Garden City, N.Y.: Anchor Books, 1979.

Grier, W. H., and Cobbs, P. M. *Black rage*. New York: Basic Books, 1968.

Guy-Sheftall, B. The women of Bronzeville. In R. P. Bell, B. Guy-Sheftall, and B. J. Parker (Eds.), Sturdy black bridges: Visions of black women in literature. Garden City, N.Y.: Anchor Books, 1979.

Hare, N., and Hare, J. Black women 1970. In J. M. Bardwick (Ed.), *Readings on the psychology of women*. New York: Harper & Row, 1972.

Hughes, L. Mother to son. In A. Bontemps and L. Hughes (Eds.), *The poetry of the Negro: 1746–1970*. Garden City, N.Y.: Doubleday, 1970.

Jackson, J. J. Black women in a racist society. In B. S. Brown, B. M. Kramer, and C. V. Willie, *Racism and mental health*. Pittsburgh: University of Pittsburgh Press, 1973.

Jones, J. S. The mature woman's re-entry into college. In press.

Kellam, S. G., Esminger, M. E., and Turner, R. J. Family structure and the mental health of children. In S. Chess and A. Thomas (Eds.), *Annual progress in child development*. 1978.

Ladner, J. A. *Tomorrow's tomorrow: The Black woman*. Garden City, N.Y.: Anchor Books, 1972.

Ladner, J. A. The women. *Ebony*, 1975, 10, 76–81.

Lawrence, M. M. *Young inner city families: Development of ego strength under stress*. New York: Behavioral Publications, 1975.

Lewis, S. D. Black women/white men: The "other" mixed marriage. *Ebony*, 1978, 3, 37–42.

Miniconsultation on the mental and physical health problems of black women. In *Mental and physical health problems of black women*. Washington, D.C.: Black Women's Community Development Foundation, 1975.

Morrison, T. *The bluest eye*. New York: Pocket Books, 1970.

Smith, M. C. Clubwoman. In A. Bontemps and L. Hughes (Eds.), *The poetry of the Negro: 1746–1970*. Garden City, N.Y.: Doubleday, 1970.

Stack, C. B. *All our kin: Strategies for survival in a black community*. New York: Harper & Row, 1974.

Staples, R. E. *The Black woman in America*. Chicago: Nelson Hall, 1973.

Staples, R. E. Black family life and development. In L. E. Gary (Ed.), *Mental health: A challenge to the black community*. Philadelphia: Dorrance, 1978.

U.S. Bureau of the Census. *Statistical abstract of the U.S.: 1980*. Washington, D.C.: U.S. Government Printing Office, 1980.

Walker, E. The Black woman. In M. M. Smythe, *The Black American reference book*. Englewood Cliffs, N.J.: Prentice-Hall, 1976.

Chapter 11

Problems of American Middle-Class Women in Their Middle Years
A Comparative Approach

BEATRICE BLYTH WHITING

How shall we define the middle years cross-culturally? Halfway between birth and death? Then life expectancy becomes a key variable. In most of the world, few women live to what we consider old age—identified here as retirement age. Their stages of life are defined by women's reproductive capacities. Thus, a female is a child until puberty, seldom nubile for long as early marriage is frequent, childbearing until menopause. Women who live past menopause may enjoy a few productive years before infirmities make it impossible for them to contribute to the daily routines of living.

In most of the Third World and later-developing countries, the major stages of a woman's life are characterized as (1) prereproductive, (2) reproductive, (3) postreproductive but productive—contributing to the survival of herself and others, and (4) postproductive—no longer able to make a contribution, dependent on others for survival. In these societies, the transition between the reproductive and the postreproductive stages usually occurs at menopause. If a woman does not have the ability to control conception and birth, her reproductive years continue until she is no longer fertile. Abstinence, abortion, and infanticide are the alternatives when there is no other means of birth control. In this

---

BEATRICE BLYTH WHITING • Laboratory of Human Development, Harvard University, Cambridge, Massachusetts 02138. Material in this chapter was originally prepared for the seminar series "Women in Their Middle Years" funded by The Social Science Research Council, 1978–1979.

perspective, the middle years as we know them are a new phenomenon, lengthened by a woman's ability to voluntarily end her reproductive career. For most American women the reproductive years are now terminated before menopause, and consequently, our women have a longer period to be productive before the aging process leads to dependency.

Since the middle years are not identical chronologically, it is difficult to compare women's lives across cultures, especially the lives of women of the Third World with those of American women, defined in this volume as "in their middle years." On an average, the latter are probably in actual physiological age at least 10 to 15 years younger. Even if it were possible, however, to identify comparable physiological stages, the comparisons would be meaningless if one did not consider this period in relation to the entire life cycle, and to preceding life experiences.

In attempting to embark on a study of women's lives across cultures, it is necessary to identify universal dimensions for comparison. We need a theoretical framework that isolates universal aspects of life experience. I will present as a framework a list of the needs or wants assumed to be shared by the members of all populations across all ages. Accepting the fact that these universal needs must be satisfied by every culture to ensure the mental and physical health of its members over the life-span, we can then contrast the ways in which different societies attempt to meet them. The list of needs is familiar to students of human development, but in our child-centered society we have concentrated on concern for the fate of infancy and the childhood years.

I will not consider here the physical needs and their fate. These pose problems being faced by the environmentalists and the epidemiologists studying infectious and lethal diseases (DeLorey, Chapter 12, and Parlee, Chapter 13, in this volume). The consideration here is of psychological needs necessary for mental health. The basic assumption is that men and women, all human beings, have five fundamental needs or wants that we will label psychological. Included are (1) the desire to reproduce oneself, to have offspring that carry on one's family line; (2) the need for physical contact that from infancy onward reduces anxiety and fear and provides comfort; (3) the need for social, cognitive, and, with puberty, sexual stimulation; (4) the need for support from other human beings who are responsive to one's overtures; and (5) the need to predict events in the physical and social world (Whiting, 1980). These are not needs in the sense of being essential for physical existence but rather wants and desires that we assume are necessary for psychological well-being.

A brief review of the fate of these psychological needs during the reproductive and postreproductive years in some Third World societies will help to place the problems of American middle-class women in perspective. The aim is to define the needs operationally, to assess the success of American middle-class culture in meeting these needs, and to evaluate some of the attempts that are being made to revise life-styles to cope with existing deprivations in the postreproductive years.

Sociobiologists have focused their attention on the first need; they have been concerned with the necessity of all species to reproduce themselves to ensure survival. As a proximate mechanism they assume that each individual member of a species wishes to have offspring, and that he or she selects either a strategy in which each strives to optimize reproductive success by having as many children as possible (r strategy) or a strategy that calls for concentrating on ensuring the well-being of a few children (k strategy) (Trivers, 1972). American middle-class families have adopted the latter strategy, some women opting out of having any children and attempting to satisfy the assumed need by investing in kin, the offspring of close relatives.

Our society has recognized the second need, the desire for physical contact. Research on primates, infants, and children has documented the psychological problems that ensue when infants are deprived of this contact. The young of a species need a secure warm body to cling to when exploration of the world is too frightening. Such body contact is comforting and quieting and often encourages needed rest. During infancy and early childhood the maternal figure responds with reciprocal feelings of well-being as she holds her infant.

In general, however, the fact that the need continues throughout the life-course is overlooked, one more indication of the child-centeredness of our society.

Our society is just beginning to recognize this continuing need of contact, as evidenced by all the new types of therapy that encourage touching, the new cult of communal bathing and the new, more crowded sitting behavior in social gatherings, and the new types of furniture that encourage close body contact.

From a comparative point of view, our society has been on the deprivation side of this need. Our babies sleep by themselves rather than with their mothers; clothes separate them from skin contact. Our children sleep alone rather than with other children or with adults. We stand apart when talking to each other (Hall, 1959). American men are particularly deprived in that physical contact with other men has been considered taboo except in the athletic arena. We are startled when we enter hospitals in Kenya and find old people sleeping together or babies in traction sharing a crib. We are confused when Kenyan village friends send someone in to sleep with a field researcher to comfort her when she shakes with malaria-induced chills.

A cross-cultural study of sleeping arrangements suggests that in most of the Third World countries adults do not sleep alone. As in Tarong, Luzon, and Juxtluhuaca, Mexico (Whiting, 1963), even the elderly have sleeping companions, children sent to share the bed of their grandparents.

Middle-class women in our culture seldom sleep together, nor do adult men; to many, such behavior would be an indication of sexual aberration, the individuals labeled as homosexual, indicating all too clearly that sleeping arrangements in our middle-class society are associated primarily with sexual behavior. "Sleeping with" is a euphemism for sexual behavior in our culture. Comparatively speaking, we are extreme in our neglect of the need for physical contact.

We are on the opposite extreme when it comes to our belief in the need for stimulation. However, the emphasis has been on the needs of infants and children and until recently has stressed cognitive stimulation. Child psychologists recommend all types of equipment, toys, games, and books to aid in the intellectual development of children. Mothers are encouraged to learn how to expand their children's concepts. At present, there is a shift to an interest in social stimulation as well, perhaps a rationalization for the new preschools for infants and toddlers. This type of stimulation is not recent in most of the world where there are large, extended, or polygynous families or close-knit communities; social stimulation is part of the life experience of young children brought up in daily association with boys and girls of all ages and with a variety of adults.

We cannot understand the fate of these needs in the postreproductive years without considering what has taken place during the previous years. In our society, research has focused on the needs of the young. How does our society meet the needs of women in the reproductive years that precede the "middle years?" Much has been written about the deadening quality of a housebound woman in an isolated nuclear family. Here we recognize a problem. The daily routine is remarkably similar from day to day. There may be little novelty, little stimulation from other adults, male or female. The ever-repeating daily routine may lead to a physical and emotional exhaustion that cannot be overcome even in the evening when the one adult with whom there is daily contact returns home. Here, too, the interaction may be habitual, ever the same.

How is the need met in other societies? In some cultures, such as that of the Indian women of Khalpur described by Minturn and Hitchcock (1966), religious rituals bring welcome variation to an otherwise uneventful life, restricted by rules of purdah, requiring married women during their childbearing years to remain inside the walls of the family compound. Weddings, birth ceremonies, the celebration of the gods and godlings are a source of stimulation, requiring planning and the coming together of women from different courtyards. They are a source of renewal and energy. Melissa Lewellyn-Davies has described a similar break in the normal routine of Masai women in Kenya as they plan and organize the ceremonies that take place at the time of important transitions in women's lives (1978). The Mixtecan women of Juxtluhuaca, Mexico, join together to provide the food for the fiestas for their patron saints, working hard but obviously enjoying the chance to interact with other women (Romney and Romney, 1966).

What is required is some sort of community or religious organization, too often lacking in modern middle-class American life. Sociability, interacting with a variety of individuals, is a source of stimulation that is more easily provided in extended families with three or four generations sharing living space, or in a well-run polygynous homestead where there is friendly interchange between co-wives, or between sisters-in-law in patrilineal groups where brothers bring their wives to live on their father's homestead. Face-to-face communities that share work and rituals provide a variety of social experiences for women in both the reproductive and postreproductive years.

Robert White (1959) has written most persuasively about the third universal need, the need for effectance. In its most primitive form it has been studied in the behavior of the developing infant as it explores away from home base, manipulating the physical world, seeking responses from other human beings. The sense that one can effectively interact with the physical and social world leads to a feeling of competence, a sense of personal worth.

Again, this need has been recognized in children and adolescents but forgotten in women. The young mother is creative in a biological sense, but in our society her feeling of competence may be confined to recognition of success in child-rearing. In this arena, confidence is easily undermined by the beliefs propounded by many psychologists, social workers, and the writers of manuals on child-rearing. They assume that the mother is all-important to her child's development, solely responsible for the molding of its development, capable of making irremediable mistakes during the first 5 years of her child's life; such a belief is an unrealistic burden for the reproductive woman. If confidence depends on success in such an impossible assignment, ill-conceived since there are so many other determinants of the child's development, the mother's sense of competence and personal worth are in peril, built on a vulnerable foundation.

A well-run household can give satisfaction, but the challenge is not great with all the modern technology and the plethora of processed and packaged foods. Perhaps the ease with which modern households can be run leads to a desire to complicate the routine, to include a myriad of outside activities for all the family members. Then the complicated scheduling requires executive ability. The whole frantic plan may be invented to break out of the house and use unchallenged organizational skills.

In many societies, women have arenas outside the home in addition to child-care and maintenance activities. In agricultural societies such as those of sub-Saharan Africa, a woman may spend four or five hours working in her garden or selling produce in the market, returning to her home with a sense of having contributed productively to her family's well-being, more receptive to her children than the housebound mother (Whiting, 1980). Although the economic rewards to be gained are undoubtedly a prime motive for working mothers, the need for another sphere in which to develop a sense of competence and productivity is obviously an important incentive.

The fourth need, the need for support, has become a recognized one for adults as well as children in the last decade. The nature of support groups and social networks is a popular subject in research. Social scientists are returning to interest in an old subject dressed in new labels. All humans need the support of other individuals and groups, but it would seem that for a period we were focusing our concern on more individualistic aspects of life.

The young middle-class mother who lives in an isolated nuclear family lacks the type of support enjoyed by a woman in a well-run extended or polygynous society or in one that has close-knit microcommunities. I do not believe in being romantic about the joys of the extended family; it has many drawbacks—one trades autonomy for support. However, our isolated nuclear family is at one end of a continuum of types of social structures furnishing support systems for childbearing women. I know of no other society where, up until very recently when infant daycare and toddler preschools have been introduced, there has been so little help for women caring for young children. The isolated middle-class woman suffers from lack of instrumental and emotional support as well as from loneliness for adult company.

Belonging to a support group, having a network of friends, requires social skills, patterns of sociability. These skills involve greeting behavior, knowledge of how to initiate and sustain friendly interaction, how to join with others in group activities, how to share—behaviors now labeled social competence by child psychologists. To master these skills one must be attuned to the needs and reactions of others, able to predict their responses to your behavior, able to attend and respond to their communications, willing to share intimacies, hopes, fears, and disappointments. In our culture these traits have been labeled feminine, dependent, intuitive, sensitive, and are identified as occurring proportionately more frequently in women than in men. The label has carried with it denigration. Why men are forbidden by our culture to have these characteristics is a research question in itself, perhaps to be explained historically. There are indications now that these taboos are becoming less widespread, perhaps no longer required in the modern industrial age.

Both historically in this country and in the Third World, there are social systems that allow for intimacy among both adult males and females. The age-graded societies of sub-Saharan Africa constitute one of the best examples. Young men who have been initiated into manhood together maintain close friendship bonds throughout life.

That American women are more skilled than men in the ability to establish support groups is suggested by the reported reaction of men whose wives or friends have joined groups. They express an interest in belonging to a group but their habits of interaction are primarily instrumental, tinged with competition and friendly aggression and joking. They find the serious, intimate exchange of women embarassing. They do not easily adopt the habit of mutual emotional help and the exchange of confidences. Cultures certainly differ on the degree to which men form solidarities. American Protestant middle-class men of Yankee descent are extreme, as their ethos proscribes seeking help or engaging in intimate exchanges with other men (Mathai, 1979). Such behavior is considered dependent and feminine, suggesting the interaction of mothers and children.

How does one come by the skills that enable one to belong to a support group? Research on women's networks suggests that skills are learned early, from mothers who have well-developed social interaction patterns with both same-sex and cross-sex groups. Most frequently, these mothers have lived in the same community for many years. Abernethy (1973) has shown that young women coming from such homes and transferred to new environments are better skilled than women from less stable backgrounds in setting up new networks. This research implies that those who grow up in motile families, the experience of many of the American middle class, have less well-developed social skills. Perhaps we have taken too lightly the teaching of these skills.

The last need, the sense of being able to predict the behavior of the physical and social world, is less clearly universal, more subject to specific cultural belief systems. Societies vary in the degree to which individuals feel competent not only to predict but to control these worlds; they vary in the degree to which they accept their perceived ability or inability to shape fate and the degree to which they feel the necessity for predicting and controlling. For many societies the locus of control is in the supernatural, and a human being's fate is in the lap of the gods. An acceptance of fate leads to less torment on the part of mothers, less self-blame for the undesirable behavior of children, a greater ability to accept the frustrations of life. Middle-class America has been taught to believe in personal efficacy, and, as discussed above, our women during the confining years of childbearing, blinded by this belief, blame themselves unduly for some of their failures.

Accepting, then, that these five needs are present at all stages in the life-course and observing that societies differ in the cultural forms that meet these needs during the reproductive years, we are ready to address the particular problems of American middle-class women in their middle or postreproductive years. What is the fate of these needs during this period and how are women attempting to revise the cultural forms they find unsatisfactory?

Our strategy for meeting the first need, investing in a few children, has drawbacks. The loss of one child is probably more devastating when the average number of offspring per reproductive middle-class woman is less than three. The focus of attention on one or two children may lead to an overcommitment, risky for both parents and child. The overconcerned and overprotective mother of the reproductive years finds it difficult or impossible to relinquish control of her children. Too often an ambivalent relationship develops. On the one hand, she wishes to be free of feelings of responsibility; on the other, she remains emotionally bonded. Since she has invested so much in her two or three children, her unrealistic expectations and unattainable standards for success may lead to loss of self-esteem and depression, impairing her relations both with her children and with her grandchildren.

We are only beginning to explore the consequences of choosing not to have children, although in Western societies, unlike most of the Third World, the role of maiden aunts and bachelor uncles has been accepted as within the cultural norm. Investing in adopted children is found in many parts of the world. Anthropologists have begun to explore in depth the adoption patterns in the Polynesian and Micronesian Islands and in West Africa. Social scientists are monitoring the outcome of the American middle-class women who eschew childbearing. To date there are few hard data on which to base an opinion, but there are no data suggesting that these women are as a group suffering from severe deprivation. A new strategy may be in the making, reducing the expense of parental investment by sharing the cost in time, money, and emotion among kin.

For women in our culture, the need for physical comfort, for body contact, has been satisfied in the childbearing and early marital years by contact with infants and children and, depending on life-style, by sleeping arrangements of husbands and wives. We have suggested that these sleeping arrangements are associated with sexual behavior. What happens when there are no small children left at home and the desire for sexual relations with one's spouse is less intense, less frequent? Is there a new perception of the function of sharing the same bed or is there withdrawal from physical contact? What of the divorced, never-married, or widowed woman? (See Luria and Meade, Chapter 17, this volume.) How will she satisfy her need for physical contact in a manner acceptable to our present middle-class norms?

As we have noted, there is a growing awareness of the deprivation. There appears to be an increase in same-sex embracing, less anxiety about being labeled sexually aberrant. As noted above, there are new therapies that involve touching, new patterns of bathing, and in general, a loosening of all the taboos on physical contact and awareness. The desire for sexual stimulation that has been associated in our culture with the desire for physical contact is also being elucidated, and is recognized as present in postreproductive and postmenopausal women. There is a revolution in progress in our sexual mores. Most controversial, perhaps, is the growing acceptance of masturbatory and homosexual forms of satisfaction.

Most attention in the literature and research on women in their middle years has been focused on the need for new arenas for developing a sense of competence and personal worth, a need for new activities. There is also concern about the need for new support networks. A new set of questions is being addressed by women in their middle years who have the desire for new activities and new associates.

As we have seen, many women in the Third World have had work outside their homes in agriculture, animal husbandry, marketing, or home industries. Their sense of personal worth and competence has not rested exclusively on the success of any one child. In their postreproductive years these women can now spend more hours in the arenas outside the home. They are freer to move into the community, their reproductive capacities no longer threatening to those who guard the sanctity of family honor based on sexual fidelity.

The West African market women, especially the wholesalers who travel distances to buy and arrange for trucking in goods from outlying districts to the central markets, are often cited in the literature for their competence and economic success. In traditional Kikuyu cultures of East Africa, postreproductive women joined the council of senior women and took over the supervision of ceremonies and responsibility for the general welfare and behavior of younger women. Older women in many societies gain political power, recognized for their wisdom in decision-making. In many societies, postreproductive women have careers as midwives, herbalists, and shamans. Some become priestesses and religious functionaries. In sum, these women pursue careers already started during the childbearing years or enter into new careers open to women of their age grade.

A look at the present scene in the United States shows that there seem to be two predominant life-styles for postreproductive women. One life-style is followed by those who adjust to the middle years by accepting their roles as wives, mothers of teenagers and grown children, and grandmothers of their children. They concentrate their energies on the needs of their husbands and their children, no matter what their age, hopefully venturing forth on some new social activities, seeking volunteer jobs that are not too demanding, and hoping to be able to enjoy the role of a benevolent grandmother. They are frequently found among travelers and shoppers. Their feelings of competence and self-worth are dependent in large part on the careers of their husbands and children and the density of the support groups they have already developed. If they have skills in establishing and maintaining friendships, they are better equipped to follow non-career-oriented life-styles. Although this was once the most prevalent life-style among American middle-class women, census data suggest that it is becoming less frequent.

The second life-style is that of women who have already embarked on careers, have never given them up during their child-rearing years, or are attempting to return to former career interests or initiate new ones. These women are becoming more numerous. It is their needs that will be the concern of the rest of this chapter. Of particular concern is a group of women, a cohort that may not exist in the new generations, who have dedicated years almost exclusively to child care, and who, when the children reach a stage in schooling that makes them less demanding, have decided to seek employment. The psychological needs for stimulation, and for a sense of competence and personal worth, combine with economic motives to influence this decision. In their hunger they often overcommit themselves. Inexperienced in predicting the demands of a job and the length of time projects take, wanting to prove their competence, they tend to demand too much of themselves, to promise more than they can deliver. Their lives become frenetic. They suffer from too much rather than too little stimulation.

Prior to these new commitments, they have attended, often in compulsive detail, to the needs of their husbands and children. Now their energies are redirected, and if they have undertaken full-time employment or study, they return to the home tired and unable to continue the type of nurturance that has nourished and reinforced their husband's needs for food, comfort, and intimacy. As they increase contacts with the outside world, they set up new social networks and transfer their nurturance to colleagues, fellow students, and workers. Left behind are the husbands, who are less able to branch out and form new networks.

There is evidence that the men whose wives seek new careers and set up new networks feel deserted. Frequently they turn to other, younger women for the intimacy and support that they are only able to establish with a sexual partner. It is the hypothesis here that the turning to another woman is more an attempt to satisfy these needs, frequently labeled dependent, than a desire for sexual novelty and pleasure. This need of men for dependence is also suggested by the frequency of divorce following the birth of the second child (Hetherington, Cox, and Cox, 1975), behavior that can be interpreted as the husband's response to feelings of having been displaced in his wife's nurturant sphere by two babies, a feeling of deprivation and loss.

A woman in her middle years, faced with divorce, is often devastated, not understanding what has happened. Research is needed to clarify the components of the situation that has led to separation. It is particularly important to contrast the women with part-time and full-time commitments outside the home, to contrast women whose husbands receive emotional support from other individuals as well as from their wives, to contrast men with varying degrees of dependency needs and women with various degrees of ambition and habits of nurturance. We need to explore the decision-making process of women when they decide on the type of commitment to make outside the home.

Of the women who choose to stay home, their satisfaction with life should be explored, and their embeddedness in social networks in relation to their talents for sociability. We need to discover which women have the ability and opportunity to play the role of a grandmother, and we must identify the behavior that brings with it a new sense of competence.

Are these problems of the middle-aged woman universal, and if so, how have other cultures met men's and women's changing needs? The transition in women's lives in the postreproductive years appears to be universal, but some societies have cultural forms that ease the transition. Polygynous societies have an advantage. The middle-aged wife is joined by a younger co-wife who takes over part of the household responsibilities, the nurturant care, and the satisfaction of the sexual desires of the husband, releasing the senior wife to pursue a career as a tradeswoman or a more productive farmer. She is not divorced for her new interests but remains the executive woman in the homestead, sharing her husband with his junior wives. The senior wife often has a special relationship with her husband that develops in her postchildbearing years. Large extended households also offer possibilities for a middle-aged woman to start on a new career. We are all familiar with the

Indian women who come to the United States in their middle years to study, leaving behind husband and children, knowing that they will be cared for by relatives in the large family compounds.

Several possible solutions to our problems suggest themselves. Would it not be possible for women desiring new areas of competence to both work and continue in a more nurturant role if there were more half-time employment opportunities? Could not men be reeducated to meet some of their needs for dependency outside their sexual partners? Could not some of the taboos on bodily contact and intimacy that have restricted men's lives be aired and through scrutiny dispelled? Could not women be encouraged to examine their ambitions, to analyze their overcommitments, and to monitor the degree to which they are deserting the men who have learned to depend upon their nurturant initiations? To implement such changes in life-styles, it is necessary to convince both men and women that there are benefits to be gained. By contrasting the lives of men and women from different subcultures in our own society, investigating the satisfaction of their needs during the various stages of the life-course, we may be able to identify those patterns that seem to offer the best insurance against feelings of loneliness, abandonment, and exhaustion, and to encourage feelings of personal worth, comfort, and support.

Already it is coming to be recognized that women who choose to have few children must have arenas for developing a sense of competence beyond the confines of child care and household maintenance. There is growing recognition that men and women need to share intimacies with individuals besides their marital partners, that they need support networks beyond the family. There is growing recognition of the need to reestablish microcommunities that share activities. Less attention has been given to how one reaches these goals. We have not given enough thought to the management of the pace of life. If we develop cognitive skills to the exclusion of social skills, if we do not learn concern for others beyond ourselves and our children, we will be ill equipped to be members of such a community. (Whiting, 1978). We may also realize that career lines for men and women who choose to invest in children and in community living may require a shorter work day, leaving time and energy for nurturance and sociability. For many societies in the Third World this combination of work and community living was a way of life, too often terminated when entrance into the industrial world, with its compulsion for the 8-hour day, put an end to the hours needed for nonwork activities. We need time and energy to ensure that we can satisfy all our psychological needs.

Our focus is on the problems of women in their middle years, but their choice of life-style must be synchronized with that of men. One must be wary of the backlash against the women's movement that seems, in part at least, to be the reaction of men who fear desertion. Our research should monitor the success of the various life-styles of subgroups in our culture in meeting the universal psychological needs of both men and women.

REFERENCES

Abernethy, V. D. Social network and response to the maternal role. *International Journal of Sociology of the Family*, 1973, *3*: 386–392.

Hall, E. T. *The silent language*. New York: Doubleday/Anchor, 1959.

Hetherington, E. M., Cox, M., and Cox, R. *Beyond father absence: Conceptualization of effects of divorce*. Paper presented at the meeting of the Society for Research in Child Development, Denver, 1975.

Llewelyn-Davies, M. Two contexts of solidarity. In P. Caplan and J. M. Bujra (Eds.), *Women united, women divided*. London. Tavistock, 1978.

Mathai, P. A. *The myth of the self-sufficient Yankee. Support systems of white Angle-Saxon Protestants in New England*. Thesis presented to the Faculty of the Graduate School of Education of Harvard, 1979.

Minturn, L. and Hitchcock, J. *The Rajputs of Khalapur, India* (Six-Culture Series, Vol. 3). New York: Wiley, 1966.

Romney, A. K., and Romney, R. *The Mixtecans of Juxtluhuaca, Mexico* (Six-Culture Series, Vol. 4). New York: Wiley, 1966.

Trivers, R. L. Parental investment and sexual selection. In B. Campbell (Ed.), *Sexual selection and the descent of man 1871–1971*. Chicago: Aldine, 1972.

White, R. W. Motivation reconsidered: The concept of competence. *Psychological Review*. 1959, *66*, 297–333.

Whiting, B. The dependency hang-up and experiments in alternative life styles. In J. M. Yinger and S. J. Cutler (Eds.), *Major social issues: A multidisciplinary view*. 1978.

Whiting, B. Culture and social behavior: A model for the development of social behavior. *Ethos*, 1980, *8*(2).

PART III

Enhancing Well-Being

Chapter 12

Health Care and Midlife Women

CATHERINE DELOREY

INTRODUCTION

Health care for midlife women in the United States of the 20th century is a complex blend of myth and reality viewed against a backdrop of rapid social change. The myths that have evolved concern women's roles, specifically older women's roles, and also include menopause, an event that occurs most often at midlife. Until recently, little information has been available concerning the health or health care of midlife women. Most research on women's health at midlife is clinically oriented and assumes that menopause is the most important aspect of women's lives and health. Although this has changed somewhat in recent years, in part due to the impetus of women's groups such as the Menopause Collective in Cambridge, Massachusetts, and the National Women's Health Network, much needs to be changed before we have research that validates women's experiences as well as providing them with the information that they can use to make appropriate decisions for their own health.

Any discussion of health care for midlife women needs to take account of the structure and beliefs underlying the way this health care is provided—that is, how the health care system functions. Health providers as well as health planners, for the most part, are outsiders observing an alien culture, the culture of midlife women. As they attempt to understand and interpret women's health needs, these observations are colored by the biases and preconceptions of a biomedical model perspective. The biomedical model of health care, based on the biosciences, sees

---

CATHERINE DELOREY • Women's Health Research Institute, Boston, Massachusetts 02113.

most health problems as exemplifying a direct cause–effect relationship. Health issues are then diagnosed and treated as scientific abstractions although, because they involve social beings, they occur in a sociocultural context. The biomedical model tends to use restricted definitions of health status without regard for social definitions; it assumes that physicians, who are the primary purveyors of health, are experts who are neutral providers, dispensing their product unaffected by social, cultural, or political forces (Mishler, Amarasingham, Hauser, Liem, Osherson, and Waxler, 1981).

Because the existing system of care is based on this biomedical model, there is in reality no "health care system," but rather a "medical care system," which by definition perceives life in medical terms. This system, bounded by societally and culturally imposed ideas of women's roles, relies on myths and stereotypes to govern the way health care is provided for women.

These myths and stereotypes impose restricted roles on women at all points throughout the life-span; women are classified as products of their reproductive system and its hormones, and normal life developmental stages or transitions are defined as medical issues. Therefore, women must then enter the medical care system for essentially normal health events such as contraception, care during pregnancy and birthing, or information about midlife transitions.

As women age, medicine continues to view them as controlled by the endocrine system, and consequently, medical care for midlife women continues to be dominated by attention to hormonal factors. Many events that occur at the same time in life as hormonal changes are not caused by hormonal changes. Association is not causation. However, many health aspects of midlife are seen as resulting from the cyclical hormonal transitions of menopause. Thus, we have midlife women being given estrogen to control hot flashes or to prevent and/or ameliorate thinning of the bones (osteoporosis) when life-style changes such as improved nutrition or more exercise may be as effective. This is particularly relevant for the cohort of women who are 40 to 60 years old today, the older women of tomorrow. These midlife women of today are the women who were given diethylstilbestrol to maintain pregnancy, the high doses of estrogen in the first contraceptive pills, and high doses of estrogen at menopause, so they could be, as one physician promised, "feminine forever" (Wilson, 1961).

Within recent years there has been an increased interest in the status and health of midlife women. What has been the impetus for this interest? During the latter part of the 20th century, midlife women have become increasingly visible partly because of their greater numbers, as well as their changing social roles. When any subgroup within the population becomes more visible or noticed, for whatever reasons, the health status of that group takes on added interest to the larger population.

Some of the demographic and social shifts that have altered the visibility of midlife women include a decreased birth rate coupled with an overall decreased maternal mortality rate, an increased expected life-span at all age levels, and changes in the structure of the work force. From 1900 to 1975 the birth rate dropped from 32.2 live births (per thousand population) to 18.4 (Department of Commerce, 1975), while at the same time the maternal mortality rate decreased from 69.5 (per 100,000 live births) in 1920 to 15.2, a decrease of 98% (Bureau of the Census, 1975). The life-span for women has increased at all ages, a result of changes in maternal mortality, medical response to infectious disease, and early detection of noninfectious diseases. Because the maternal mortality rate for women over 40 has consistently been nine times greater than for women under 30 (Bureau of the Census, 1975), the decrease in maternal mortality has had a great impact on life-expectancy statistics for women 40 and older. These changes further increased female life expectancy so that in 1970 a (white) woman at 40 could expect to live for 39 more years, whereas her 40-year-old counterpart in 1900 could anticipate 29 more years.

These and other demographic changes have resulted in a population in which the median age increased from 22 years in 1900 to 30 years in 1970, and the proportion of midlife women increased from 13% of the population to 21%. By 1980 over 50% of midlife women were in the work force, a substantial increase from the 38% of 1950. Thus, the increased visibility and prominence of midlife women results not only from numerical changes but from role changes as well, making the health status of midlife women a significant issue for the whole society.

MAJOR HEALTH ISSUES FOR MIDLIFE WOMEN

Although mortality figures are at best a crude indication of the health status of a population, they do provide a basis for comparison and present one aspect of the total picture. Tables 1 and 2 indicate the major causes of death for midlife women. One can see that the major killers of midlife women are not gynecological conditions. Mortality from cancer of the breast, cervix, and uterus is at the rate of 50.1 (per 100,000) for white women and 63 (per 100,000) for nonwhite women, whereas heart disease and cerebrovascular disease account for the largest number of deaths for both white and nonwhite women (Table 1).

Looking at women divided according to white and nonwhite categorizations provides some very important information. It illustrates that heart disease, cerebrovascular diseases, and malignancies are major kill-

Table 1. Ten Leading Causes of Death for Midlife Women[a,b]

Cause of death	Rate[c]
White women	
Malignant neoplasms	264.9
Heart disease	159.7
Cerebrovascular diseases	37.6
Cirrhosis	22.6
Accidents	22.0
Diabetes	14.1
Suicide	11.3
Influenza, pneumonia	10.1
Bronchitis, emphysema, asthma	8.5
Benign neoplasm	2.9
Nonwhite women	
Heart disease	324.1
Malignant neoplasms	301.0
Cerebrovascular diseases	97.3
Diabetes	42.0
Cirrhosis	39.4
Accidents	31.9
Influenza, pneumonia	20.0
Nephritis, nephrosis	15.5
Homicide	9.1
Septicemia	6.9

[a]Based on data from National Center for Health Statistics (Dunn, 1981).
[b]Midlife defined as 45–55 years old for this table.
[c]Rates per 100,000.

ers of all women. The mortality rates for nonwhite women are greater in all categories, but the white/nonwhite designation does not tell us if a Native American woman has the same risks as a Hispanic woman; it does not tell us how socioeconomic factors influence the data. Frequently it is assumed that a racial breakdown for health data is a surrogate for socioeconomic influences, since many nonwhite persons in United States culture are relegated to lower socioeconomic status as a result of discriminatory practices. But making this assumption does not give much information concerning the risk factors for the middle-class black woman or the poor white woman, and it can serve to further the perpetuation of cultural stereotypes not based on fact.

Regarding the mortality studies in Table 1, what does it mean that the mortality rate from suicide for white women is 11.3/100,000, yet suicide is not listed in the 10 major killers of nonwhite women? The higher rates for nonwhite women of heart disease and malignant neo-

Table 2. Causes of Death from Malignant Neoplasms for Midlife Women[a,b]

	45–49	50–54	55–59	60–64
Breast				
White	41.0	60.3	76.3	92.3
Nonwhite	43.5	59.1	72.2	82.4
Cervix uteri				
White	6.7	7.3	8.6	10.4
Nonwhite	15.3	19.0	22.4	25.9
Corpus uteri				
White	2.4	4.4	8.3	14.6
Nonwhite	4.0	7.2	13.7	24.2

[a]Based on data from National Center for Health Statistics (Dunn, 1981).
[b]Rates per 100,000.

plasms (cancers) may reflect greater stresses because of environmental influences or, conversely, may reflect the poorer-quality health care often available to persons in lower socioeconomic groups. Kidney diseases, nephritis and nephrosis, are major killers of nonwhite women but are not among the 10 major killers of white women.

Nonwhite women may have less access to preventive health/medical care or may encounter more toxins in the workplace, occupational hazards with which poorer women are more likely to come into contact.

Other approaches used to determine the health status of a population include looking at the use of health services, including physician visits and hospitalizations, and at how much illness interferes with daily activities, the assumption being that one can infer the health status of the total group from this information. Although there are slight increases in use of health services associated with age for midlife women, the predominant differences, as throughout the life-span, are between men and women. Midlife women make 5.9 visits to physicians a year, 25% more than the 4.7 visits of midlife men (Givens, 1979), as well as having an incidence of acute conditions 24% greater than men of the same age. Midlife women's activities are restricted by illness 46% more than for midlife men, although this is 8% less than for women in general.

There has been speculation that this type of information may reflect sex biases on the part of physicians, but this view has not been substantiated by available data. In a rigorous analysis using National Ambulatory Medical Care Study (NAMCS) data, Verbrugge could find no examples where the differences in care could be attributed to physician bias (Verbrugge and Steiner, 1981). But it does not seem likely that only a biological or biomedical model is sufficient to explain these differences.

Other explanations for these differences take sociocultural aspects of women's roles into consideration, such as that it is more acceptable for women to report illness; that because of women's role responsibilities, they can assume a sick role more easily than men; that women may indeed have more illness because their roles are more stressful; or that because of interviewing techniques of large surveys, women have a greater probability than men of being interviewed directly but as a proxy for men, thus recalling greater illness for themselves and less for men (Nathanson, 1975; Verbrugge, 1976).

Finding the explanation for these sex differences in health experiences will provide significant information but will not directly approach the issue of whether care given to women is appropriate to their needs. Sex bias in health care may be impossible to measure because it is grounded in societal assumptions concerning women that are commonly held by providers, researchers, and often women themselves. Because of this it becomes difficult to evaluate the data that are available. How do we evaluate the fact that up to the present most research on heart disease, stress-related illness, or occupational health was done with male subjects and the results extrapolated to women? How do we evaluate the information that when men and women visit a physician or a clinic, women have fewer diagnostic tests and procedures done than men (Hadden, 1981)? Thus, although heart disease is a major killer of women, only 27% of women receive cardiograms compared to 41% of men. This may reflect sex bias or it may reflect physicians' perceptions of actual gender differences. It does not seem to reflect adequate assessment of the risk-factor profile. Assessment of health in midlife women becomes even more difficult because the effect of stereotypes about aging need to be added to the picture. Thus, the biases from age stereotypes as well as those of the medical model influence the way health care is planned and provided for midlife women. One result of this is that the literature presents a narrow view of midlife women's health by seeing menopause as the most important issue—a view that is often in conflict with what women themselves want or think.

In a random community survey of 120 midlife women and their physicians conducted by this author in 1981, no woman thought that menopause was a major health problem, but 21% of the physicians responded that menopause was the major health problem for midlife women. Moreover, 60% of the women replied that menopause was of no concern to them, while 83% of the physicians thought it was a major concern to them (DeLorey, 1981). In follow-up discussions with some of the physicians, they consistently asked for any available information on midlife women, saying that the only information about midlife women they received in their medical training had been in pathophysiology courses, where menopause was discussed. There is clearly a need for major changes in the existing structure of the medical education system.

Looking again at the leading causes of death in Table 1, we find that some are more relevant than others to a discussion of health for midlife women. Heart disease and cerebrovascular disease are relevant because they account for a larger number of deaths as women age, and also because many people are unaware of their importance to women. Cancer of the uterus, cervix, and breast are relevant because they are specifically women's issues that begin to show their significance at midlife, particularly breast cancer, the largest single cause of death for midlife women.

Two other health issues of major importance to midlife women are menopause and occupational health. Menopause is important because it is a physiological transition that usually occurs at midlife. Occupational health is important because 54% of midlife women are employed outside the home. Insufficient attention has been given to the health hazards of the workplace in general, and those that relate specifically to midlife have been ignored completely.

Menopause

Menopause becomes a major issue for discussion in any consideration of health and midlife women because it is experienced by most women at midlife and because it overwhelmingly dominates the medical literature. In addition, there is a growing awareness that traditional ideas concerning the experience of menopause are not accurate and that inferences are therefore made without adequate justification.

A major reason for inaccurate assessments of menopause is that much research concerning menopause and midlife is biased and fragmented. It is biased because most studies are conducted with clinical populations; it is fragmented because many studies are done assuming only a biological, psychological, or sociocultural model of explanation with little integration of the models or awareness of how each relates to the other when attempting to explain the totality of the experience for women.

Over the last 20 years menopause has gained increased recognition as an acceptable area of scientific research, with the most dramatic increase occurring in the last decade. Recognition has been stimulated by developments in hormone research as well as the increasing numbers of women experiencing menopause or postmenopausal stages of life. Although behavioral and clinical aspects of menopause are studied, these two components are not related to each other or to the health care provided to midlife women.

With a few exceptions, research on menopause lacks clarity of design and methodological rigor. Definitions of menopause vary, for example. Menopause usually refers to physiological aspects of change in the ovary, or cessation of the pituitary–ovarian feedback mechanism, which in turn results in the cessation of menstruation. Climacterium usually refers to a sociocultural period of time of change occurring in the middle years of life. In many studies, menopause and climacterium are used interchangeably (Dalton, 1976; Taich, 1978), with climacterium often defined as the time period in which menopause occurs (Neugarten, 1963; Goodman, 1976; Utian, 1976). Frequently menopause loosely refers to the time of the last menstruation (Neugarten, 1963; McKinlay and Jefferys, 1974; Utian, 1976; Eskin, 1980) and is subdivided into premenopause, menopause, and postmenopause. These categories are defined by the time elapsed since the most recent menstrual cycle (Thompson, 1973; McKinlay and Jefferys, 1974), as well as subjective response of women (Maoz, 1970). Even reports from conferences specifically focused on menopause may fail to provide consistent or objective definitions of menopause (Ryan and Gibson, 1973; Beard, 1976; Campbell, 1976; van Keep, 1976).

The vagueness of definition not only prevents a clear understanding of the event, it precludes a definition of the true "population at risk." A standard definition of menopause would permit a clearer understanding of the etiology of any problems, of the processes involved in the genesis of such problems, and of diagnosis and treatment issues.

The fact that menopause occurs at the time in a woman's life when other biological and social changes take place intensifies problems involved in conducting research. Not only must the effects of menopause be separated from those of chronological aging, but the biological aspects of menopause need to be separated from the psychosocial to understand the role of each. Because menopause is both a biological and a sociocultural event, this separation is even more difficult.

BIOLOGICAL ASPECTS OF MENOPAUSE. Although separating biological and social factors is difficult, some aspects of menopause are considered as strictly biological. The biological changes are those directly involved in alterations of the ovary and circulating estrogen supply. It is not clear whether symptoms reported around the time of menopause are biological events of menopause, biological events of other processes in the body (e.g., aging), or psychosocial events such as reactive depression to life events.

Estrogen. Because cessation of menstruation is a result of a diminished, but not eliminated, supply of cyclical ovarian estrogen, there is much controversy concerning estrogen's function in the menopausal/postmenopausal woman. A small number of researchers and practitioners consider menopause an estrogen deficiency disease and therefore suggest the use of estrogen as a therapeutic agent to alleviate symptoms associated with midlife. Discussion of the function of estrogen in the body and the use of estrogen replacement therapy must acknowledge that different substances are considered. The first are endogenous estrogens, natural steroids produced by the body. The others are exogenous estrogens, which are either synthesized in the laboratory or extracted from animals. There is no definitive evidence in the literature to indicate that exogenous estrogens have the same effect as those estrogens naturally produced by the body.

Treatment for the changes at midlife that get labeled as symptoms of menopause varies according to how menopause is defined, how symptoms are evaluated, and how effective treatment is thought to be (Midwinter, 1976; Shoemaker, 1977). There are natural regimens for these "symptoms" that include exercise, nutritional changes, and various vitamin programs (Prensky, 1974; Seaman and Seaman, 1977; Siegal and Michaud, 1980). Many women are prescribed tranquilizers, antidepressants, or antianxiety medications to alleviate problems, but the most prescribed and used treatment for menopause is exogenous estrogens. Three to four million women in the United States take exogenous estrogens, with an estimated two to three million taking it for more than 3 months (Wolfe, 1977). The total number of prescriptions for estrogen replacement increased by 35% from 1970 to 1975, but then decreased by 29% from 1975 to 1977. This decrease reversed a trend that began in the 1930s and increased dramatically in the 1960s. The reversal that began in 1975 may be associated with the publication of research suggesting a causal link between endometrial cancer and estrogen use (Mack, Pike, Henderson, Pfeffer, Gerkins, Arthur, and Brown, 1976; Smith, 1975; Ziel and Finkle, 1975). Even with this decrease in total prescriptions, a Food and Drug Administration Bulletin of 1976 concludes that estrogen is misused to an extent that cannot be explained (Food and Drug Administration, 1976). Although there is general consensus that hot flushes, or flashes, and dryness of vaginal mucous membranes are the only symptoms altered by the administration of exogenous estrogens, estrogen is often prescribed for "general well-being" and just for "the menopause," with no clear criteria for prescribing it. Those practitioners who believe menopause is an "estrogen deficiency disease" suggest it be given to all menopausal women (Wilson, 1961; Greenblatt, 1977; Lebich, 1976; Notelovitz, 1976; Wenderlein, 1980), whereas other practitioners suggest using it sparingly and judiciously, specifically for hot flushes/flashes that are bothersome to the individual woman (Connell, 1977; Coope, 1976).

A number of unwanted effects of, and contraindications for, prescribing estrogen are recognized (Reitz, 1977; Seaman and Seaman, 1977; Utian, 1976). Those receiving the most attention concern the carcinogeneity of estrogen replacement therapy. Cancer of the breast is one type of cancer linked with estrogens (Burch, 1971; Trichopoulos, 1972; Hoover, 1976; Lawson, Jick, Hunter, and Madsen, 1981). This hypothesis linking estrogen with cancer of the breast is complex and not yet definitively demonstrated. The hypothesis suggests that the exposure of breast-duct epithelium to unopposed estrogen results in changes that are precursors to cancer. Estrogens have been a causative factor of breast tumors in mammals (Cutts, 1964), and groups of women at high risk of breast cancer have higher plasma levels of estrogen (Henderson, and Canellos, 1980). Two major recent studies have indicated a greater risk of breast cancer with the use of menopausal estrogen, particularly at higher doses over long periods of time (Hoover, 1976; Ross, Paganini-Hill, Gerkins, Mack, Pfeffer, Arthur, and Henderson, 1980; Lawson, Wick, Hunter, and Madsen, 1981). The study by Ross et al. indicates that women who still had their ovaries and received estrogens had a 2.5-fold higher risk for breast cancer, and the study by Lawson et al. showed a two-fold increase for women who use exogenous estrogen at midlife.

Even though the relationship of estrogens and breast cancer is now receiving attention, most discussion and research on the carcinogeneity of estrogens relate to cancer of the endometrium. Recent epidemiological research suggests that women taking estrogen over a period of time have a greater risk of cancer of the endometrium (Smith, 1975; Ziel and Finkle, 1975; Mack et al., 1976; Antunes, 1979). Though there has been disagreement as to the analytical procedures of the research for the mechanisms involved in the causality, there is agreement that some causal link exists between endometrial cancer and estrogen (Weiss, Szekely, and Austin, 1976; Mack et al., 1976; Proudfit, 1976). Some research suggests that a causal link exists but only in women who are cancer-prone, and that the dangers of estrogen replacement therapy might be mitigated by prescribing cyclic estrogen with progesterone (Gambrell, 1976; Greenblatt, 1977).

In any studies linking cancer with estrogen use, the relationship between large doses and long-term use is highlighted. This is particularly relevant when we think of the women who are at midlife in the United States in late 20th century. These are the women who received the synthetic estrogen diethylstilbestrol in the 1950s and 1960s as a protective intervention in what were defined as high-risk pregnancies, who received the high-estrogen birth control pills in the 1960s, and/or who received high doses of estrogen replacement therapy to keep them "feminine forever." The outcome of these estrogen interventions will be difficult to determine because there are so many other factors that can confound the cause and progression of cancers.

Symptoms Attributed to Menopause. In discussing what are often designated as the symptoms of menopause it is necessary to remember the stage in a woman's life when menopause occurs. It is a time of many physical changes that can influence both somatic and psychological experiences. A more realistic approach in assessing the health of midlife women would be to define the various signs of midlife, naming menopause as one of them.

There is no accurate assessment of how many midlife women have symptoms of menopause, and of those women who do, to what extent. This is because most studies relating to health and menopause are conducted using clinical groups of women and because few prospective studies have been conducted.[1]

Information on the symptoms of menopause or how many women experience them is lacking because there is no precise definition of the symptoms, because distinctions are not made between symptoms of menopause and symptoms of other phenomena, and because researchers measure symptoms in different ways (Kaufert, 1981). Some studies include such diverse experiences as insomnia, diarrhea, and skin-crawling as symptoms, whereas many researchers now believe that only two symptoms can be attributed to menopause: hot flashes and dryness of vaginal mucosa. In obtaining the data on symptoms, some studies report clinical data while others report women's perceptions after the fact. Estimations of the proportion of women who have "symptoms" of menopause reflect this lack of clarity in the research. These estimates range from 20% (Jern, 1973) to 37% (DeLorey, 1981) to 62% (Council of the Medical Women's Federation, 1933) and up to 80% (Wilson, 1962; Thompson, 1973; McKinlay and Jefferys, 1974; Weideger, 1977). Most estimations of the proportion of women who see a physician for menopausal symptoms report 50% or less (Weideger, 1977; Studd, 1981; Evans, 1982).

There is no clear-cut evidence of a causal link between symptoms associated with menopause and a decrease of cyclical ovarian estrogen. That is not to deny the existence of symptoms or to deny the experience of women who report them. But further research is needed from the biological and experiential perspectives before the significance of these symptoms can be evaluated. From the biological perspective, more in-

---

[1]Two recent exceptions to this offer exciting prospects for future results and future research. Sonja McKinlay is conducting a prospective study on midlife women in the United States and expects to replicate the study with a Canadian cohort. Maryanne Golnalons-Nicolet and Elizabeth Markson are planning a prospective study on midlife that will compare women in Switzerland, France, and the United States. These studies will provide more information on the midlife experience as well as highlight the factors most relevant to women's health in old age.

formation is needed on the clinical and epidemiological manifestations of the symptoms and the women who experience them. From the experiential perspective, more information is needed concerning which women do and do not report symptoms, to determine antecedents that influence their health status, including their experience of menopause, at midlife.

PSYCHOSOCIAL ASPECTS OF MENOPAUSE. Menopause is a biological process that takes place within a particular social and cultural setting. Thus, the psychosocial aspects of menopause are as important a consideration as the biological aspects. Because of the symbolic representation of menopause, the social aspects produce profound changes in the way women at menopause view themselves and in turn are viewed by society.

Menopause is discussed and evaluated as a social event in both professional and nonprofessional literature (Patrick, 1970; Crawford, 1973; Boston Women's Health Book Collective, 1976; Gray, 1976; Parlee, 1976; van Keep, 1976; Reitz, 1977; Bart, 1967; McCarter, 1982). The influence of different cultural settings and different cultural backgrounds on a woman's perception of menopause is well documented (Maoz, 1970; McKinlay and Jefferys, 1974; van Keep, 1976; Griffin, 1978; Datan, 1981; Frey, 1981) and is further evidence that a biological explanation is not sufficient to explain the varied experiences of menopause.

Although there is evidence that class differences influence a woman's perception of menopause (McKinlay and Jeffreys, 1974), as does how a woman experiences her parental role (Bart, 1967), little is known about other social factors. One interesting cross-cultural perspective is that of Marsha Flint, who has carried out anthropological studies of women of the Rajput caste in the Indian states of Rajasthan and Himachel Pradesh. These women had none of the symptoms Western women often associated with menopause. If they had not yet achieved menopause they were looking forward to it, while those women who had already reached menopause were very positive about it.

Flint's explanation is that these Rajput women live in purdah and are not allowed in the company of men prior to menopause, when they are released from these restrictions and allowed to publicly visit and socialize with men. The women view menopause as raising their status. Flint contrasts the elevation of status in these Indian cultures with the changing roles of menopausal women in the United States, whose status declines as they age, and suggests that the rewards, or lack of them, can influence women's experiences of menopause or midlife (Flint, 1982).

Other recent research is exploring cross-cultural differences (Griffin, 1978; Datan, 1981) as well as sexuality and role norms (McCarter, 1982).

Heart Disease and Midlife Women

Much of the information concerning heart disease and midlife women assumes a connection with menopause, a connotation perpetuated by a misinterpretation of the data, a denial of the multifactorial causes of heart disease, and a lack of relevant research on women and heart disease.

If menopause were responsible for increased heart-disease mortality, then we would expect to see a sharp increase at the time of menopause, but instead the reality is that there is a gradual increase with age, with no acceleration at menopause (Ryan and Gibson, 1973; Sauer, 1980). It is the *ratio* of deaths from heart disease between men and women that changes. For all ages, the female : male ratio for heart-disease fatalities is 2 : 36 for white women (1 : 47 for black women) but by 60 years of age it becomes 1 : 71 for all groups. This change in the ratio reflects the steadily increasing rate for women as well as a diminishing of the acceleration of men's rates. The sharp difference in the male : female ratios between blacks and whites should be noted. Black men and black women have higher death rates from heart disease throughout the life-span, but the ratio of black men to black women is almost half that of their white counterparts. There is yet no evidence that hormonal factors in black and white women differ, and if indeed hormonal influences were protective for women against heart disease, we would expect to see the ratios similar for black and white persons. The role of estrogens in heart disease risk is not yet known.

It is more reasonable to assume that genetic, dietary, and life-style factors are more relevant to heart disease fatalities than menopause status. The linear increase with age may not be from aging factors or hormonal changes but instead may reflect prolonged exposure to high risk factors. In looking at heart disease, midlife women, and menopause, we need to separate out those activities that confound each other such as body size, smoking, and alcohol consumption, all of which are associated with both an early menopause and cerebrovascular disease (Hill, 1979; Gordon, Kannell, Hjortland, and McNamara, 1978).

Coronary risk factors for women have received scant attention compared to men. This is particularly striking for sociocultural factors. Recent work by Haynes and others in the Framingham Study indicate that midlife women classified as high in Type-A behavior (emotional lability, aging worries, tension, and anger symptoms) have an increase in the rate of coronary heart disease compared to women who show less Type-A behavior. Employed women showed more Type-A behavior than their homemaker sisters and were similar to the Type-A men (Haynes, Levine, Scotch, Feinlab, and Kannell, 1978); overall, only clerical workers with family responsibilities actually had a higher coronary risk than homemakers.

Further epidemiological research is needed to explain male–female differences in cardiac mortality. But if the evidence is not yet available to explain these differences, neither is it available to demonstrate that menopause is a cause of heart disease in midlife women.

Cancer and Midlife Women

Next to heart/cerebrovascular diseases, cancer is the leading killer of midlife women. Cancers of the uterus, cervix, and breast account for approximately 40% of all female cancer deaths (see Table 2).

Cancer of the breast is responsible for 26% of all diagnosed cancers and 19% of cancer mortality, or 30,000 deaths in the United States, higher than for any other site in women. Although breast cancer mortality has declined in past decades for women under 50 years of age, it is on the rise for women over 50 (Tishler, 1978; Kopstein, 1972), with both incidence and mortality greater in black women.

The specific causes of breast cancer are unknown, and it is unlikely that there is one single etiological factor. Instead, it appears to be dependent upon a number of factors, including age, familial history, environment, and exogenous hormones. A woman's risk of breast cancer increases by 80% to 150% if her mother or sister has had breast cancer, but it is not clear whether this increased risk is primarily inherited or is a reflection of common environmental experiences (Bain, Speizer, Rosner, Belanger, and Hennekens, 1981). The use of exogenous estrogens at midlife increases a woman's risk of breast cancer at least twofold (Ross *et al.*, 1980; Lawson *et al.*, 1981). Fibrocystic disease of the breast is another factor thought to be associated with a higher risk of breast cancer, but recent research questions this belief. It seems more likely that those other factors that put a woman at risk for breast cancer influence precancerous changes in the breast; these factors, rather than fibrocystic changes, influence the risk status for breast cancer (Love, Gilman, and Silen, 1982).

The term *breast cancer* is in reality a general phrase used to designate a heterogeneous group of cancers of the breast residing in a heterogeneous group of women. Thus, to think of the natural history of breast cancer as a single phenomenon is fallacious (Fisher, Redmond, and Fisher 1978). This makes research on the progress of the disease and therapeutic interventions complex and often confusing. The complexity in research can be addressed by doing prospective randomized clinical trials in which, by design, women in different groups will be as similar as possible, and any differences will therefore be from what is being evaluated. The complexity in deciding upon treatment for individual women is made even more difficult by rapid changes of information regarding diagnostic procedures and therapeutic decisions. Screening programs and breast self-examination are responsible for detecting the majority of breast tumors. The success of any screening program depends on the stage of the lesions detected (Strax, 1978), but even this is now the subject of some controversy. Screening may not actually influence the survival rate by early detection. Instead, a tumor detected in a screening program may just be diagnosed earlier in its natural history, and thus the longer survival time is an artifact of early detection. There is also some consideration of another bias, in that slow-growing tumors are more likely to be detected at screening while fast-growing tumors will be detected in the times between. Slow-growing tumors are less life-threatening and respond to treatment better than fast-growing tumors (Henderson and Canellos, 1980).

Screening for breast cancer relies on three major components: clinical examination (including palpation and inspection), mammography, and thermography. Because of a high rate of false diagnoses and disagreement on criteria of normalcy, thermography is not widely used at present (Moskowitz, Milbrath, Gartside, Zermeno, and Mandel, 1976). Mammography is a form of X ray specifically designed for breast examinations. Its efficacy and safety have been challenged (Bailer 1976; Strax 1978), but with improvement in mammographic technique and the use of mammography only for women over 50 years or in high-risk categories, the possible dangers are mitigated.

There are few remaining standards for the treatment of breast cancer. Factors that must be considered in planning therapeutic intervention include the stage of the cancer at diagnosis, the natural history of the tumor, and the type of tumor (Henderson and Canellos, 1980). In the past, radical mastectomy (complete removal of the affected breast, underlying tissue, and lymph nodes) and chemotherapy were the major treatments for breast cancer. The value of using such major interventions on a routine basis is now questioned by some researchers and practitioners on the grounds that the results are not any better than other forms of treatment (Kohn, 1982). Alternative treatments for early stages include primary irradiation after biopsy, lumpectomy (excision of the tumor) with endocrine therapy, or combined chemotherapy for recurrence or advanced disease.

With the rapid changes in therapies as well as the resulting disagreements among practitioners, what is an individual woman to do when confronted with the possibility of breast cancer? Because it is a complex disease manifested differently in each woman, there is no one correct form of treatment. A woman must insist that her physician discuss all relevant options and their outcomes with her so that together they may make the decisions concerning her care. If her physician is reluctant, she should get a second opinion, now covered by most insurances. If she cannot get the information she needs, she can contact her nearest women's health center or consumer health information service.

To the physician, breast cancer is seen as a life-threatening concern, but for the woman involved, it means not only confronting a life-threatening illness but the possible loss of a very significant part of her body, with grief at this loss (Notman, 1979). It is therefore essential that a woman have full information so she can then make the most appropriate decisions for herself.

Cancer of the endometrium (*corpus uteri*) is not a major killer of women, but its relevance for midlife women has increased since a causal link between estrogen use and endometrial cancer has been proposed. Although some researchers suggest that the reported increase is an artifact of closer surveillance or lack of differentiation of cellular changes (Campbell, 1976), most researchers indicate an increased risk of endometrial cancer from four- to eightfold with the use of exogenous estrogens (Weiss, Srekely, and Austin, 1976; Sartwell, 1976; Spengler, Clarke, Worlever, Newman, and Osborn, 1981).

Cervical cancer is not a major cause of death among United States women, accounting for only 3% of cancer deaths, and the mortality from it has been decreasing rapidly. Even though the mortality is decreasing, there is wide disparity among groups, with black women three times more likely to die from cancer of the cervix than white women.

The availability and use of the Papanicolaou (Pap) test has often been credited with the declining mortality from cancer of the cervix. Recently, debate on this issue has centered around the fact that the decline may have started before Pap tests were routinely administered, that the decline exists where Pap tests are not done, and that increasing numbers of hysterectomies mask the epidemiological data since a woman cannot get cancer of the cervix if she has no uterus. Although debate on the issue continues, particularly concerning the costs of screening a total population, even critics concede that screening according to high-risk groups is appropriate (Kleinman, 1979). Women at high risk are those who have had sexual intercourse, particularly with early onset of sexual activity and multiple sexual partners (Canadian Task Force, 1976). Because screening programs can detect lesions before they have progressed, and because cervical cancer can be effectively treated when detected early enough, the most appropriate use of resources would be to screen those groups at high risk for cervical cancer and to educate women and physicians concerning the value of selective screening.

Occupational Health Issues for Midlife Women

If a paucity of information characterizes other aspects of health for midlife women, then it completely defines what we know about work and health and midlife women. Most of the attention to occupational health issues has been directed to young male workers and, to a lesser degree, to young female workers; typically, concern about females has centered around reproductive issues. Occupations that are predominantly female, such as clerical work and household work, have been consistently neglected in the determination of health hazards. Additionally, nontraditional occupations for women have been neglected in considering differential effects of health hazards on women. An important point for the group of women who are at midlife today is that these women 55–60 years old in the 1980s entered the work force in the 1940s, during World War II. These women are the Rosie the Riveters, who were exposed to all the hazards of the workplace usually considered relevant only to men.

Little research has been done on the hazards of the workplace that primarily affect women, and further research is needed to identify the epidemiology of work-related health conditions, rates of occupational illness, and occupational disabilities specific to midlife women.

A 1981 American Public Health Association report on older women and their health (Rathbone-McCuan and Dunn, 1981) suggests the following priorities for older women and occupational health:[2]

1. As more women enter craft-skill jobs and hazardous occupations that have yet to design equipment for women workers, the protective equipment needs of women must be investigated.
2. Working conditions such as ventilation inadequacies, excessive temperature ranges, and exposure to noise, dust, fume levels, and chemical substances should be investigated for their relationship to chronic diseases and related disabilities that have an impact on women.
3. Occupational stress and work-related crisis events should be examined in relation to the mental health of women as they age in a combined life-style of work and family.
4. The interrelationship of job satisfaction, economic status, job status, and future life-style decisions should be studied in the context of women's retirement planning and postretirement adaptations.

---

[2]The priorities are quoted from the report, *The Surviving Majority: Older Women and Their Health*, with permission of the authors.

5. Studies of employee health services are needed to assess their relevance to the special needs of older women and to identify specific programs or modifications of services that will meet their health needs for prevention and early diagnosis and follow-up.

Conclusion

The American Public Health Association project on Older Women's Health Issues (1981) reported on social and physical health, aging, occupational health hazards, and research issues (Rathbone-McCuan and Dunn, 1981). The researchers reported that they were hindered by huge gaps in the information that they needed to make realistic assessments of the health of older women. This implies that the existing "medical model" health care system is inappropriate and ineffective to meet the health needs of older women. A new system with new perspectives is needed, one that considers all factors that relate to health. Because a person's life-style and past experiences are integral components of health status, it is crucial that health care include a life-style perspective. Events in women's lives do not follow a predetermined staircase pattern, as much of the biomedical literature assumes. Life-style factors such as a woman's work history, her reproductive history, or her nurturant responsibilities, as well as other role relationships, and the timing of each of these in her life cycle all need to be considered.

One cornerstone of the present medical system is the assumption that the gynecologist is the primary care provider for women. This is inappropriate as well as impractical, because gynecological health problems are not the major health problems or causes of death for women. Heart disease (*not* a gynecological problem) is the leading cause of death for women, accounting for 38% of all deaths (Kleinman, 1979). The fact that gynecology is a surgical specialty also argues against gynecologists being the primary providers for midlife women. In addition, it is conceptually and politically inappropriate to have gynecologists as the primary health providers for older women because it perpetuates the reductionist attitude of seeing women only as products of their reproductive organs and of prescribing surgery as the obvious solution of choice for many common health issues.

Furthermore, many gynecologists are out of step with women's genuine health needs. One indication of this lack of congruity between women and gynecologists is that almost all medical literature concerning midlife women focuses on menopause, whereas in reality menopause accounts for only 3% of physician visits made by midlife women (45 to 65 years old). Hypertension accounts for the largest number of visits, 8.8%—almost three times as many visits as for menopause-related reasons. Not surprisingly, gynecologists attribute the reasons for women's visits to menopausal reasons at a 64% higher rate than women themselves do (Cypress, 1980).

In a survey of medical literature it became clear that the information currently available to physicians perpetuates negative attitudes toward menopause and midlife women (DeLorey, 1981). Of over 30 textbooks concerning women, not one discusses midlife women without menopause as the predominant subject, and few even mention other aspects of health (Romney, 1975; Martin, 1978; Taylor, 1969; Wilson, 1979; Baden and Thornton, 1980). Less than one-third of the texts present menopause as a normal, nonpathological process (Beeson and McDermot, 1971; Jeffcoate, 1975; Novak, 1975; Romney, 1975; Martin, 1978; Parson and Sommers, 1978; Wilson, 1979; Baden and Thornton, 1980). By presenting menopause as negative and by focusing on menopause as the major midlife health issue, the authors perpetuate the reductionist perspective that women's reproductive organs are the central focus of their life and health.

If the existing system of health care is not appropriate for midlife women, what would an adequate health system include? Both as individuals and as a group, women need to be listened to and heard, and as a group they need to be given the opportunity to implement their ideas of good health care. Women need encouragement to seek and demand information concerning their own health, so that they themselves may make the decisions for, and have control of, their health and their bodies. In such a health care system prevention of disease would be stressed.

There already exists a strong movement of women of all ages concerned with health who are incorporating these ideas into actions. These women, part of the women's self-help health movement, are often associated with women-controlled health centers, and focus on menopause issues, midlife issues, and health for older women. This women's self-help movement goes beyond discussions of how or why the medical care system does not meet their needs; members view self-help as an action-oriented concept, with major goals being (a) to demystify health/medical care through sharing and translating medical literature, (b) to demedicalize health care for women, and (c) to empower women to reclaim control of their health and bodies through validation of their own experiences.

These goals are actualized through groups and centers that midlife women themselves control. These include such diverse groups as the Menopause Collective in the metropolitan Boston area, the Midlife and Older Women's Committee of the National Women's Health Network, the Older Women's League, and the Gray Panthers Health Project

Fund. It is from these older women's self-help groups, more than from medical sources, that valuable information has been generated and disseminated. This new information includes various ways to ameliorate hot flashes, why exercise continues to be important for women as they get older, and the continued importance of nutrition for older women. These groups also emphasize the need to separate normal aging from illness and the need to consider women's lives in totality.

Because the nature of the phenomena of midlife, women, and health make these difficult to study, the myths more than the realities of each have guided providers, policy-makers, and researchers. The implications of this lack of accurate information and perpetuation of stereotypes are far-reaching. The immediate implication is that midlife women cannot receive adequate and appropriate health care if every aspect of their health is seen as related to menopause. The long-term implication is that by the attribution of all symptoms or complaints of midlife to the diminution of ovarian estrogen, the possible consequences of these complaints and their relation to the aging process are ignored, perhaps to manifest themselves as chronic disease processes of old age that could have been alleviated with appropriate attention at midlife.

To provide appropriate health services for midlife women, both the structure of the existing services and the dearth of accurate information need to be addressed. To accomplish this we must do the following:

1. Establish priorities of health care that address women's priorities derived from their own experiences and that are based on the sociological and behavioral as well as the biomedical sciences.
2. Establish an information base that considers the precursors of health at midlife. For example, one could focus on how nutrition and exercise throughout the life-span affect osteoporosis, rather than focus on medical intervention issues after the process has already begun.
3. Redefine research priorities so that nonclinical and prospective studies are conducted that give a more accurate assessment of midlife.
4. Present a more realistic, less pathological view of midlife women to health providers. This perspective is not readily available in the medical literature but is available in the literature from the behavioral sciences (Bart and Grossman, 1976; Parlee, 1976; Koeske, 1977; Bart, 1967; Notman, 1979; Rubin, 1979; Datan, 1981), as well as in the literature written by and for women (Boston Women's Health Book Collective, 1976; Clay, 1977; Reitz, 1977; Weideger, 1977; Sommers and Shields, 1980; Santa

Fe Health Education Project, 1980; Block, Davidson, and Grambs, 1981).
5. Support environments in which women can develop realistic expectations about midlife health issues. These environments already exist through many self-help groups and workshops conducted at women's health centers, and in other women's groups where women learn through sharing and validating their experiences with each other.

Midlife is an important stage of women's lives, but from the perspective of health issues, the domination of menopause has obscured our understanding of the totality of women's health experiences. Only when we look at all the facets of this rich experience can we begin to make valid statements and assessments relating to the health of midlife women. The task now is to hear what women themselves say of their experiences of midlife, including menopause, so that both the social and biological significance of midlife can be seen as it really is, not as it is assumed to be. Then, attention can be redirected to look at all the factors influencing women's health at midlife and women themselves will then have accurate and appropriate information when they make choices about their own health care.

REFERENCES

Antunes, C. M. F. Endometrial cancer and estrogen use. *New England Journal of Medicine*, 1979, *300*, 9–13.

Baden, W. F., and Thornton, D. R. (Eds.). *Primary health care for obstetricians and gynecologists*. Baltimore: Williams and Wilkins, 1980.

Bailer, J. V. Mammography: A contrary view. *Annals of Internal Medicine*, 1976, *84*, 77–84.

Bain, C., Speizer, F. E., Rosner, B., Belanger, C., and Hennekens, C. H. Family history of breast cancer as a risk indicator for the diseases. *American Journal of Epidemiology*, 1981, *111*, 301–308.

Bart, P. *Depression in middle-aged women: Some sociocultural factors*. Doctoral dissertation, University of California at Los Angeles, 1967.

Bart, P., and Grossman, M. Menopause. *Women and Health*, 1976, *1*, 3–11.

Beard, R. J. (Ed.). *The menopause: A guide to current research and practice*. Baltimore: University Park Press, 1976.

Beeson, P. B., and McDermot, W. *Cecil-Loeb textbook of medicine*. Philadelphia: Saunders, 1971.

Block, M. R., Davidson, J. L., and Grambs, J. D. *Women over forty: Visions and realities*. New York: Springer, 1981.

Boston Women's Health Book Collective. *Our bodies, ourselves*. New York: Simon & Schuster, 1976.

Burch, J. C., and Byrd, B. F. Effects of long-term administration of estrogen on the occurrence of mammary cancer in women. *Annals of Surgery*, 1971, *174*, 414–418.

Bureau of the Census. *A statistical portrait of women*. Current Population Reports, Special Studies: Series P-23 No. 58, Washington, D.C., 1975.

Campbell, S. (Ed.). *The management of the menopause and post-menopausal years.* Baltimore: University Park Press, 1976.

Canadian Task Force. Cervical cancer screening programs. *Canadian Medical Association Journal,* 1976, *114,* 1003–1033.

Clay, U. S. *Women: Menopause and middle age.* Pittsburgh: Know, Inc., 1977.

Connell, E. Estrogen: What to do until the results are in. In L. Rose (Ed.), *The menopause book.* New York: Hawthorn Books, 1977.

Coope, J. Double blind cross over study of estrogen replacement therapy. In S. Campbell (Ed.), *The management of the menopause and post-menopausal years.* Baltimore: University Park Press, 1976.

Council of the Medical Women's Federation. An investigation of the menopause in one thousand women. *Lancet,* 1933, *1,* 106.

Crawford, M., and Hooper, D. Menopausal aging. *The Family* 1973, *7,* 464–482.

Cutts, J. H., and Noble, R. L. Estrone-induced mammary tumors in the rat. *Cancer Research,* 1964, *24,* 1116–1123.

Cypress, B. K. *Office visits by women.* Vital and Health Statistics: Series 13; No. 45 (DHEW Publication No. (PHS) 80-1796). Hyattsville, Md.: 1980.

Dalton, K. Menopause: A clinician's view. *Royal Society of Health Journal,* 1976, *96,* 75–81.

Datan, N. *A time to reap.* Baltimore: Johns Hopkins University Press, 1981.

DeLorey, C. *Health care for midlife women.* Unpublished doctoral dissertation, Harvard University, 1981.

Department of Commerce. *Historical statistics of the United States* (DHEW Publication No. 004-024-00120-9), Washington, D.C.: U.S. Government Printing Office, 1975.

Dunn, L. National Center for Health Statistics, personal communication, December 1981.

Eskin, B. A. *The menopause: Comprehensive management.* New York: Masson, 1980.

Evans, B. *Life change.* London: Pan Books, 1982.

Fisher, B., Redmond, C., and Fisher, E. R. Clinical trials and the surgical treatment of breast cancer. *Surgical Clinics of North America,* 1978, *58,* 723–735.

Flint, M. Male and female menopause: A cultural put-on. In A. M. Voda, M. Dinnerstein, and S. R. O'Donnell (Eds.), *Changing perspectives on menopause.* Austin: University of Texas Press, 1982.

Food and Drug Administration. *FDA drug bulletin.* February/March 1976.

Frey, A. K. Middle-aged women's experience and perceptions of menopause. *Women and Health,* 1981, *6,* 25–36.

Gambrell, R. D. Estrogens, progestogens and endometrial cancer. In P. A. Van Keep, R. B. Greenblatt, and M. Albeaux-Fernet (Eds.), *Consensus of menopause research.* Baltimore: University Park Press, 1976.

Givens, J. D. *Current estimates from the health interview survey.* Vital and Health Statistics: Series 10, No. 130 (DHEW Publication No. (PHS) 80-1551). Hyattsville, Md.: U.S. Government Printing Office, 1979.

Goodman, M. *Menopause: A pilot study.* University of Hawaii Women's Studies Program, Working Paper Series, 1976, *1,* 1–23.

Gordon, T., Kannell, W. B., Hjortland, M. C., and McNamara, P. M. Menopause and coronary heart disease. *Journal of the American Medical Association,* 1978, *89,* 157–161.

Gray, R. H. The menopause—Epidemiological and demographic consideration. In R. J. Beard (Ed.), *The menopause.* Baltimore: University Park Press, 1976.

Greenblatt, R. B. Estrogens and endometrial cancer—Gross exaggeration or fact? *Geriatrics,* 1977, *32,* 60–72.

Griffin, J. A cross-cultural investigation of behavioral changes at menopause. In K. O'Connor-Blumhagen and W. D. Johnson (Eds.), *Women's studies: An interdisciplinary collection.* Westport, Conn.: Greenwood Press, 1978.

Hadden, W. C. *Basic data on health care needs of adults ages 25–74 years, United States,*

1971–1975. Vital and Health Statistics: Series 11, No. 218 (DHEW Publication No. (PHS) 81-1668). Hyattsville, Md.: U.S. Government Printing Office, 1981.

Haynes, S. G., Levine, S., Scotch, N., Feinlab, M., and Kannell, W. B. The relationship of psychosocial factors to coronary heart disease in the Framingham study. *American Journal of Epidemiology*, 1978, *107*, 384–401.

Henderson, I. C., and Canellos, G. P. Cancer of the breast: The past decade. *New England Journal of Medicine*, 1980, *302*, 17–30.

Hill, J. *Menopause and cardiovascular disease.* Paper presented at the Interdisciplinary Research Conference on Menopause, Tucson, 1979.

Hoover, R. Menopausal estrogens and breast cancer. *New England Journal of Medicine*, 1976, *295*, 401–405.

Jeffcoate, N. *Principles of gynecology.* Boston: Butterworths, 1975.

Jern, H. *Hormone therapy of the menopause and aging.* Springfield, Ill.: Charles C Thomas, 1973.

Kaufert, P. Symptom reporting at the menopause. *Social Science and Medicine*, 1981, *151*, 173–184.

Kleinmann, J. C. Death rates from cervical cancer by health service area 1968–72. *Statistical Notes for Health Planners*, No. 8, August 1979 (DHEW Publication No. (PHS) 79-1237). Washington: U.S. Government Printing Office, 1979.

Koeske, R. K. *Theoretical perspectives on menstrual cycle research.* Paper presented at the Menstrual Cycle Conference, Chicago, 1977.

Kohn, J. Treating breast cancer conservatively: Dissension, contention continue. *Journal of the American Medical Association*, 1982, *248*, 1793–1802.

Kopstein, A. N. Breast cancer death rates by health service area, 1968–72. *Statistical Notes for Health Planners*, No. 30, July 1978 (DHEW Publication No. (PHS) 78-1250). Washington: U.S. Government Printing Office, 1972.

Lawson, D. H., Jick, H., Hunter, J., and Madsen, S. Exogenous estrogens and breast cancer. *American Journal of Epidemiology*, 1981, *114*, 710–713.

Lebich, P. E. Effects and side effects of estrogen therapy. In D. A. Van Keep, R. B. Gesenblatt, and M. Albeaux-Fernet (Eds.), *Consensus of menopause research.* Baltimore: University Park Press, 1976.

Love, S. M., Gilman, R. S., and Silen, W. Fibrocystic "disease" of the breast—A nondisease? *New England Journal of Medicine*, 1982, *307*, 1010–1014.

Mack, T. M., Pike, M. C., Henderson, B. E., Pfeffer, R. I., Gerkins, V. R., Arthur, M., and Brown, S. E. Estrogens and endometrial cancer in a retirement community. *New England Journal of Medicine*, 1976, *294*, 1262–1267.

Maoz, B. Female attitudes to menopause. *Social Psychiatry*, 1970, *5*, 35–40.

Martin, L. L. *Health care of women.* Philadelphia: Lippincott, 1978.

McCarter, S. S. Physical changes related to menopause. In S. L. Tyler and G. M. Woodall (Eds.), *Female health and gynecology across the lifespan.* Bowie, Md.: Robert J. Brady, 1982.

McKinlay, S. M., and Jefferys, M. The menopausal syndrome. *British Journal of Preventive and Social Medicine*, 1974, *28*, 108–115.

McKinlay, S., Jefferys, M., and Thompson, B. An investigation of the age at menopause. *Journal of Biosocial Science*, 1971, *4*, 161–173.

Midwinter, A., Contra-indications to estrogen therapy and management of the menopausal syndrome in these cases. In S. Campbell (Ed.), *The management of the menopausal and post-menopausal years.* Baltimore: University Park Press, 1976.

Mishler, E. G., Amarasingham, L. R., Hauser, S., Liem, R., Osherson, S. D., and Waxler, N. E. *Social contexts of health, illness, and patient care.* New York: Cambridge University Press, 1981.

Moskovitz, M., Milbrath, J., Gertside, P., Zermeno, A., and Mandel, D. Lack of efficacy of thermography as a screening tool for minimal and Stage I cancer. *New England Journal of Medicine,* 1976, *295,* 249–252.

Nathanson, A. Illness and the feminine role: A theoretical review. *Social Science and Medicine,* 1975, *9,* 57–62.

Neugarten, B. L. Women's attitudes toward the menopause. *Vita Humanae,* 1963, *6,* 140–146.

Notelovitz, M. The effect of long term estrogen replacement therapy on glucose and lipid metabolism in post-menopausal women. *South African Medical Journal,* 1976, *50,* 2001–2003.

Notman, M. Midlife concerns of women: Implications of the menopause. *American Journal of Psychiatry,* 1979, *136,* 1270–1274.

Novak, E. R. *Novak's text book of gynecology.* Baltimore: Williams and Wilkins, 1975.

Parlee, M. B. Social factors in the psychology of menstruation, birth, and menopause. *Primary Care,* 1976, *3,* 477–490.

Parson, L., and Sommers, S. C. *Gynecology.* Philadelphia: Saunders, 1978.

Patrick, M. L. A study of middle-aged women and menopause. Unpublished doctoral dissertation, University of California at Los Angeles, 1970.

Prensky, J. *Healing yourself.* New York: Bantam, 1974.

Proudfit, C. D. Estrogens and menopause. *Journal of the American Medical Association,* 1976, *236,* 939–940.

Rathbone-McCuan, E., and Dunn, T. *The surviving majority: Older women and their health* (APHA Project No. 440032). Washington, D.C.: American Public Health Association, 1981.

Reitz, R. *Menopause: A positive approach.* Radnor, Pa.: Chilton, 1977.

Romney, S. *Gynecology and obstetrics: The health care of women.* New York: McGraw-Hill, 1975.

Ross, R. K., Paganini-Hill, A., Gerkins, O. R., Mack, T. M., Pfeffer, R. I., Arthur, M., and Henderson, B. E. A case-control study of menopausal estrogen therapy and breast cancer. *Journal of the American Medical Association,* 1980, *243,* 1635–1638.

Rubin, L. B. *Women of a certain age: The midlife search for self.* New York: Harper & Row, 1979.

Ryan, K. J., and Givson, D. C. *Menopause and aging* (DHEW Publication No. (NIH) 73-319). Washington: U.S. Government Printing Office, 1973.

Santa Fe Health Education Project. *Menopause: A self care manual.* Santa Fe, N. Mex.: Santa Fe Health Education Project, 1980.

Sartwell, P. Estrogen replacement theory and endometrial carcinoma: Epidemiologic evidence. *Clinical Obstetrics and Gynecology,* 1976, *19,* 817–823.

Sauer, H. I. *Geographic patterns in the risk of dying and associated factors, ages 35–74, United States, 1968–1972.* Vital and Health Statistics: Series 3: No. 18 (DHHS Publication No. (PHS) 80-1402). Hyattsville, Md.: U.S. Government Printing Office, 1980.

Seaman, B., and Seaman, G. *Women and the crisis in sex hormones.* New York: Rawson Associates, 1977.

Shoemaker, S. Estrogen treatment of post-menopausal women: Benefits and risks. *Journal of the American Medical Association,* 1977, *238,* 1524–1530.

Siegal, D., and Michaud, A. Exercise at menopause. *WomanWise,* 1980, *3,* 7.

Smith, D. Association of exogenous estrogen and endometrial cancer. *New England Journal of Medicine,* 1975, *293,* 1164–1167.

Sommers, T., and Shields, L. Older women and health care. In *Gray paper no. 3.* Oakland, Calif.: Older Women's League, 1980.

Spengler, R. F., Clarke, E. A., Worlever, D. A., Newman, A. M., and Osborn, R. W. Exogenous estrogens and endometrial cancer: A case-control study and assessment of potential biases. *American Journal of Epidemiology,* 1981, *114,* 497–506.

Strax, P. Evaluation of screening programs for the early diagnosis of breast cancer. *Surgical Clinics of North America*, 1978, *58*, 667–679.
Studd, J. W. W. *The menopause*. London: Guideway, 1981.
Taich, A. Social implications of menopause. Paper presented at the American Women in Psychology Conference, Pittsburgh, 1978.
Taylor, E. S. *Essentials of gynecology*. Philadelphia: Lea and Febiger, 1969.
Thompson, B. Menopausal age and symptomatology in a general practice. *Journal of Biosocial Sciences*, 1973, *71*, 1973.
Tishler, S. L. Breast disorders. In M. T. Notman and C. C. Nadelson (Eds.), *The woman patient*. New York: Plenum Press, 1978.
Trichopoulos, D. Menopause and breast cancer risk. *Journal of the National Cancer Institute*, 1972, *48*, 605–613.
Utian, W. H. The scientific basis for post-menopausal estrogen therapy: The management of specific symptoms and rationale for long-term replacement. In R. J. Beard (Ed.), *The menopause*. Baltimore: University Park Press, 1976.
van Keep, P. A., Greenblatt, R. B., and Albeauz-Fernet, M. (Eds.). *Consensus on menopause research*. Baltimore: University Park Press, 1976.
Verbrugge, L. M. Females and illness: Recent trends in sex differences in the United States. *Journal of Health and Social Behavior*, 1976, *17*, 387–403.
Verbrugge, L. M., and Steiner, R. P. Physician treatment of men and women patients: Sex bias or appropriate care? *Medical Care*, 1981, *19*, 609–632.
Weideger, P. *Menstruation and menopause*. New York: Dell, 1977.
Weiss, N. S., Szekely, D. R., and Austin, D. F. Increasing incidence of endometrial cancer in the United States. *New England Journal of Medicine*, 1976, *294*, 1259–1262.
Wenderlein, J. M. Psychotherapeutic effects of estrogen substitution during the climacteric period. In N. Pasetto, R. Paoletti, and J. L. Ambrus (Eds.), *The menopause and postmenopause*. Baltimore: University Park Press, 1980.
Wilson, J. *Obstetrics and gynecology*. St. Louis: C. V. Mosby, 1979.
Wilson, R. A. *Feminine forever*. New York: M. Evans, 1961.
Wilson, R. J. Roles of estrogen and progesterone in breast and genital cancer. *Journal of the American Medical Association*, 1962, *82*, 327–331.
Wolfe, S. M. Affidavit of Sidney M. Wolf, M.D., United States District Court for the District of Delaware: *Pharmaceutical Manufacturers Association* vs. *Food and Drug Administration*, September 22, 1977.
Women's Bureau. *Mature women workers*. Washington, D.C.: U.S. Department of Labor, 1976.
Ziel, H. K., and Finkle, W. D. Increased risk of endometrial carcinoma among users of conjugated estrogens. *New England Journal of Medicine*, 1975, *293*, 1167–1170.

Chapter 13

Reproductive Issues, Including Menopause

MARY BROWN PARLEE

Scientific and clinical knowledge about the psychology of female reproduction has expanded rapidly over the past 15 years. Not only is there more research on the psychology of menstruation, pregnancy, birth, and menopause, it is better: more grounded in empirical data and more reflective of the complexity of the phenomena.[1]

A good deal of credit for this progress belongs to feminist researchers, scholars, and health care workers, both inside and outside academia and traditional health care institutions. Beginning with the groundbreaking *Our Bodies, Ourselves* (Bosten Women's Health Book Collective, 1973), these investigators reexamined and reevaluated literature on female health and reproduction, identifying implicit assumptions in the traditional work and pointing at gaps in knowledge where further research was needed. Such critiques—analyses of underlying assumptions and their implications for research—have played a central role in advances in research on the psychology of female reproduction, particularly in research on the psychology of menstruation (Dan, Graham, and Beecher, 1981; Komnenich, McSweeney, Noack, and Elder, 1981; Friedman, 1982; Golub, in press).

Despite significant progress in psychological research on menstruation and menarche, research and thinking about the psychology of menopause does not appear to have progressed as far (Voda, Dinnerstein, and O'Donnell, 1982). Why is that? Why should the psychological

---

MARY BROWN PARLEE • Center for the Study of Women and Society, Graduate School and University Center, City University of New York, 33 West 42nd Street, New York, New York 10036. This work was supported in part by a grant from the Ford Foundation to the Center for the Study of Women and Society, Graduate School and University Center, City University of New York.

aspects of menopause have proved so much more intractable to conceptual and empirical analysis than have other stages of the female reproductive life cycle?

Part of the answer may be that menopause is psychologically significant in different domains of experience and behavior from those of the menstrual cycle or pregnancy, and that psychological researchers, including feminists, have been working with assumptions that do not usually lead them to explore these domains fruitfully.[2] These assumptions may be resistant to change, furthermore, because they reflect and are embedded in an important set of social processes that not only shape the experience and actions of women in midlife but also serve to maintain the stable functioning of society as a whole. Catherine DeLorey (Chapter 12, this volume) discusses some of these significant social processes related to menopause—among them, how middle-aged women interact with health care systems. Other potentially fruitful domains for menopause research will also be suggested as the following line of reasoning is developed.

In brief, I would like to suggest that feminist critiques of research on the psychology of menopause point to the importance of what will be called here a *psychological* rather than a *biological* perspective. This distinction does not coincide with one between social/psychological and biological *causation*. Such critiques have not so far led to programmatic research, however, because of a further general problem pervading scientific thinking about the psychology of female reproduction, a problem that the topic of menopause represents in a particular acute form. The problem is that the language and concepts of psychological research on female reproduction tend to mirror the language and thought of society as a whole, and these linguistic/conceptual patterns are an integral part of a set of important social processes whose equilibrium depends upon them. To change scientific thinking and research about the psychology of female reproduction, then, means that researchers would need to step outside everyday ways of thinking, a bootstrap operation that is perhaps never completely possible.[3] If this operation were successful,

---

[2]As will become apparent, my analysis in no way resembles, in content, in tone, or, I think, in rigor, Judith Posner's disparaging commentary on the caricature she presents as feminist research on menopause (Posner, 1979). While I agree with her observation that "the relationship of political ideology to research into human behavior" is crucial, I do not think conceptual clarity on the issues is likely to emerge from the "straw man" she constructs and then labels "the feminist position."

[3]As research on the psychology of female reproduction has improved (including that on menopause and the climacterium), investigators increasingly point to the importance of studying biological–psychological–social *interactions* (e.g., van Keep and Humphrey, 1976). The problem is that no one does it or, seemingly, can point to a body of exemplary research. It is issues that still may be blocking the development of those appropriate new paradigms to which the present chapter is addressed.

furthermore, it would inevitably raise questions about—perhaps posing challenges to—the social processes in which the usual patterns of thought are embedded.

If this analysis is correct, then it follows that research on the psychology of female reproduction will be successful (1) to the extent that everyday ways of thinking about the phenomenon are compatible with fruitful paradigms for empirical research and/or (2) to the degree to which alteration of these ways of thinking can be absorbed without disruption of the social processes of which they are a part. I think one reason psychological research on menopause has not developed satisfactorily is that scientific concepts based on everyday thinking are highly inappropriate: They incorporate assumptions about the usefulness of a biological perspective in studying domains of behavior and experience for which adoption of a psychological perspective would probably be useful. For a variety of reasons, two of which will be discussed in detail, this mismatch between the research perspective adopted and the domain of psychological phenomena being investigated is greater for menopause than for other events in the female reproductive life cycle. This argument will now be elaborated in greater detail.

In Chapter 12, DeLorey rightly points to the fragmented and biased nature of previous research on menopause and to the lack of a conceptual model integrating biological, psychological, and sociocultural processes. DeLorey and others have, further, identified several key assumptions underlying traditional psychological research on menopause. Their analyses, together with the related research supporting them, appear to converge on the following four points: (1) Judging from self-reports, menopause and the symptoms traditionally thought to be associated with it do not seem to be dominant or universal features of the experience and behavior of middle-aged women in the United States (Neugarten, Wood, Kraines, and Loomis, 1963; Neugarten and Kraines, 1965; Greene, 1976; Polit and LaRocco, 1980; Townsend and Carbone, 1980). (2) Women's experience and behavior are affected by midlife changes in their social roles as well as those of others with whom they are emotionally involved—husband, children, parents, friends (Ballinger, 1975; Flint, 1975; Bart and Grossman, 1976; van Keep and Kellerhals, 1976; Barnett and Baruch, 1978; Nadelson, Polonsky, and Mathews, 1979; Severne, 1979; Greene and Cooke, 1980). (3) The psychological significance of menopause as an event in a continuing process (the climacterium) is difficult to disentangle from the psychological significance of more general age-related physiological changes (Ballinger, 1976; Goodman, Stewart, and Gilbert, 1977). (4) Menopause is often invoked by physicians and by laypeople as an implicit or explicit explanation for symptoms or behaviors arising from other causes (Donovan, 1951; Osofsky and Seidenberg, 1970; Eisenberg, 1979; Weissman, 1979; Cowan, in press). These four claims, arising largely from feminist analyses of traditional research, seem sufficiently obvious and well documented by now to serve as assumptons, as starting points for further research. That investigators have tended to reiterate these points rather than use them as the basis for new research suggests that additional, still implicit assumptions must be operating that impair the development of programmatic research and theory.

Elsewhere I have suggested that researchers interested in the psychological aspects of female reproductive processes tend to approach the problem in one of two ways (Parlee, 1981, 1982). If they approach the study of psychological phenomena from a *biological* perspective, their conceptual starting point is the *biological process* (menstrual cycle, pregnancy, menopause). The psychological question asked from this perspective is: What are the psychological consequences of these particular biological changes?

This is a reasonable way to study biological influences on behavior and experience. Its success depends upon the investigator's being able to identify those psychological phenomena that are in fact fairly directly influenced by underlying biological changes, with minimal individual differences arising from current social influences and/or personality structure. In research on the psychology of the menstrual cycle, for example, phenomena related to basic sensory processes appear to be a domain of psychological functioning for which a biological perspective is fruitful (Baker, 1975; Parlee, 1982). Similarly, in psychological research on menopause, it may well be the case that psychological phenomena related to and including hot flashes are best studied from a biological perspective (Nelson, 1979).

On the other hand, researchers can also adopt a *psychological* perspective in studying the psychology of female reproduction. From this perspective, the conceptual starting point is *psychological change over time.* The research question is: What is the nature of the processes—biological, social, and psychological—that produce psychological changes?

In the study of the psychology of women at midlife, researchers are adopting what is here called a psychological perspective when they hypothesize and examine the ways in which changes in social roles might cause psychological changes in middle-aged women (Barnett and Baruch, 1978). Such psychological changes might or might not also be influenced by the biological changes of the climacterium. From a psychological perspective, then, researchers can in principle take into account multiple, covarying causal processes of different kinds (biological, social, psychological). As with the biological perspective, the success of research conducted from a psychological perspective depends upon the investigator's being able to find an appropriate fit between the kind of psychological phenomenon being studied and the kind(s) of causal process(es) by which it is influenced. This is very difficult to do, particularly when the psychological phenomenon under investigation (changes in depression, for example) may be subject to different causal influences operating at the same time and also to primary causation by one kind of process (biological changes) at one time and another kind of process (role loss) at another.

In addition to the inherent difficulty of the subject matter, psychological research on female reproduction in general, and on menopause in particular, is made more difficult by the way in which everyday language and thought highlight some features of the phenomenon and mask others. According to stereotypes popular in much of the United States, certain aspects of women's behavior under particular conditions tend to be causally attributed to their reproductive biology. As Randi Koeske has pointed out and demonstrated (Koeske, 1981; Koeske and Koeske, 1975), premenstrual changes in physiology are often taken to be the cause for negative, out-of-role behavior for women (e.g., anger, aggression). Stereotypes about a "premenstrual tension syndrome," regardless of the extent to which they are descriptively accurate, can thus serve as a cohesive explanatory framework, assimilating within it actions and experiences that might also have nonbiological causes.

For the present argument, it is important to note that *everyday thought and language tend to impute a causal role to female reproductive biology at major transition points in the social life cycle.* It is also at such points that deviancy from role expectations might be predicted by sociologists to trigger social labeling and other social processes that either produce conformity or isolate the deviant individual as mad (sick) or bad (Scheff, 1966). The phrase "postpartum depression," for example, serves to highlight and isolate a physiological event (birth) as the implicit cause of the psychological phenomenon to be explained (depression). "New mother depression," of course, would be an equally accurate description of the concurrent biological, psychological, and social events. A woman who is depressed after the birth of a child, however, departs from the general social expectation that motherhood is usually a pleasurable and fulfilling role. Deviancy theory would predict that when such behavior threatens the smooth functioning of an important social institution (in this case, the family), the deviant individual is labeled and becomes a focus of social processes (or social interactions shaped by roles within institutions) that serve to protect the integrity of society as a whole (Lemert, 1964).

Thus, the new mother who is depressed is described as suffering from "postpartum depression." Her behavior will be tolerated because of her "illness" until she is ready to take up her nondepressing role as mother. In extreme cases, doctors may prescribe drugs for her or recommend hospitalization to cure her "postpartum depression." Social changes that might make the role of mother less depressing are not considered, since the assumption (incorporated in the label) is that the individual woman is suffering psychological problems as a result of changes in her postpartum reproductive biology. Some postpartum depressions may, in fact, as the label implies, have fairly clear and direct biological causes. The important point for the present argument, however, is that the labeling and social processes mobilized in response to it make no effort to discriminate women with such biologically caused postpartum depression from those whose depression arises from role changes and thus, if understood and acted upon, might represent a threat to the stability of social roles within the family.

As with other labeling phenomena studied by deviancy theorists, it is particularly striking that the social responses to potential deviance are usually initiated and carried out by decent, well-meaning, caring people. The husband, family, friends, and doctors of the depressed mother are not conspiring to disregard or mask the real sources of her depression by making causal attributions to reproductive biology. They genuinely want to help. The fact is, however, that ordinary language and thought focus attention exclusively on biology, and these thought patterns are deeply implicated in both social roles and institutions and in the psychology of individuals in them. The acquisition of culture by the individual through language makes it unlikely that he or she will focus on (think about) the presence and properties of phenomena that are unnamed in everyday language and thought (Scribner and Cole, 1974), or that different names and meanings will be given to those that are named.

Researchers as well as laypeople have found it difficult to break away from an everyday explanatory framework that attributes postpartum psychological changes to reproductive biology. One consequence of this has been an inability to develop a cumulative body of psychological research and theory on the postpartum period (Parlee, 1978). Everyday thought has encouraged a biological perspective in the research when a psychological perspective seems also to be appropriate and necessary if scientific progress is to be made.

Labeling and thinking about certain psychological phenomena as "menopausal" has had much the same effect, both in life and in research. The word's reference to biological changes highlights their potential causal significance and implicitly masks concomitant changes in social roles and in age-related psychological development. It is applied to women at a transition point in the social life cycle when several major roles are likely to be changing, either because they have run their natural course or because of general physical changes of the aging process.

While it is not clear what the role expectations for a "menopausal woman" are, it is fairly clear that, as deviance theory would predict, labeling her in this way has consequences for the way others treat her, and perhaps also for the way she regards herself and her possibilities in life. The biological label may thus serve to reduce the likelihood that she and others will examine her experiences in light of possible social and psychological causes.

The problem of linguistic/conceptual bias toward exclusively biological causes is much more acute with menopause, however, than with any of the other major stages of the female reproductive life cycle, One reason is that a much broader range of psychological phenomena are causally attributed to the menopause than to either the recurring changes of the menstrual cycle or to pregnancy, birth, and postpartum. Stereotypes about the "menopausal woman" not only encompass emotional and perhaps cognitive changes but also seem to carry with them a subtle pejorative reference to her inconsequential social status and perhaps also to her physical appearance. Research concepts arising from everyday language and thought, then, seem implicitly to assimilate multiple domains and levels of psychological functioning within the single explanatory framework of changes in reproductive biology. This seems implausible on the face of it, and no body of research has been accumulated to date that would suggest that this biological perspective alone will prove adequate.

There is a second, related reason why research based on concepts from everyday language and thought is more problematic for menopause than for other phases of the reproductive life cycle, It is that the time scales of the psychological, social, and biological changes are not coincident in the way they are for the menstrual cycle and for pregnancy and birth. The biological changes of pregnancy, for example, are temporally concomitant with the psychological changes. Regardless of whether one adopts a psychological or a biological perspective in psychological research on pregnancy, it makes sense to examine biological influences on all the psychological processes occurring over the given time period.

In psychological research on menopause, however, the situation is different. If one adopts a biological perspective, the task is to identify the domain(s) of psychological functioning that are causally influenced by biological changes occurring over a time period defined in terms of biological markers. If one adopts a psychological perspective, the task is to identify a relatively limited domain of psychological functioning that changes over a given time period (defined by psychological markers) and then to ask what biological, psychological, and social processes might account for these changes. Many of the areas of psychological functioning that one might want to explore in women in midlife occur over a different time scale—longer, shorter, or at a different time altogether—from physiological changes of the climacterium (including menopause). For example, one might be interested in changes in depression or self-esteem in women at midlife. Such changes could occur in conjunction with major changes in social roles, with menopause as a discrete event marking the end of fertility, with difficulty in separating from children or parents, with the physical changes of the climacteric, with repeated social encounters with those disdainful of "menopausal women." One needs to discover the major causal influences on clearly defined psychological changes through psychological research. But it obviously need not be assumed at the start that the psychological changes of interest will be concomitant in time with the psychological changes of the climacteric and menopause.

As psychologists interested in women at midlife, we need to identify those psychological issues and processes we think are of greater significance or interest according to whatever criteria we choose to use. My hunch is that from this psychological perspective, the significant psychological issues at midlife are not greatly affected by physiological changes of the climacterium. Most psychologists are probably more interested in specific aspects of psychological changes and development in personality and behavior over the course of the middle years than in the more limited class of psychological events that present evidence suggests is fairly directly caused by the climacterium (Nadelson et al., 1979; Notman, 1979).

The conclusions from feminist research and critique (outlined above) all point to the same inference. The ongoing changes in behavior and experience occurring in midlife women are not very closely related to the climacteric or to menopause. Yet too often researchers interested in midlife have continued to focus on menopause as the conceptual starting point for the research, attempting to assimilate within its potential explanatory domain relatively large arenas of behavior extending over long periods of time. It is of course difficult to avoid in research the patterns of language and thought in the culture that have conflated middle age and menopause. But it can and must be done if scientific psychological research and theory are to proceed beyond critiques.

The fragmented, noncumulative state of the psychological literature on menopause continues unambiguously to suggest that a biological perspective is not appropriate, except in research on the psychological nature and consequences of hot flashes and flushes (Nelson, 1979; Feldman, Postlethwaite, and Glenn, 1976). If researchers interested in specific psychological changes occurring in women in the middle years consistently adopt a psychological perspective, they may well find that menopause plays little or no causal role (Barnett and Baruch, 1978; Notman, 1979; Wood, 1979). The time has surely come when investigators studying middle-aged women can respond to the implicit or explicit query "But what about menopause?" with "What *about* menopause?" And let it go at that. The stereotypes imputing causal significance to menopause need be granted no scientific standing. The burden of proof can now be placed on those who want to argue that menopause is psychologically significant in such-and-such (and let them specify) domains of behavior and experience.

In fact, I think menopause may be psychologically significant in at least the following two domains: (1) It may be the stimulus for application of a social label (stigma) that triggers social interactions having negative consequences for women. DeLorey describes some that occur in one very important social institution, the health-care system. It is clear, however, that it is the application of the label and not the physiological event that is psychologically significant. Women who are or ought to be menopausal may be treated in certain ways (and we need to know what these are), regardless of their actual biological status. (2) Menopause may be psychologically significant as one marker of the cessation of fertility, an event that seems likely to have different meanings for different women. It is important, however, to note here, too, that menopause is only one event that may trigger psychological concern with and resolution of issues related to fertility. Some women may deal with such issues when they have a hysterectomy, others when they are diagnosed by a physician as infertile.

In both of these potential areas of research, it is the psychological processes and issues that are the main focus. Menopause plays a role, but not the direct causal role implied in the biological perspective. Consistently adopting a psychological perspective in research on midlife women, then, may even enable us to learn more about the genuine psychological significance of menopause—and a great deal more about psychological changes in midlife.

REFERENCES

Ballinger, C. B. Psychiatric morbidity and the menopause; screening of general population sample. *British Medical Journal*, 1975, 2, 344–346.
Ballinger, C. B. Subjective sleep disturbance at the menopause. *Journal of Psychosomatic Research*, 1976, 20, 509–513.
Barnett, R. C., and Baruch, G. K. Women in the middle years: A critique of research and theory. *Psychology of Women Quarterly*, 1978, 3, 187–197.
Bart, P. B., and Grossman, M. Menopause. *Women and Health*, 1976, 1, 3–11.

Boston Women's Health Book Collective. *Our bodies, ourselves.* New York: Simon & Schuster, 1973.
Cowan, G. Medical perceptions of menopausal symptoms. *Psychology of Women Quarterly,* in press.
Dan, A. J., Graham, E. A., and Beecher, C. P. (Eds.). *The menstrual cycle (Vol. 1): A synthesis of interdisciplinary research.* New York: Springer, 1981.
Donovan, J. C. Menopausal syndrome: A study of case histories. *American Journal of Obstetrics and Gynecology,* 1951, *62,* 1281–1286.
Eisenberg, J. M. Sociologic influences on decision-making by clinicians. *Annals of Internal Medicine,* 1979, *90,* 957–964.
Feldman, J. M., Postlethwaite, R. W., and Glenn, J. F. Hot flashes and sweats in men with testicular insufficiency. *Archives of Internal Medicine,* 1976, *136,* 606–608.
Flint, M. The menopause: Reward or punishment? *Psychosomatics,* 1975, *16,* 161–163.
Friedman, R. C. (Ed.). *Behavior and the menstrual cycle.* New York: Marcell Dekker, 1982.
Golub, S. (Ed.). *Menarche.* Boston: Heath, in press.
Goodman, M. J., Stewart, C. J., and Gilbert, F., Jr. Patterns of menopause: A study of certain medical and physiological variables among Caucasian and Japanese women living in Hawaii. *Journal of Gerontology,* 1977, *32,* 291–98.
Greene, J. G. A factor analytic study of climacteric symptoms. *Journal of Psychosomatic Research,* 1976, *20,* 425–430.
Greene, J. G., and Cooke, D. J. Life stress and symptons at the climacterium. *British Journal of Psychiatry,* 1980, *136,* 486–491.
Koeske, R. D. Theoretical perspectives for menstrual cycle research. In A. J. Dan, E. A. Graham, and C. P. Beecher (Eds.), *The menstrual cycle (Vol. 1): A synthesis of interdisciplinary research.* New York: Springer, 1981.
Koeske, R. D., and Koeske, G. F. An attributional approach to moods and the menstrual cycle. *Journal of Personality and Social Psychology,* 1975, *31,* 473–478.
Komnenich, P., McSweeney, M., Noack, J. A., and Elder, S. N. (Eds.). *The menstrual cycle, (Vol. 2): Research and implications for women's health.* New York: Springer, 1981.
Lemert, E. M. Social structure, social control, and deviation. In M. B. Clinard (Ed.), *Anomie and deviant behavior.* New York: Free Press of Glencoe, 1964.
Nadelson, C. C., Polonsky, D. C., and Mathews, M. A. Marriage and midlife: The impact of social change. *Journal of Clinical Psychiatry,* 1979, *40,* 292–298.
Nelson, S. B. Flooding, flashing, and flushing: Emotional repercussions. *Arizona Medicine,* 1979, *36,* 675–678.
Neugarten, B. L., and Kraines, R. J. "Menopausal symptoms" in women of various ages. *Psychosomatic Medicine,* 1965, *27,* 266–273.
Neugarten, B. L., Wood, V., Kraines, R. J., and Loomis, B. Women's attitudes toward the menopause. *Vita Humana,* 1963, *6,* 140–151.
Notman, M. Midlife concerns of women: Implications of the menopause. *American Journal of Psychiatry,* 1979, *136,* 1270–1274.
Osofsky, H. J., and Seidenberg, R. Is female menopausal depression inevitable? *Obstetrics and Gynecology,* 1970, *36,* 611–615.
Parlee, M. B. Psychological aspects of menstruation, childbirth, and menopause. In J. A. Sherman and F. L. Denmark (Eds.), *The psychology of women: Future directions of research.* New York: Psychological Dimensions, 1978.
Parlee, M. B. Gaps in behavioral research on the menstrual cycle. In P. Komnenich, M. McSweeney, J. A. Noack, and S. N. Elder (Eds.), *The menstrual cycle, (Vol. 2): Research and implications for women's health.* New York: Springer, 1981.
Parlee, M. B. The psychology of the menstrual cycle: Biological and psychological perspectives. In R. C. Friedman (Ed.), *Behavior and the menstrual cycle.* New York: Marcel Dekker, 1982.

Polit, D. F., and LaRocco. Social and psychological correlates of menopausal symptoms. *Psychosomatic Medicine*, 1980, *42*, 335–345.

Posner, J. It's all in your head: Feminist and medical models of menopause (strange bedfellows). *Sex Roles*, 1979, *5*, 179–190.

Scheff, T. J. *Being mentally ill: A sociological theory.* Chicago: Aldine, 1966.

Scribner, S., and Cole, M. *Culture and thought.* New York: Wiley, 1974.

Severne, L. Psycho-social aspects of the menopause. In A. A. Haspels and H. Musaph (Eds.), *Psychosomatics in peri-menopause.* Baltimore: University Park Press, 1979.

Townsend, J. M., and Carbone, C. L. Menopausal syndrome: Illness or social role—A transcultural analysis. *Culture, Medicine, and Psychiatry*, 1980, *4*, 229–248.

van Keep, P. A., and Humphrey, M. Psycho-social aspects of the climacteric. In P. A. van Keep, R. B. Greenblatt, and M. Albeaux-Femet (Eds.), *Consensus on menopause research.* Baltimore: University Park Press, 1976.

van Keep, P. A., and Kellerhals, J. M. The ageing women: About the influence of some social and cultural factors on the changes in attitude and behavior that occur during and after the menopause. *Acta Obstetricia et Gynecologica Scandinavica, Supplement*, 1976, *51*, 19–27.

Weissman, M. M. The myth of involutional melancholia. *Journal of the American Medical Association*, 1979, *242*, 742–744.

Wood, C. Menopausal myths. *Medical Journal of Australia*, 1979, *1*, 496–499.

Chapter 14

The Midlife Woman as Student

NANCY K. SCHLOSSBERG

A learning explosion is under way in this country. According to a study conducted by the College Board's Future Directions for a Learning Society, "half of all Americans 25 years and older (over 60 million adults) learned one or more topics in the past year" (Aslanian and Brickell, 1980, p. 43). Women constituted over half (52%) of this group of learners. The definition of *learning* used in the college board study was broad, encompassing informal and independent learning activities as well as organized, formal instruction. Hence, the estimated participation rate is unusually high.

Other estimates of adult participation in learning are more modest. For example, the National Center for Education Statistics (NCES) reports that in 1978 over 18 million people participated in adult education, defined as "courses and organized educational activities other than those taken by full-time students in programs leading toward a high school diploma or an academic degree and in occupational programs of six months or more duration" (Dearman and Plisko, 1980, p. 230). Thus, of the age-25-and-over population, about 12% were involved in adult education. Of these 18 million participants, 36% were 25–34 years old, 34% were 35–54 years old, and 2.4% were age 65 and older. Women outnumbered men in all age groups among adult-education participants, constituting 57% of the total. Their predominance was particularly evident in the older groups: They account for 61% of the 55–64-year-olds and 69% of the age-65-and-older group of adult education participants.

Because of recent definitional changes, reliable trends are difficult to calculate from NCES data for 1978. Earlier statistics show, however, that

---

NANCY K. SCHLOSSBERG • Department of Education, University of Maryland, College Park, Maryland 20742.

between 1969 and 1975, the number of adults particpating in continuing education activities increased by 30.8%, while the total adult population increased by only 12.6%. This growth in the number of adult education participants was much greater among women (an annual average of 6.4%) than among men (an annual average of 1.9%), though it was smallest for women between 35 and 54 years old (2.5% annually) and largest for women aged 55 and over (7.6% annually) (Entine, 1978, p. 156). The proportion of the population aged 17 and older who participate in adult education seems to have stabilized at about 12.5% since 1975, but the actual number has continued to increase as the adult population has increased. Moreover, "the size of the adult population is projected to grow further throughout the 1980's, suggesting that if the participation rate remains constant, the number of adult education participants will continue to grow" (Dearman and Plisko, 1980, p. 231).

The number of adults enrolling in the *collegiate* sector has increased even more dramatically. Indeed, according to an article by Magarrell (1981), "institutions concerned about maintaining their enrollment levels are looking to the older groups to offset, at least partially, a decline in the population of 18-year-olds during the 1980s" (p. 3). Although the number of students aged 35 and older attending the nation's colleges and universities increased by 36.8% between 1975 and 1979, only a small proportion of the total adult population aged 35 and older were attending higher education institutions. To summarize, "over 18 million adults participated in . . . formal education . . . in 1978 . . . [while] over 136 million adults did not participate" (Charner, 1981).

Granting that more adults are becoming involved in formal education programs, what else do we know about who they are, besides the fact that more are women? We know that relative to the general adult population, adult education participants tended to be well educated, to have high incomes, to live in the suburbs rather than the central city or rural areas, and to hold high-status jobs; underrepresented are the blue-collar and farm workers, the unemployed blacks and Hispanics (Dearman and Plisko, 1980, p. 232).

We know that of those women participating in higher education, the majority still "have more marginal status and stand on more tenuous educational ground than men" (Randour, Strasburg, and Lipman-Blumen, 1981, p. 33). They are still concentrated in female-intensive fields whose status and market value is low, they are less well-represented at each higher degree level, and they are more likely than men to be enrolled in public institutions and to attend college on a part-time basis. Randour *et al* deplore the increasing tendency of women to enter community colleges, which have been shown negatively to affect degree aspirations and persistance (see Astin, 1975; Karabel, 1972). Thus, women have not yet achieved parity with men in higher education. Despite these reservations, the authors agree that older women have made rapid strides in recent years.

This theme is sounded again in a recent release from the Project on the Status and Education of Women: "Re-entry women—women over 25 who have interrupted their education for at least a few years and are now entering or re-entering postsecondary institutions—comprise the largest potential source of students, and their participation in higher education is expected to increase for some time to come" (Hall and Gleaves, 1981, p. 1).

In short, statistics show and observers agree that increasing numbers of adult women engage in learning activities and pursue formal education, although the number of nonparticipants far exceeds the number of participants. This background provides the context for the remainder of this chapter, which is based on a series of questions: (1) Is there such an entity as the adult learner? (2) What factors motivate women to become learners? (3) What are the barriers hindering women from pursuing education? (4) What can be said of the learning experience itself for those women pursuing education? The following sections address these questions.

THE ADULT LEARNER: SOME ASSUMPTIONS

Is there such an entity as "the adult learner"? As evidenced by the growing number of articles and books on the subject, adult learners have special needs and capacities that distinguish them from traditional-aged students. At the same time, the group is very diverse. Adult learners are a heterogeneous group, just as younger learners are. Some are bright, others dull; some are knowledgeable, other ignorant; some are energetic, others apathetic; some are anxious, others self-confident.

Either position gives rise to certain difficulties. To say that the adult learner is a distinctive category feeds into the agism of our society and evokes other stereotypes that bear little relation to reality. For instance, many minority women (and other special populations) are hesitant to enroll in reentry and continuing education programs because they have a "gilded cage" image of such programs, seeing them as aimed primarily at "bored, middle-class, middle-aged housewives" (Hall and Gleaves, 1981, p. 5). Similarly, adult and continuing education is often denigrated on the grounds that it consists chiefly of such courses as basket weaving and flower arranging. Even if one avoids these oversimplifications, making age the central variable still carries some dangers. One is apt to overlook other important characteristics of the adult learner or, worse, to conclude that some people are simply too old to learn.

On the other hand, denying the existence of adult learners as a distinct category may well lead to overlooking some of the special needs of that population, needs that should be addressed by policy-makers and educators.

In brief, age may be a salient but not the central defining variable. Given these caveats, we will examine two issues: (1) the relationship between age and learning capacity and (2) the categorization of midlife women.

The Relationship of Age to Learning Capacity

Though few people in this day and age would subscribe to the notion that "you can't teach an old dog new tricks," the conventional wisdom seems to be that intellectual functioning slows down with age. For instance, Cattell (1963) differentiated *fluid intelligence* (the ability to process information rapidly in problem solving) from *crystallized intelligence* (stored information such as vocabulary and general knowledge). The former seems to decline with age, whereas the latter seems to remain stable and even to improve (Gallagher, Thompson, and Levy, 1980, p. 23). While brain cells are continually being destroyed as a person ages, there are more than enough active brain cells to ensure that the intellectual functioning of most men and women will remain adequate until they die, except in cases of illness where, for instance, the circulatory supply to the brain is disturbed (Ramey, 1981).

Reviewing issues connected with the study of adult intelligence, Willis and Baltes (1980) conclude: "Chronological age per se accounts for a relatively modest amount of the variance observed in intellectual aging during late adulthood up to the 60s or early 70s" (p. 263). According to Willis and Baltes, one must take into account three sets of influences on intellectual functioning.

> *Age-graded influences:*—those biological and environmental determinants that are correlated with chronological age; "their occurrence, timing, and duration are fairly similar for all individuals of a given set of aging cohorts" (p. 267).
> *History-graded influences*—those biological and environmental events correlated with historical change: "Their degree of generality and predictability varies. Some of them, however, are fairly normative, in that they apply to most members of a given set of aging cohorts in similar ways" (p. 267). For instance, people who grew up during the Great Depression may differ in consistent ways from people

who grew up in the post-World War II era of economic expansion, and these differences may be reflected in their cognitive functioning. Similarly, intergenerational differences in labor force participation or family life may result in intergenerational differences in intellectual development.

Nonnormative critical life events—those events in the life of the individual that are relatively idiosyncratic: e.g., usual opportunities for learning, illness, unemployment, bereavement. Such events may affect intellectual development directly (as in the case of disease that results in brain damage) or indirectly, through stress.

Willis and Baltes maintain that, if investigators are to arrive at an understanding of intellectual development over the life-span, they must give greater attention in their research designs to history-graded influences and nonnormative critical life events.

Learning capacity may improve rather than decrease over time in certain situations. Kohn (1980) and his associates identified more than 50 job dimensions or occupational conditions, 12 of which were found to have significant positive effects on psychological functioning, after all other pertinent factors were statistically controlled. The most important of these dimensions is *substantive complexity*, defined as "the degree to which the work, in its very substance, requires thought and independent judgment. Substantively complex work by its very nature requires making many decisions that must take into account ill-defined or apparently conflicting contingencies. . . . The index of substantive complexity that we have generally employed is based on the degree of complexity of the person's work with things, with data, and with people" (Kohn, 1980, p. 197). Kohn further asserts that substantive complexity is a central structural characteristic of the work experience; that it is related to a wide range of psychological factors including job satisfaction, occupational commitment, self-direction, self-esteem, authoritarian conservatism, and intellectual flexibility; and that the causal relation is reciprocal—that is, one's psychological functioning affects the substantive complexity of the work one does, and the substantive complexity of the work one does affects one's psychological functioning. Looking in particular at intellectual flexibility, as indicated by performance and behavior on tests and during interviews, Kohn states:

> If two men of equivalent intellectual flexibility were to start their careers in jobs different in substantive complexity, the man in the more complex job would be likely to outstrip the other in further intellectual growth. This, in time, might lead to his attaining jobs of greater complexity, further affecting his intellectual growth. Meantime, the man in the less complex job would develop intellectually at a slower pace, perhaps not at all, and in the extreme

case might even decline in his intellectual functioning. As a result, small differences in the substantive complexity of early jobs might lead to increasing differences in intellectual development. (Kohn, 1980, p. 203)

Moreover, similar results emerged from a study of 269 employed married women. Those women whose work was substantively complex and, in addition, nonroutinized (i.e., involved a variety of unpredictable tasks) demonstrated greater intellectual flexibility than those women performing relatively simple, routine work (Miller, Schooler, Kohn, and Miller, 1979, p. 80).

How do these findings apply to the topic of midlife women and education? Women who have been continuously exposed to stimulating and complex environments that exercise their problem-solving abilities may be more intellectually flexible—and thus more likely to benefit from learning activities—than those women who work in environments where they perform only routine and repetitive tasks. Although the research of Kohn and his associates has been limited to employed adults, one could argue that many women who do not hold outside jobs nonetheless perform work—in the home and in the community—of considerable substantive complexity. Further, those women who do play occupational, as well as conjugal and maternal, roles may live substantively complex lives even if their jobs are relatively low-level.

In brief, age is not the sole, or even the primary, determinant of learning capacity. History-graded influences, nonnormative critical life events, and the substantive complexity of the environment must also be considered in assessing the individual's learning capacity. These points deserve emphasis because many midlife women (and men as well) are victims of the age stereotypes that pervade our society. Because they feel they have slowed down intellectually, they may be fearful of committing themselves to educational activities. The evidence cited here indicates that such fears are probably groundless.

Categorizing Midlife Women

Two ways to classify women as students are in terms of cognitive development (Perry, 1970) and in terms of role involvement (Campbell, Wilson, and Harrison, 1980; Lowenthal, Thurnher, and Chiriboga, 1975). Both these classificatory schemes seem particularly well-suited to studying the midlife women as learner because they touch on aspects of her life and personality that are directly connected with her response to education, and they may be useful for planning curricula and advising midlife students.

COGNITIVE DEVELOPMENT. Perry's model of cognitive development (1970) grew out of his empirical work with several cohorts of Harvard undergraduates, who were studied longitudinally from their freshman to their senior years. In interviews at the end of each year, the students were asked a broad general question about what had "stood out" for them during the year and then were questioned in more detail. Their responses were found to reflect attitudes about the nature of knowledge and thinking, the function of educational institutions and teachers, the responsibility of the learner, and so forth. Perry defined a set of hierarchical stages, which are as follows:

Basic Duality. The world is seen in terms of such polarities as good–bad, right–wrong. Knowledge is absolute, and Authority (the teacher) has the Right Answer, which will duly be revealed to the hardworking and obedient student.

Multiplicity Prelegitimate. Differences of opinion exist, but they are attributable to confusion on the part of the teacher or are an exercise set by the teacher so that students can find the Right Answer for themselves.

Multiplicity. Uncertainty and differences of opinion are acceptable in some areas where the Right Answer simply has not been discovered yet. At the extreme, the student believes that "anyone has a right to his own opinion" and that all opinions have equal validity.

Relativism. All knowledge and values, including those of Authority, are contextual and relativistic.

Commitment. Although absolute certainty is impossible, some kind of personal commitment or affirmation is needed. The student makes such a commitment. As this commitment develops, the student affirms his or her own identity.

Not all students progress through the stages easily and smoothly to attain the highest level. Most difficult for both traditional-aged and adult students is the shift from Multiplicity to Relativism, which involves "discarding the view that knowledge is a quantitative accretion of discrete rightness, including the kind of discrete rightness in which everyone has a right to his own opinion, and adopting a conception of knowledge as the qualitative assessment of contextual observations and relationships" (Weathersby and Tarule, 1980, p. 34). In addition, Perry's model resembles Kohlberg's (1970) theory of moral development and Loevinger's (1976) theory of ego development in that all three view development as progression from the simple to the complex, from an external orientation (where the individual is dependent on authority or on the judgment of others) to an inner orientation (where the individual takes responsibility for the consequences of his or her own actions), from absolutism and dogmatism to increasing tolerance for ambiguity and uncertainty, from a tendency to perceive those outside one's own immediate group in stereotypic terms to increasing awareness of individual differences and greater empathy with others, and "from a strong self focus to a posture of conformity to the group and then to a mature focus on mutual interdependence on others. The individual is truly autonomous and inner-directed when she arrives at the point of acknowledging her interdependence on others in her life" (Knefelkamp, Widick, and Stroad, 1976, p. 16).

Perry's model is useful because of its direct applicability to understanding adult learners. It is more useful to know whether a learner is a dualist or a relativist rather than whether he or she is age 20, 40, or 60. Teaching and curriculum development should be geared to the individual's style of learning and not the individual's chronological age.

ROLE INVOLVEMENT. Some attention needs to be given to the midlife woman student's involvement in other roles and activities as one way of understanding her attitudes toward and response to education. The role-involvement typology most directly related to adult learners was developed in a study of age-25-and-over undergraduates at the University of Texas in 1979 (Campbell *et al.*, 1980). On the basis of time spent in various activities (e.g., working at a paying job, doing schoolwork, doing things with the family), these adult students were classified into five types:

Type 1. These were full-time students who were not employed and who spent more than 40 hours a week with their families and had little free time. This group was largely women (75%), most of whom had at least one child at home.

Type 2. This category comprised full-time students who were not employed and who had few family responsibilities and a considerable amount of free time. Forty-two percent were women. Over half of the total group were single or divorced.

Type 3. These were part-time students who were employed full time, spent little time with their families, and had considerable free time. Again, women constituted a little under half of this group (47%).

Type 4. In this group were full-time students who were not employed and who, despite their family ties, spent little time in family or social/recreational activities but a great deal of time (an average of over 60 hours a week) on schoolwork and had little free time. About half of this group (42%) were women; about a third of the total group had at least one child at home.

Type 5. This type were students who were employed full time, had signed up for one or two courses, spent a great deal of time in family activities, and had very little free time. Forty-nine percent were women; 49% had one child.

Campbell and his associates found that the five types of adult learners differed "on a number of background characteristics, on the degree of difficulty they had in deciding to return to school, and on the kind of problems they had after enrollment. . . . Members of one type were as likely as members of another to have difficulties adjusting to student life; however, the reasons for these difficulties varied by type" (Campbell et al., 1980, p. 85).

This discussion of role involvement points out that there is no single category of midlife women. Women have many kinds of role involvement. To some degree, those involvements will determine whether a particular midlife women will decide to pursue education at all. The next section examines in more detail the various "push" and "pull" factors that may motivate the midlife woman to return to school.

MOTIVATION FOR LEARNING

Reviewing the literature on motivation for learning, Cross (1981) distinguishes those investigators who deal with types of learners from those who deal with clusters of learning motives. A broad perspective on learning motives is offered by Kuhlen (1963), who suggests that adult behavior in general is impelled by two "meta-motives": The first is a positive drive for expansion and growth; the second is a self-protective drive, based on anxiety and insecurity, to compensate for perceived inadequacies. Obviously, both motives may be present in the pursuit of education; that is, adult learners may be motivated by a desire to achieve in their careers, to improve their social skills and interpersonal relations, or simply to expand their knowledge of the world; or they may be "pushed" by the fear that, without further education, they will lose their jobs, their friends, or their cognitive powers.

Like Kuhlen, White (1976) believes that people have a lifelong drive for competence, a need to expand, explore, and achieve mastery over the world and over themslues. As they grow older, they continually try out new coping mechanisms that will facilitate "successful transaction with the environment." Empirical support for this view comes from a study of the wives of coal miners (Giesen and Datan, 1980), women between the ages of 47 and 62 who had fewer resources than most women in this age group. Contradicting the stereotype of older women as "dependent, passive, incompetent, and generally unable to deal with the problems and crises of life" (p. 57), this study found that most of the women interviewed gave evidence of being able to "interact effectively with the environment" and "to cope with and solve problems" (p. 60). Moreover, most of them felt they had gained in competence and were better able to handle life than they had been at a younger age. Similarly, a study of women who lead complex lives found that those who were satisfied with their multiple roles also showed gains in competence and in sense of well-being (Baruch and Barnett, 1980).

Obviously, there are many possible approaches to the question of what motivates midlife women to pursue learning. In the remainder of this section, two recent contributions to the literature will be presented. The first, by Aslanian and Brickell (1980), see life changes as providing the impetus for adult learning. The second, while not dealing directly with adult education, is nonetheless highly suggestive; it is Marjorie Fiske's (1980) view of changes in value commitments over time.

Life Changes

Aslanian and Brickell (1980) attribute the learning explosion currently under way in the United States to the aging of the population; the greater labor force participation of women; the growth in the proportions of part-time workers and of professional, managerial, and service workers and the concomitant decline in the proportions of laborers, factory operatives, and craft workers; and the increase in leisure time. More adults are seeking and will continue to seek learning opportunities as a means of facilitating their adaptation to these transitions.

Aslanian and Brickell define a *transition* as a "change in status . . . that makes learning necessary. The adult needs to become competent at something that he or she could not do before in order to succeed in the new status" (pp. 38–39). It should be noted that learning can be informal and self-directed; it need not involve formal, organized instruction. The authors further distinguish between a transition and a *trigger*, defined as the specific life event that precipitates "the decision to learn at that point in time" (p. 39). The trigger is not necessarily related either to the transition or to the topic studied. For instance, an unemployed woman who is suddenly widowed may enroll in a medical technology course in order to become qualified for a job. The transition is the change of status from nonworker to worker; the triggering event is the husband's death.

Finally, Aslanian and Brickell identify seven life areas into which both transitions and triggers may be classified: career, family, health, religion, citizenship, art, and leisure. Within this theoretical framework, they examine the data collected through personal and telephone interviews with a national sample of approximately 1500 subjects who were 25 years of age or older. Among the most notable findings to emerge from this survey were the following:

1. Close to half the sample indicated that they were engaged in

some kind of learning activity at the time of the survey or had been so engaged during the previous year.
2. Over four in five of the learners (83%) said that they were motivated to learn by some transition in their lives; only 17% were learning simply for the sake of learning.
3. Of those who said that some life transition had motivated them, 56% cited career transitions, 16% cited family transitions, and 13% cited leisure transitions.
4. Sex differences in reasons for learning were evident: 71% of the men, but only 42% of the women, mentioned career transition. Twice as many women (21%) as men (10%) mentioned family transitions. Women were also more likely than men to mention transitions in the areas of leisure, health, religion, art, and citizenship. In short, women show greater variation in their reasons for learning.

Looking more closely at the various life areas, career transitions—the top-ranked reasons for both men and women—include moving into a new job, adapting to a changing job, and advancing in a career. Specific triggers included such events as technological or organizational changes demanding the acquisition of new skills, an offer of advancement, job termination, and retirement. The triggering event for many women who engage in learning for career-related reasons often lies in family life: The youngest child enters school or leaves home, the couple is divorced or separated, the husband dies.

In the area of family life, many women pursue education to learn how to can food, how to prepare special cuisines, how to make household repairs, how to sew. Other transitions in this area include adapting to shifts in family income or changes in the health of a family member. Family-centered events that may trigger learning activities include marriage, pregnancy, children's progress through school, divorce, residential moves, the retirement or death of a family member, and changes in family income.

Transitions in the area of leisure involved acquiring "skills in sports, crafts, hobbies, and social activities, for the sole purpose of making constructive use of free time" (Aslanian and Brickell, 1980, p. 77). Triggers for these changes always occurred in some other areas: For instance, retirement from a job, a reduction in the work week, or a child's entering kindergarten may all lead to an increase in the leisure time of an adult; similarly, a residential move or a divorce may lead to a change in one's social circle and thus to the development of new interests. Closely related to leisure are changes in artistic life that prompt the adult to take piano lessons (for instance) or to take a course in art appreciation. Transitions in the area of personal health take two forms: recovering from illness or injury and maintaining physical fitness. Transitions in religious life include religious conversions; transitions in citizenship including becoming a citizen and becoming a volunteer worker.

Clearly, career transitions are the primary reasons behind learning for both sexes, while changes in family life are much more likely to be triggers for women (52%) than for men (20%). Aslanian and Brickell suggest, "To know an adult's life schedule is to know an adult's learning schedule" (p. 61).

Changes in Commitments

A look at changing commitments—or what gives meaning to one's life—throws some additional light on why many midlife women pursue education. According to Fiske (1980), the individual's value hierarchy does not remain constant over the life-span; rather, major changes or reorientations in commitment may occur. As she grows older, the woman may become increasingly concerned with mastery, competence, and dominance. Even if such a value shift does not take place, she may find that her interpersonal and altruistic commitments can no longer be fulfilled by family life. In either case, she may be motivated to pursue education as a means of giving expression to her value commitments.

BARRIERS TO LEARNING

What of the other side of the coin? With the various life and commitment changes that may be pushing her to pursue education, what factors prevent the midlife woman from reentering an educational program? Cross (1981) identifies three types of barriers:

Situational—those barriers "arising from one's situation in life at a given time" (p. 98): e.g., lack of time, lack of funds.
Institutional—"all those practices and procedures that exclude or discourage . . . participation" (p. 98): e.g., financial aid policies, scheduling of classes.
Dispositional—those barriers "related to attitudes and self-perceptions about oneself as a learner" (p. 98): e.g., lack of confidence in academic ability, lack of energy, fear of being too old to begin.

Carp, Peterson, and Roelfs (1974) surveyed "potential learners" (i.e., those who indicated that they had a desire to learn but that they were not currently engaged in any kind of organized educational program) to find out the relative importance of various barriers (Table 1), which will be discussed in the following section.

Table 1. Perceived Barriers to Learning[a]

Barriers	Percent of potential learners[b]
Situational barriers	
Cost, including tuition, books, child care, etc.	53[c]
Not enough time	46
Home responsibilities	32
Job responsibilities	28
No child care	11
No transportation	8
No place to study or practice	7
Friends or family don't like the idea	3
Institutional barriers	
Don't want to go to school full time	35
Amount of time required to complete program	21
Courses aren't scheduled when I can attend	16
No information about offerings	16
Strict attendance requirements	15
Courses I want don't seem to be available	12
Too much red tape in getting enrolled	10
Don't meet requirements to begin program	6
No way to get credit or a degree	5
Dispositional barriers	
Afraid that I'm too old to begin	17
Low grades in past, not confident of my ability	12
Don't enjoy studying	9
Not enough energy and stamina	9
Tired of school, tired of classrooms	6
Don't know what to learn or what it would lead to	5
Hesitate to seem too ambitious	3

[a]Source: Cross, 1981, p. 99. Adapted from Carp, Peterson, and Roelfs, 1974, p. 46.
[b]Potential learners are those who indicated a desire to learn but who are not currently engaged in organized instruction.
[c]Respondents were asked to check all items that applied.

Situational Barriers

Situational barriers—especially costs and lack of time—are mentioned most frequently as impediments to learning in most studies (Table 1). The situational barriers vary somewhat by subgroup: For instance, low-income adults most frequently identify costs as a major barrier, whereas young mothers are more inclined than other groups to mention lack of child care.

The costs of education include not only direct costs (such as tuition and books) but also indirect costs (foregone income, child care, transportation). Given these high costs, it is not surprising that one finds socioeconomic class differences with respect to participation in adult education. For instance, persons with annual incomes of under $10,000 constituted 30% of the U. S. population but only 17% of adult education participants. Conversely, 60% of those persons enrolled in adult education, but only 44% of the U.S. population aged 17 and over, come from families with incomes of $15,000 or more (Dearman and Plisko, 1980, p. 244). Clearly, the affluent find it easier to pay for education. But there is more to it than that.

According to Boaz (1978), about one-third of all blacks enrolled in adult education are supported by public funds, and about one-third of all white males are supported by their employers; "this leaves white females the only population subgroup presented in NCES data in which a majority of learners (66 percent) are supporting educational costs from their own or family funds" (Boaz, 1978, p. 73). This no doubt explains why more women than men say that the cost of education constitutes a barrier for them. Another problem may be that women feel guilty about spending money on themselves; education may seem like an indulgence (Cross, 1981, p. 101).

Other frequently mentioned situational barriers include lack of time (mentioned by 46% of the potential learners in the Carp et al., 1974, survey), home responsibilities (32%), and job responsibilities (28%). Obviously, these items overlap to some extent—that is, the individual with home or job responsibilities often does not have enough time to pursue education, especially the woman with children. Ages of the children, rather than the number of children, seems to be the decisive factor in limiting education (Westervelt, 1975).

As was reported earlier, participation in adult education has increased much more among women than among men, but the rate of increase between 1969 and 1975 was smallest among women in the 35–54 age group. Soldo (1980) suggests one possible reason for their lower rate: For women, middle age may be "a time of maximum responsibility" (p. 1). Middle-aged women are often caught in a "dependency squeeze" caused by the "competing pressures of employment, . . . children, home life *and* older relatives" (p. 1), especially aging parents who require care. As the life-span has lengthened, and as four-generation families have become more common, midlife women often find themselves having to provide care not only for grandchildren but also for older relatives. To demonstrate more clearly the impact of these responsibilities, Soldo divided middle-aged women into two age groups: the 40–49-year-olds and the 50–59-year-olds. Only 7% of the younger group, but 55% of the older group, were providing care for an older relative. By age 60, nearly 1 million women are involved in kin care. Moreover, given the exorbitant cost of nursing care, women in upper-income brackets are just as likely to be faced with these responsibilities as are low-income women.

The seriousness of this problem was brought home to me by the situation of a client, a 42-year-old woman who had just been elected to the city council. At about the same time, her husband's mother broke her hip and was incapacitated to the extent of requiring constant nursing care. Because there were four children in the family, three of them in college, money was an issue, even though the family was relatively well off in absolute terms. Moreover, the husband strenuously objected to the idea of placing his mother in a nursing home. Thus, my client was caught in a no-win situation: She was the only one who could stay home to care for the older woman, so she was expected to resign her membership on the city council.

This case illustrates several points: (a) The middle-aged wife is the family member who is expected to care for children, grandchildren, and aging relatives. (b) The woman is more likely than the man to require care as she ages. (c) Thus, the women—especially the married woman in her middle years—is less likely to be able to take advantage of learning opportunties.

Other situational constraints include lack of a private place in which to study, a particular problem for married women with children. Moreover, transportation to and from the educational institution may be difficult unless the institution is relatively close to home, which may account in part for the overrepresentation of adult women in community colleges; these tend to be more geographically accessible than other types of institutions.

Institutional Barriers

Numerous reports have proposed recommendations designed to reduce or eliminate the institutional barriers that women encounter as they seek education. These categories include admissions practices, financial aid practices, institutional regulations, curriculum planning and student personnel services, and faculty and staff attitudes.

Examples of barriers in the form of admissions practices include the imposition of higher standards (high school grade-average, aptitude test scores) for female applicants than for male applicants; age restrictions (many graduate schools will not accept applicants who are over 35 or 40 years of age, a practice that discriminates against women, who are more likely to delay their education than are men; and regulations governing the transferability of credit (many institutions do not accept credits after a certain number of years have lapsed or limit the junior-college credits that can be transferred).

Most financial aid is targeted to full-time students. Thus, midlife women (and others) who must attend school part time because of job or family responsibilities are denied access to such funds. Women may also find themselves ineligible for financial assistance because they are married or pregnant and because they are concentrated in "soft" fields—e.g., education, arts, and humanities—which receive less support than the sciences and engineering. Moreover, even when women do receive grants, the amounts are typically smaller than the amounts awarded to men, even when their income levels are the same. The lack of aid to pay for child care constitutes another financial barrier for adult women.

Among the institutional regulations that seem to work a particular hardship on women are time limits on certain kinds of certificate and degree programs that make full-time study a necessity.

In the area of curriculum planning and student personnel services, the location and scheduling of classes may constitute a formidable barrier for many adult women, especially those who have to travel some distance if they are to attend classes. Similarly, adult women may find it hard to make full use of such academic resources as libraries, laboratories, and computer centers, or of such student services as administrative offices, health centers, and counseling centers.

Finally, faculty and staff attitudes, including subtle forms of sex and age discrimination, may discourage midlife women from pursuing education. The lack of female role models among faculty and administrators is another aspect of the institutional environment that has received much attention as a possible deterrent to potential learners among adult women.

These and other institutional barriers are regularly addressed in reports from the Project on the Status and Education of Women. For instance, Hall and Gleaves (1981) examine the needs of special populations of reentry women (including minority women, single parents, displaced homemakers, older women, and disabled women) and offer a series of recommendations covering the categories discussed above, as well as recruitment and basic skills programs.

As the traditional-aged college population continues to shrink, it seems likely that higher education institutions will make greater efforts to attract "nontraditional" students, including midlife women, and that many of the institutional barriers discussed above will be eliminated.

Dispositional Factors

As Table 1 indicates, dispositional factors were less frequently perceived to be a barrier to education than were situational and institutional factors, although 17% of the potential learners indicated they were afraid they were too old to learn, and 12% said they had made low grades in the past and lacked confidence in their academic ability. It should be pointed out, however, that "potential learners" were defined by their desire to learn; many adults may lack this desire because of dispositional factors. Moreover, even those people who have a desire to learn may not be able to recognize the psychological characteristics that prevent them from pursuing education. Thus, it seems probable that dispositional factors constitute more of a barrier to learning than the figures in the table suggest.

For instance, many older people, influenced by the age stereotypes prevalent in American society, may tacitly accept the assumption that learning ability declines with age and thus may not even consider enrolling in an educational program. Others may feel anxious about competing with younger students but may be unwilling to express their anxiety.

Similarly, because of internalized sex-role stereotypes, many women may not see education as a viable option. Lipman-Blumen (1972) has pointed out that our society socializes women to "vicarious achievement" (i.e., through the men in their lives) rather than "direct achievement." While norms have changed somewhat in recent years and while younger women are likely to reject the "vicarious achievement ethic," it may still influence the thinking and behavior of many middle-aged women, especially those from low socioeconomic backgrounds where college-going is not a tradition.

Hall and Gleaves (1981) cite a number of other dispositional factors that are particularly likely to prevent minority women and other "special populations" from pursuing education. First, as was mentioned earlier, these women may have a "gilded cage" image of reentry and continuing education programs, seeing them as directed at affluent white women with ample leisure time. Second, they may fear that such courses will not be related "to their employment, community, and cultural needs" and "will serve to divorce them from their own cultural background" (pp. 5–6). Third, they may suffer from a "fear of 'chilly waters,'" feeling that they will be the only ones from their particular population to enroll in a given program.

Other dispositional factors listed in Table 1 as barriers to the pursuit of education seem more idiosyncratic. Thus, some people indicated simply that they did not enjoy studying or that they were tired of school.

The Final Equation

Having considered some of the motivations for and barriers to learning, we are still left with the question of why some midlife women

Table 2. Motivators and Barriers

Motivators
   Life changes occurring primarily in the areas of career and family
   Changes in value commitments
   Desire for mastery/competence and a need to fulfill interpersonal and altruistic commitments outside the home

Barriers
   Situational factors, including economic contraints and multiple family responsibilities such as the care of aging relatives
   Institutional factors that work a particular hardship on midlife women, such as various kinds of discrimination against part-time students
   Dispositional factors that may in part represent the internalization of societal norms regarding sex and age

choose to pursue education and others do not. To arrive at some kind of final equation that will help to explain this difference, one has to balance the various factors discussed above. Table 2 outlines the motivators and barriers that can simultaneously push and pull an individual to return to school.

As was pointed out earlier, participants in adult education tend to be relatively well educated already. For instance, in 1978 they were almost twice as likely as adults in the total population to have at least some college experience (57% vs. 30%; Dearman and Plisko, 1980, p. 242). What accounts for the greater tendency of the well educated to seek more education? Cross (1978) suggests three hypotheses by way of explanation.

> First, the more people experience [education] the more they like it—either for its intrinsic or extrinsic rewards. A second hypothesis is that those who have been successful in the fairly narrow demands of the educational system stay in it longer and also wish to return to the scene of their earlier success. A third hypothesis is that human beings are basically curious and enjoy learning, but that the "haves" possess the information and wherewithal to pursue learning that interests them, whereas the "have nots" are handicapped and thwarted in attaining what all people basically desire. . . . [Thus,] those with high motivation, high past success, good information networks, and adequate funds get more and more education while those already dragging in the educational race fall farther and farther behind. (Cross, 1978, p. 12)

But is this gloomy conclusion justified? Are certain groups destined to remain have-nots insofar as education (and its rewards) are concerned? Recent data on freshmen enrollments suggest that this is not necessarily the case: In the fall of 1980, close to half of all full-time freshmen entering the nation's colleges and universities indicated that their parents had not gone beyond the high school level; thus, they were first-generation college students (Astin, King, and Richardson, 1981).

Moreover, as the statistics cited earlier show, adult women account for an increasing proportion of both part- and full-time enrollments in regular college courses, as well as making up the majority of adult education participants; the implication is that a large number who for some reason did not enter or complete postsecondary education at traditional college age are now catching up. Finally, the proportions of minority women who go on to college or participate in adult education have increased somewhat over the last decade or so and are projected to continue to increase in the decades ahead (Fisher-Thompson and Kuhn, 1981). Thus, many former have-nots are becoming haves, at least insofar as education is concerned. Although progress is indicated, the number of returning women is still a relatively small proportion of the potential pool.

THE EXPERIENCE OF EDUCATION

So far, the discussion has dealt with the bare fact of participation in education. But what of the actual experience? Once the adult woman has made the decision and actually entered a formal education program, what happens then?

Campbell *et al.* (1980), studying the adjustment process for adults (25 years and older) returning to school as undergraduates at the University of Texas, take an ecological approach in assessing the educational experience: "The focus is on the degree of fit between the characteristics of the individual student and the properties of the student's environment. Psychological adjustment is conceived in terms of person–environment fit" (p. 1). The authors first identified four stages in the return to school (represented diagramatically in Figure 1).

Balance. The person is in a state of equilibrium, "neither enrolled in school nor actively considering a return to school," but employed full time, taking care of the home and raising children, or whatever. "The overall degree of person–environment fit may range, however, from very good to poor" (p. 4).

Conflict. The equilibrium is threatened, and the person actively contemplates returning to school. The motivating forces may be personal (e.g., need for intellectual stimulation) or environmental (e.g., job requirements, need for a second income in the family). Other forces act as barriers to the return (e.g., lack of confidence in academic ability, financial constraints, family opposition). "Thus, individuals considering re-enrollment are typically in a state of conflict" (p. 4).

Transition. The person makes a commitment to enroll in school, "a major decision having impact on all realms of the person's life and . . . therefore, potentially a highly stressful period" (p. 5).

I. Balance	II. Conflict	III. Transition	IV. Outcome (New Balance)
	Environmental Forces Toward and Against Return to School	Environmental Mediators of Psychosocial Adjustments	Good P–E Fit
State of Person– Environment Balance	State of Indecision	Decision to Return	Potentially Stressful Situation
	Personal Forces toward and against Return to School	Personal Mediators of Psychosocial Adjustment	Poor P–E Fit

Figure 1. Four-stage process model of psychosocial adjustment of returning adult students. Source: Campbell, Wilson, and Hanson (1980, p. 5).

Outcome. The person achieves a new state of equilibrium incorporating the return to school. Again, the person–environment fit may range from very good to poor.

Next, Campbell and his associates categorized the 440 adult students in their sample into five groups, on the basis of time spent in various activities (e.g., paid employment, school work, family life). (The five types were discussed earlier, in the section entitled Role Involvement). To assess the person–environment fit in both the balance and the outcome stage, they used an Index of Well-Being (Campbell, Converse, and Rogers, 1976), an instrument predicated on the assumption that

> the optimum "fit" occurs . . . when (1) the particular combination of social settings provides multiple opportunities for fulfilling a wide range of personal needs; (2) the person is accommodating to the demands of each social setting; (3) in negotiating the environment to meet these needs and social demands, the individual is experiencing a degree of challenge that stimulated personal growth but is not overwhelming; and (4) in addition to satisfying personal needs the person is progressing toward fulfillment of higher-order needs. (Campbell *et al.*, 1980, p. 134)

Some of the major findings to emerge from this particular study provide a useful summary for the entire discussion of midlife women and education:

1. Most adults returned to school because they were dissatisfied with their lives and regarded education as a way to a better life. The majority had definite career-related goals in mind: "They want training that will help them develop a career, advance in a current career, or change to a better career" (p. 89).

2. Two-thirds of these adults had wanted to enroll sooner than they actually did but were impeded by institutional barriers (chiefly a univer-

sity requirement that students get special permission to enroll for fewer than 12 credit hours and the lack of evening courses) or situational barriers (family and job responsibilities).

3. Their greatest apprehensions prior to returning to school were connected with lack of funds, multiple responsibilities, academic performance, the impact of the return on their families, and their own ability to adjust. "A lack of information about what to expect after enrollment seems to have contributed to the conflict" (p. 81).

4. Most found that their life-style was disrupted considerably by returning to school.

5. Background characteristics such as age and sex bore little relation to ease or difficulty of adjustment.

6. Adjustment was most difficult for those who were coping with other major life changes (e.g., a divorce, a job change), those who had been anxious about the return, those whose life-styles were changed most drastically, and those with heavy family responsibilities (e.g., single parents).

7. Of the adult students saying they needed campus services, those who experienced the most adjustment difficulty were least likely to make use of such services. The implication is that "those students who used campus resources when problems arose were able to reduce the overall levels of stress and difficulty associated with the transition process" (p. 83).

8. For most students, the person–environment fit was better, and the sense of well-being greater, 4 months after enrollment than prior to enrollment.

9. All five types of students experience some difficulty in adjusting to the return to school, but the sources of the difficulty differed by type:
   a. Type 1 students (mostly married women with children) had "the greatest difficulty deciding to return to school; they were the most apprehensive, yet they were also looking forward to school more than the other types" (p. 85), and the chief source of their difficulty was balancing the demands of school and family.
   b. Type 2 students most closely resembled traditional-aged students in that few were either married or employed. They had a fairly easy time adjusting to the return to school. Their difficulties stemmed chiefly from "adjusting to a lowered standard of living and maintaining an adequate social life" (p. 86).
   c. Type 3 students (most unmarried adults employed full time and attending school part time) had considerable difficulty adjusting because of financial and academic problems; many dropped out after one semester.

d. Type 4 students (mostly full-time students who were married but spent little time with their families and devoted a great deal of time to their studies) experienced few academic problems but nonetheless reported "high levels of difficulty and stress during the adjustment period," probably because they "were not able to fulfill important social needs" (p. 87).
   e. Type 5 students (mostly married, employed full time, and enrolled in only one or two courses) indicated that returning to school did not change their life-style but nonetheless experienced some stress, chiefly because "they had trouble fitting school in their already busy lives" (p. 87).

In summary, ease of adjustment and sense of well-being seemed to depend on the student's particular situation following enrollment. Competing demands on time were a greater source of stress than were academic demands *per se*.

Conclusion and Recommendations

In the foregoing discussion, a series of questions related to midlife women and education have been raised. To the overriding questions: What use does the midlife woman make of education? What value does it have for her? My answer must be: It all depends. It depends on the woman's particular situation, on her level of cognitive development, her role involvements, the motives that drive her, and the barriers that impede her. Although one can, for convenience, differentiate adult learners from traditional-age learners, one cannot talk about the "midlife woman" without doing violence to reality. To some women, midlife is a period of greater freedom and opportunity; to others, it is a period of greater constraint and responsibility. To the former group, education may be a vehicle for growth and renewal; to the latter, it might simply constitute an added burden.

Even though the number of adult learners—particularly women—has increased dramatically, it is important to remember that a far greater number do not participate in formal learning activities. Projections indicate that by the year 2010 there will be 36 million women between the ages of 45 and 64 in this nation. Will most of them be so preoccupied with their roles as workers and caretakers that they will be unable to utilize education?

Earlier, situational, institutional, and dispositional factors that impede midlife women's participation in education were outlined. The following two recommendations would help remove all three sets of barriers.

1. *Postsecondary educational institutions should initiate policies more responsive to the needs of adult students.* These policies would include (a) granting credit for life experiences that have been appropriately evaluated; (b) giving financial aid to part-time as well as full-time students; (c) establishing internships (paid and unpaid) that will give adult students a chance to explore a new field before making a full commitment to it; (d) revision of schedules; (e) revision of admissions procedures (Charner, 1981, p. 2).

2. *Regional Adult Counseling Centers should be established, to serve both as model centers and as resources for satellite centers throughout the region.* These centers would offer a comprehensive array of services, including individual and group counseling, career planning, skills training, and special-interest workshops. Satellite centers might offer only some of these services, referring clients to the regional center for other services as necessary. Despite the proliferation of counseling centers serving adults of both sexes, such services are not universally available. So far, there is no systematic delivery system to assure that the ordinary adult woman in any given community will have somewhere to go for help in uncovering educational and other options.

Until we have social policies that offer opportunities for education throughout life and provide help in caring for children or aging relatives, many midlife women will continue to be excluded from the learning opportunities now enjoyed by only a few of this age group.

REFERENCES

Aslanian, C. B., and Brickell, H. M. *American in transition: Life changes as reasons for adult learning.* New York: College Entrance Examination Board, 1980.

Astin, A. W. *Preventing students from dropping out.* San Francisco: Jossey-Bass, 1975.

Astin, A. W., King, M. R., and Richardson, G. T. *The American freshman: National norms for fall 1980.* Los Angeles: Cooperative Institutional Research Program, 1981.

Baruch, G. K., and Barnett, R. C. On the well-being of adult women. In L. A. Bond and J. C. Rosen (Eds.), *Competence and coping during adulthood.* Hanover, N.H.: University Press of New England, 1980.

Boaz, R. L. *Participation in adult education: Final report, 1975.* Washington, D.C.: National Center for Education Statistics, 1978.

Campbell, A., Converse, P., and Rodgers, W. *The quality of American life.* New York: Russell Sage Foundation, 1976.

Campbell, M. D., Wilson, L. G., and Hanson, G. R. *The invisible minority: A study of adult university students.* (Final report submitted to the Hogg Foundation for Mental Health). Austin: Office of the Dean of Students, University of Texas, 1980.

Carp, A., Peterson, R. E., and Roelfs, P. J. Adult learning: Interests and experiences. in K. P. Cross, J. R. Valley, and Associates, *Planning non-traditional programs.* San Francisco: Jossey-Bass, 1974.

Cattell, R. B. Theory of fluid and crystallized intelligence: A critical experiment. *Journal of Educational Psychology,* 1963, 54, 1–22.

Charner, I. Motivating adult learning through planned change. *National Center for Educational Brokering Bulletin,* 1981, 6 (7), 1.

Cross, K. P. A critical review of state and national studies of the needs and interests of adult learners. In C. B. Stalford (Ed.), *Conference report: Adult learning needs and the demand for lifelong learning.* Washington, D. C.: National Institute of Education, U.S. Department of Health, Education and Welfare, 1978.

Cross, K. P. *Adults as learners.* San Francisco: Jossey-Bass, 1981.

Dearman, N. B., and Plisko, V. W. *The condition of education, 1980 edition.* Washington: National Center for Education, 1980.

Entine, A. D. The role of continuing education. In *Women in mid-life: Security and fulfillment, Part I.* A compendium of papers submitted to the Select Committee on Aging, U.S. House of Representatives, 95th Congress. Comm. Pub. No. 95-107, 1978.

Fisher-Thompson, J., and Kuhn, J. A. *Re-entry women: Relevant statistics.* Washington, D.C.: Project on the Status and Education of Women, Association of American Colleges, 1981.

Fiske, M. Changing hierarchies of commitment in adulthood. In N. J. Smelser and E. H. Erikson (Eds.), *Themes of work and love in adulthood.* Cambridge, Mass.: Harvard University Press, 1980.

Gallagher, D., Thompson, L. W., and Levy, S. M. Clinical psychological assessment of older adults. In L. W. Poon (Ed.), *Aging in the 1980's: Psychological issues.* Washington, D. C.: American Psychological Association, 1980.

Giesen, C. B., and Datan, N. The competent older woman. In N. Datan and N. Lohmann (Eds.), *Transitions in aging.* New York: Academic Press, 1980.

Gutmann, D. C. The cross-cultural perspective: Notes toward a comparative psychology of aging. In J. E. Birren and K. W. Schaie (Eds.), *Handbook of the psychology of aging.* New York: Van Nostrand Reinhold, 1977.

Hall, R. B., and Gleaves, F. D. *Re-entry women: Special programs for special populations.* Washington, D.C.: Project on the Status and Education of Women, Association of American Colleges, 1981.

Karabel, J. Community colleges and social stratification. *Harvard Educational Review,* 1972, 42, 521-562.

Knefelkamp, L. L., Widick, C. C., and Stroad, B. Cognitive-developmental theory: A guide to counseling women. *Counseling Psychologist,* 1976, 6, 15-19.

Kohlberg, L. Stages of moral development as a basis for moral education. In C. Beck and E. Sullivan (Eds.), *Moral education.* Canada: University of Toronto, 1970.

Kohn, M. L. Job complexity and adult personality. In N. J. Smelser and E. H. Erikson (Eds.), *Themes of work and love in adulthood.* Cambridge, Mass.: Harvard University Press, 1980.

Kuhlen, R. G. Motivational changes during the adult years. In R. G. Kuhlen (Ed.), *Psychological backgrounds of adult education.* Chicago: Center for the Study of Liberal Education for Adults, 1963.

Lipman-Blumen, J. How ideology shapes women's lives. *Scientific American,* 1972, 226, 34-42.

Loevinger, J. *Ego development: Conceptions and theories.* San Francisco: Jossey-Bass, 1976.

Lowenthal, M. F., Thurnher, M., and Chiriboga, D. *Four stages of life: A comparative study of men and women facing transitions.* San Francisco: Jossey-Bass, 1975.

Magarrell, J. The enrollment boom among older Americans: 1 in 3 college students is now over 25 years old. *Chronicle of Higher Education,* May 4, 1981, p. 3.

Miller, J., Schooler, C., Kohn, M. E., and Miller, K. A. Women and work: The psychological effects of occupational conditions. *American Journal of Sociology,* 1979, 85, 66-94.

Perry, W. G. *Forms of intellectual and ethical development in the college years.* New York: Holt, Rinehart & Winston, 1970.
Ramey, E. *Anatomy—Destiny: Is burn-out inevitable?* Paper presented at the 6th Annual Conference of Helpers of Adults, University of Maryland, May 1981.
Randour, M. L., Strasburg, G., & Lipman-Blumen, J. *Women in higher education: Trends in enrollments and degrees earned.* Unpublished manuscript, 1981.
Soldo, B. *The dependency squeeze on middle-aged women.* Paper presented to the Secretary's Committee on the Rights and Responsibilities of Women, Department of Health, Education and Welfare. Washington, D.C.: Center for Population Research, Georgetown University, 1980.
Weathersby, R. P., and Tarule, J. M. *Adult development: Implications for higher education* (AAHE-ERIC Higher Education Research Report No. 4). Washington, D.C.: American Association for Higher Education, 1980.
Westervelt, E. M. *Barriers to women's participation in postsecondary education: A review of research and commentary as of 1973–1974.* Washington, D. C.: National Center for Education Statistics, 1975.
White, R. Strategies of adaptation: An attempt at systematic description. In R. Moos (Ed.), *Human adaptation: Coping with life crises.* Lexington, Mass.: Heath, 1976.
Willis, S. L., and Baltes, P. B. Intelligence in adulthood and aging: Contemporary issues. In L. W. Poon (Ed.), *Aging in the 1980's: Psychological issues.* Washington, D.C.: American Psychological Association, 1980.

Chapter 15

The Anxiety of the Unknown—Choice, Risk, Responsibility
Therapeutic Issues for Today's Adult Women

ROSALIND C. BARNETT

Within the last several years we have seen a plethora of research findings and demographic data describing current social changes, especially as they affect women. The changes that have received greatest attention include the lengthening life-span, the widespread movement of women into the labor force, the rising divorce rate, and steadily growing inflation. These massive changes in our social environment have undoubtedly affected women's views of themselves and their life satisfaction. Yet explicit work on exploring the implications of these widely discussed social shifts on the psychological experiences of women and on the issues they bring into therapy has not kept pace. Several recent reviews (Maracek and Johnson, 1980; McMahon, 1980) focus on the process of therapy—the form, not the content. Other overviews deal with the psychiatric aspects of particular and frequent presenting problems, such as abortion, sexual dysfunctions, eating disorders (see, for example, Notman and Nadelson, 1978). These efforts, however, rarely address the impact that the sweeping changes in the social and political definitions of women's roles have had on the issues with which adult women are grappling, especially in their middle years.

Research in such diverse fields as life-span developmental psychology and social gerontology has illuminated such relevant topics as (1) individual adjustment to a longer life-span and, in particular, to in-

---

ROSALIND C. BARNETT • Wellesley College Center for Research on Women, Wellesley, Massachusetts 02181.

tergenerational relationships over the life-span (Hagestad, 1981; Hagestad, Smyer, and Stierman, 1982); (2) the psychological well-being of women in the middle years as it relates to women's employment and family statuses (Barnett and Baruch, 1981); and (3) the influence of social-historical events on individual adjustment (Elder, 1979; Hareven, 1976; Pearlin, 1975).

The Social Context

This chapter is an attempt to articulate several pressing therapeutic issues for mature women in the 1980s that grow out of this new social context and to view them against the backdrop provided by pertinent research findings. These issues reflect women's growing realization that they need to shape their lives actively, to take risks, and to be responsible for their own happiness. Underlying these issues are the dual concerns over establishing one's sense of femininity and of sexuality in a time when old prescriptions are shattered and newer ones are not yet in place.

My comments pertain predominantly to middle-class Caucasian women and to the concerns they are bringing into therapy. These concerns are not necessarily new; however, they have a new urgency and intensity that calls for special attention from therapists.

For mature women, the last decade has been one of radical departures. The steady stream of demographic statistics makes it absolutely clear that the life patterns of today's women differ dramatically from the pattern that their mothers followed and for which they were socialized. Compared to their mothers, today's women are far better educated, are more often in the paid labor force for their entire adult lives, are marrying later or not marrying at all, are having fewer children later or none at all, and are dissolving bad marriages rather than preserving them "at least until the children are grown up." As a percentage of the female population, women who live out over the long term the idealized life pattern of being married and at home with children are now a minority.

Awareness that the old norms no longer apply is only the first step in accepting that diversity and normlessness are the new norms. Understandably, yet sadly, full acceptance of alternative life patterns as "right," "fitting," or "fulfilling" lags, creating a psychological gap. For many women, this gap results in anxiety, depression, and painful soul-searching, particularly as they approach the middle years.

For a long time educated women have acknowledged intellectually that freedom to choose one's life pattern is essential. Awareness of demographic shifts, of the need to prepare for future goals, is reflected in the growing numbers of women completing higher education and committing themselves to continuous employment. For many women, however, these alternative patterns have been experienced as largely irrelevant for defining their core identities and for fulfilling themselves as women. While intellectually championing the importance of nontraditional roles, most middle-class women have difficulty embracing them as means of satisfying their basic personal needs. This difficulty grows in part out of their upbringing and is sustained by the realization of what their mothers' lives have been and what their own expectations therefore are. With the demise of the old norms and the new emphasis on alternative life patterns comes the need to reevaluate nontraditional roles for their capacity to fulfill basic needs. And conscious reevaluation of alternative life patterns raises the issue of choice.

Making Choices

Resistant to planning ahead, reared to believe that the future will be taken care of by the man of their dreams, women are now grappling with the need to plan for themselves and to take responsibility for their own lives. These needs are very anxiety-producing, raising concerns about essential femininity, responsibility for oneself, relations to one's mother. Hard-hit by the demands of the changing social situation are women in their 30s and 40s. These women have been reared by mothers embodying the Feminine Mystique and have absorbed the expectation that at midlife they too would be in a similarly stable family situation.

Many women struggling with these issues enter therapy. For some there is still conflict, even when knowing consciously that they value their independence and their time alone, that they do not want to be married, that they do not want children, that the ideal relationship for them is one that is free of long-term commitments. Conflict arises because their feelings don't quite match their conscious beliefs. They agonize over whether they are emotionally ready to live out the new "patterns" they may have chosen or that may seem desirable. They both know what they want and aren't sure whether they want it. How do I know these things? Am I perhaps still rebelling against my mother? Was I perhaps caught up in the politicization of women's issues and am still banner-waving? Conflict leads to questioning. How can I want such a different life pattern from the one my mother chose and the one I am supposed to "want"?

Departures from known patterns also have consequences for the parental generation. Mothers watch as their daughters mature under social conditions with which they have a difficult time identifying. The Feminine Mystique mother never had to deal consciously with the array of choices confronting her daughter. She may not understand or be able to support her daughter who postpones marriage to finish a degree, chooses to have an abortion rather than drop out of school, brings someone in to care for her young children so that she may resume work, or divorces her husband when her children are still young. Under these pressures, mothers may feel useless, incompetent, and rejected as models. Hence, they may retreat, criticize, or in other ways fail to acknowledge their daughters' choices, thus inadvertently adding to their daughters' anxiety about the "rightness" of the life choices they are making. The potential for a sense of betrayal on both sides is great, fueling the daughter's concern over being someone her mother can approve of on the one hand, and, on the other, generating tension over inadequacies in knowing how to parent an adult daughter whose life bears so little resemblance to her own.

The following vignette illustrates how a mother's behavior can unwittingly add to her daughter's anxiety.

> Alice, a 34-year-old married professional woman, has an infant daughter. She continued to work actively until the day before her daughter was born and returned to work shortly thereafter. She managed her new role by arranging to work from her home office part of the time, and she hired a live-in maid to assist with the baby. Her colleagues and professional women friends had made similar arrangements and were supportive of the pattern she had worked out. However, Alice had a nagging sense that her choices would not be approved of by her mother, and this realization increased her uncertainty about the "rightness" of the life-style she was developing. Her uncertainty and anxiety predated the birth of her child. She is from a large traditional family and is the first child and grandchild to have completed a professional degree. As a woman and as a member of this family she was an anomaly; none of her close relatives had life experiences that were, in critical ways, at all similar to hers. Within her own family she first began to feel a lack of understanding and a distance during her college years, when it became clear to her that she wanted to pursue advanced training. Her parents had fully supported her in completing a college education. However, graduate school was another thing. They had never known anyone who had gone to graduate school and certainly never expected their daughter to make that choice.
>
> The difference between what they had expected for her and her actual choices began to mount. She did not get married when all her friends did. She explained to her parents that she wasn't ready to marry because she had not decided what to do with her life. They had a difficult time understanding what she meant.
>
> She completed her program and got married. She decided to postpone having children until her career was established. Again, her parents, who had expected her to marry and start a family years before, were unable to comprehend. They never openly confronted her on these issues, but they made their disappointments known largely by not asking personal questions and never inquiring about her professional life. Alice knew that they were having trouble understanding the life choices she was making. Nevertheless, her mother's inability, or lack of effort, to understand served as a constant reminder of her own uncertainty about the new pattern she was following. In

therapy she related the following incident, which reflected the various strains in her relationship with her mother: Her parents came to visit her when the baby was just a few weeks old. Alice brought the baby over so that her mother could hold her. Her mother was delighted and took the baby in her arms. After just a few seconds, she turned to Alice and said, "No, you take her; after all you don't get to hold her too often."

This interchange underscored the attempts these two women were making to connect with one another as well as the tension, implicit criticism, and consequent anxiety generated by these attempts.

The remainder of this chapter focuses on several sources of anxiety in today's women—specifically, concerns over being feminine and being sexual—and how therapists can understand the related issues of choice, risk, and responsibility. Women caught in these struggles come into therapy with questions such as the following: Why am I not married? What is wrong with me? What will happen to me if I never marry, if I get divorced? What will my life be like if I never have a child? How can I possibly have a child when my professional life is so unsettled?

The intensity of affect around these concerns—all of which touch on definitions of femininity—gives striking evidence of the hold traditional ideas about femininity have on the psyches of today's women. There is an acute intrapsychic struggle being waged within many women patients (and nonpatients) over these issues, and the struggle takes several forms.

Among never-married women, for example, many who enjoy their life-style wonder whether their ability to enjoy life without a permanent partner reflects a personality deficit. And they fear that the happiness they now enjoy will be short-lived—that the price of deviating from social and maternal norms will have to be paid eventually. Those who are anguished about not being in a permanent relationship feel rejected, passed by, "out of synch." They experience themselves as deviant, unfeminine, essentially unlovable—and the proof lies in their unmarried state. Women approaching 40 who are childless—whether married or not—wrestle painfully with feelings of being incomplete, of being less than a whole female.

Rarely do women patients experience these life dilemmas as choices. Why then did I use the word *choice* in the title of this chapter? Clearly, the word needs some clarification. Hard as it may be for many women to acknowledge their part in creating the dilemmas in which they find themselves, they inevitably did make choices—consciously or unconsciously—and understanding that they did so is crucial to any resolution.

One recently married 37-year-old women patient was acutely depressed over the realization that her husband refused to have a child. She entered the marriage knowing his feelings, but wanting so much to be married that she discounted his resolve. Two years later, painfully aware of her approaching 40th birthday, she again raised the issue. From her husband's point of view there was nothing to discuss. He understood how she felt, but he had been perfectly clear about his feelings at the outset and they had not changed.

She was desperate. She yearned to have a child, to care for a baby, to nurture, to fulfill her own expectations, yet she did not want to divorce her husband. On balance, her life was happier than it had been before she married, and realistically the possibility of establishing another relationship and having a child was negligible. Her initial depression was accompanied by feelings of being incomplete and of blaming her husband for impeding the fulfillment of her femininity.

Treatment centered around disentangling her sense of her own femininity from that of being a mother, and accepting responsibility for the marital choice she had made. As her anger at her husband dissipated, she was able to recognize that prior to her marriage, she was a vivacious, independent, outgoing woman with lots of friends who, while lonely at times, was not burdened by a sense of her inadequacy as a female. As a single woman she had no assumptions about the necessary conditions for fulfilling herself as a woman and was able to "put on hold" all the expectations and social pressures that surfaced after her marriage. However, being married, the only role for which her early rearing prepared her, carried with it emotionally charged prescriptions. She was now in a position to have a child, thereby "completing" her femininity and fulfilling what she perceived as her mother's expectations for her.

In therapy she worked through the various meanings she had attached to having a child and realized that her feelings about herself and her relationship with her mother were essentially independent of whether she had a child or not. Certainly her sense of loss was real; she was not going to be a mother, and she came to accept that she might always experience some pain around that loss. But the life she had chosen offered many opportunities for her to meet other needs, and her fulfillment depended on developing and enjoying those opportunities.

Taking Risks

As with any choice, there are costs as well as benefits. One cost is the anxiety of the unknown, of being on a path untraveled by one's mother or maybe by anyone else in one's immediate circle. (The rarity of role models for "deviant" life patterns will undoubtedly be less an issue for tomorrow's mature women.) This anxiety is often associated with a need for affirmation. And one's mother is the primary person from whom that affirmation is sought.

For patients, the abstract knowledge that mature women can lead highly rewarding lives in alternative patterns is reassuring but inadequate. The road to the end point of full acceptance is often very difficult, as is illustrated by the following case:

> The issues of choice, risk, and responsibility came together for a 40-year-old patient who, after years of a stagnant marriage, acknowledged that she was miserable. Ostensibly things were going well. She had two preteenage sons and a husband who earned a good living. Unlike the situation in her own family while she was growing up, her husband did not drink, there were no brawls, there were no disagreements or arguments, calm reigned, albeit at the cost to her of subordinating the fun-loving, vibrant parts of her personality. Like her mother, she conformed to the depressive life-style dictated by her husband's moodiness. Unlike her mother, she could not blame her misfortune on her husband's drinking. In fact, she could not begin to explain to her mother why she felt so miserable; her mother would never have understood. The religious/moral/social beliefs that kept her mother in a terrible marriage also kept her from any understanding of her daughter's desire to break out of her marriage and to live her own life. She stayed away from her mother in part because she accused herself of the same selfish motives she was sure her mother would accuse her of: Bob makes no demands, he is so easygoing, why can't you go along? What is wrong with you? Is what you want important enough to destroy your family?
>
> Underneath all these accusations was the fear that her mother would accuse her of not being feminine—not supportive, self-denying, patient, undemanding—an accusation with which she tormented herself. But times and attitudes had changed, and being a socially aware woman, she knew she had to get out of her marriage; she had to do what she had wished her mother had done. And she did. It took her three years of procrastinating, of changing lawyers, of not making her needs clear. During this period, she learned how to stand up for herself at work, how to ask her friends for what she needed; she reached out to her mother, was rebuffed, and recovered. She learned that her mother's limitations made it impossible for her to be the mother she wanted—to affirm her decision to divorce and to appreciate her as a worthwhile person. She learned that her own growing sense of her worth was what counted, and she took responsibility for cultivating her self-esteem. She began to feel confident enough to accept herself as a female and as a divorced woman. With her newly grounded sense of self, she tackled the divorce process with conviction, completing in a few months what otherwise would have taken years.

Ironically, the greater the departure from her mother's model, the greater a daughter's need for affirmation and the harder it may be to obtain. Interestingly, findings from recent research (Barnett and Baruch, 1982) lend support to this formulation. This study was designed to explore the relationship between psychological well-being and varying patterns of work and family status among women 35 to 55. The women in the study ($N = 238$) were in one of four family statuses: never-married, married with children, married without children, and divorced with children. For most of the women, a close relationship to their mothers was associated with high self-esteem and a sense of psychological well being (Baruch and Barnett, 1983). For the divorced women, however, all of whom were employed and had children, a negative association was found. That is, the closer they were to their mothers, the lower was their sense of well-being. One interpretation of this finding is that the mothers of divorced women may not be able to shed their negative views about divorce; they may not know how to mother a daughter who has done something they were reared to believe was "wrong," "shameful," or "immoral." By extension they may feel that they have failed as mothers and may take on the shame that they associate with their daughter's divorce. Thus, for the divorced daughters, closeness to their mothers may result in exacerbating the very anxiety that motivated the desire for closeness.

Further evidence supporting this conjecture comes from a descriptive study of recently divorced middle-aged parents (mean age, 48.6 years for the women). A focus of the study was on the intergenerational impact of the divorce experience. The researchers (Hagestad et al., 1982) report that about one-fourth of the women who had parents living at the time of the marital disruption never discussed their marital situation with their parents, typically because they expected disapproval or lack of understanding. One woman said, "I am ashamed to say it, but at fifty I am still afraid of what my mother thinks—she intimidates me. I was divorced almost a year before I told her." And a few of the people interviewed admitted that the "divorce had been delayed because of the anticipated negative reactions from parents."

The process of accepting oneself as a complete and acceptable female in an atypical life pattern is itself experienced with anxiety. Full acceptance involves taking the risk of presenting oneself both privately and publicly as, for example, a divorced woman, a successful never-married professional, or a voluntarily childless married career woman. The successful career woman who refuses an opportunity that would make her more visible professionally may be acting out her anxiety over making clear her choice of a life pattern radically different from the idealized one that she assumed she would be following. Such a public statement would make impossible future retreat into the safety of that which is known.

Fortunately, the risks involved are most often greater in prospect than they are in actuality. For women who are struggling with achieving maternal approval, images of a powerful, threatening, difficult-to-please mother, reminiscent of childhood perceptions of larger-than-life-parents, still abound. And in these times of change, it is tempting for daughters to attribute the lack of maternal approval they feel to life pattern differences. Old images die hard. They do not allow for changes mothers may have made in the course of their own lives or in response to witnessing their daughter's experiments with new patterns.

When appropriate, I ask mature women patients to bring their mothers with them into therapy. Typically they react with dread. Competent, successful women are terrified at the prospect of talking openly with their mothers. Most often, this initial resistance is overcome and the mother in invited. Almost always she accepts. Initially the session is tense—the daughter is on guard for signs that her mother really doesn't value her; the mother is defensive. As the session progresses, it becomes clear to the mother that she is a very significant person in her daughter's life and that is why she was asked to be part of the therapy. Thus reassured, mothers relax and participate. Outcomes vary, of course, but at the very least, old images are shaken up or destroyed. The "rigid, demanding mother" is often just as eager to be accepted by her daughter as the daughter is to be accepted by her mother.

The basic lesson is that opting for one life pattern over another in order to gain maternal approval is a strategy that is doomed to fail. Many adult patients struggle to free themselves of the need for approval from their mothers. Many are engaged in a reexamination of their goals in light of what they see as their own values, not merely extensions of what they perceive their mothers want for them. This process takes on special poignancy today because of the assumed relationship between the goals women choose and their need to see themselves as "feminine." Not long ago there was a certain consensus and therefore comfort for women in the knowledge that they would follow their mothers' path—they would marry and have children—thereby automatically establishing their femininity.

Now it is more difficult. There is no longer a reasonable certainty that women will take this path, nor that, given the choice, they will find that it meets the needs many adult women are expressing. However, issues highly relevant to the content of therapy with today's women arise from serious questioning about relinquishing marriage and/or motherhood. As women contemplate alternative life patterns, the question of how one defines oneself as feminine becomes salient.

THE QUESTION OF FEMININITY

We all need to see ourselves as being like others of our sex (Kagan, 1964; Kohlberg, 1966); that is, women need to see themselves as being feminine. Historically, this was accomplished by marrying and rearing children. Thus, a woman was reassured that she was feminine because she was caring for a husband and children—following her mother's model and engaged in the same nurturing activities as her female peers. Reliance on this once widely available and accepted behavioral resolution of an essentially psychological issue is no longer viable.

Many women in nontraditional as well as traditional patterns reject the view of femininity as a status ascribed only to those who have married and have had children. Rather, they view femininity as a status to be attained. Thus, they ask: Does a woman need to be in a long-term relationship with a man to prove to herself or others that she is truly feminine? Can a woman feel completely feminine if she devotes her energies to her career? How does her definition of herself as a female relate to her sense of herself as a sexual being? The sense of loneliness and the questioning of choices expressed in therapy by women who have alternative life patterns often masks the underlying fear that the price of these choices goes beyond feeling "out of sync." The price, they fear, may be living with perpetual doubt about their adequacy as females.

How does one go about achieving femininity? Is it possible? How will I ever know if I'll feel complete as a woman? This anxiety-laden, self-questioning process is rendered more painful because it is being conducted on an individual basis. In the absence of social consensus, women have to arrive at idiosyncratic definitions of femininity.

I envision a future in which individuals will separate definitions of feminity from behavioral prescriptions; where a woman's femininity will not be called into question, by herself or by others, because she chooses not to marry or not to have children. I would like to see girls and boys reared in an environment in which adult women are portrayed as complete and feminine, independent of their marital and parental roles. However, the psychological reality for today's women is that these two are entangled. In fact, the persistent scrutiny, the external and internal doubts about the independence of femininity and life pattern constitute a major obstacle to achieving separation of the two.

The goal of feeling comfortable with oneself as a female apart from one's life choices is far from trivial. How can therapists be helpful to women caught in the struggle to attain it? One answer comes from an unexpected source. Years ago, Harvard sociologist Alex Inkeles addressed the question "What is sociology?" (Inkeles, 1964). He approached this question in several ways. One intriguing approach was to define sociology as "what sociologists do." By analogy, femininity may not best be defined directly. Rather, femininity can be thought of as what females are or describe themselves as, including feelings, traits, attitudes. This approach can be useful if the temptation is resisted to turn it into another quest for what is typically "feminine," and then to define *that* as what females "ought" to do or be. If we as females can accept our own feelings, traits, and attitudes as feminine by definition, we can resist our need to obtain external approval. Such acceptance would also help us disarm social criticism.

Acknowledging One's Sexuality

A related issue, that of acknowledging and actualizing one's sexuality, is particularly problematic for today's women. Growing awareness of their own sexual needs often creates monumental problems for women in nontraditional life patterns, as well as for married women. In the current climate, mature women "know" they have sexual needs, yet learning what those sexual needs are and how to fulfill them, and growing to accept oneself as a "sexual being," requires a revolution in thinking.

The first lesson most adult women learned as children was not to think about sex at all. Good girls didn't. Then, during their late teen years, sexual standards loosened dramatically. The sexual revolution affected women differently, depending in large part on when in their development they experienced its impact. For many women, experimenting with sexuality was just that; they felt their behavior was "wrong," more like play-acting than learning how to create a mutually satisfying sexual relationship. Most women brought to their early sexual encounters the lesson of their youth—that sexual performance meant meeting their partner's needs. Following this prescription affirmed a woman as nurturant, supportive, caring, and loving. These qualities were supposed to assure her satisfaction, but they obviously could not because her needs were not addressed. As sexual taboos loosened, women became aware that they were not alone in their frustration and that dissatisfaction, anger, and resentment grew out of culturally sanctioned denial of their own sexual needs. Now adult women are discovering their own sexuality. Along with this discovery is the need to engage their partners in fulfilling their needs. These efforts are often initiated painfully, shyly, with great difficulty, and with women not knowing how to ask, anxious over having expectations and needs, and fearing that their needs will be condemned as illegitimate and will therefore not be met.

The presence of a marital sexual partner does not and certainly has not automatically provided for the satisfaction of women's sexual needs; the absence of a marital partner, however, creates additional problems for today's women. The nonmarried woman who tries to have her sexual needs met has few choices: She can defy old prohibitions and permit herself to become sexually involved with one or more men with whom she is not in a committed relationship. In this action she is supported by current social mores, yet her internal struggle goes on. Seeing herself through her mother's eyes, she feels guilty over being promiscuous, over feeling like a whore. These feelings are part of her heritage. Again, women grapple individually with this issue and there is no easy solution. A classic case of this struggle is the sophisticated divorced woman involved romantically with a married man. Loving him, she is caught between two sexual moralities. She agonizes over how to remain in this fulfilling, yet clearly limited relationship; she is already overinvested, and dreams a monogamous dream, yet she knows the relationship will never meet those needs. And her basic sexual-moral feeling is that she has to be loyal to him, to a married man who is being unfaithful. The reality of the situation does not elude her, yet neither does it point clearly to a way out. She sees the irrationality of her predicament, yet she can't make the emotional leap. Monogamous sexual feelings are part-and-parcel of her makeup—the psychological gap is still too wide.

Of course, not all women can or want to work out their sexual needs with a man. Some prefer to take care of their needs themselves; learning to nurture and pleasure themselves puts them safely in charge of their sexuality. Again, overcoming guilt is a necessary step before this course becomes viable. Other women turn to female partners. And these alternatives are not mutually exclusive. Whatever route one takes reflects an affirmation of one's sexuality and an acknowledgment that sexual needs are not to be denied. This is a mammoth undertaking, particularly for midlife women, one fraught with anxiety, self-doubt, recrimination, and enormous fear of the consequences.

The Role of the Therapist

The therapist alert to the centrality of these issues can help separate them from the manifest context in which they are raised. Thus, a presenting problem—for example, the sense of failure experienced around an impending divorce—can be hypothesized as arising in large part from the threat a woman experiences to her sense of femininity. What does her divorce imply about her femininity? How can she establish a sense of femininity when she is no longer in a marital relationship? By addressing these basic questions we can help our women patients redefine femininity as an inherent attitude, not an achieved status. Their essential femininity is then not threatened by divorce. Once this issue is dealt with, the risks inherent in contemplating a nontraditional life pattern are greatly reduced.

The position that femininity is independent of one's life pattern is supported by several research findings. Of all the "choices" today's women are contemplating, the one that calls up the issue of femininity most acutely is that of choosing not to have children. Women who make that choice are open to being stigmatized as unfeminine, i.e., selfish, immature, irresponsible, unnatural. To explore the personality traits of voluntarily childless women, psychologist Judith Teicholtz (1978) compared a group of 38 married women who had decided never to bear children (the age range was 23 to 38; the mean age was 30 years) to a group of 32 unmarried women who planned to have children (the age range was 24 to 37; the mean age was 28 years). While hers was not a random sample and the findings must therefore be taken only as suggestive, she found no significant differences between the two groups of women on measures of adjustment, social responsibility, maturity, and most important—femininity. These two groups of women described themselves in essentially identical ways on several measures assessing "conscious or unconscious" feminine identity.

In their interview study, based on a random sample of somewhat older women, 35 to 55, Barnett and Baruch (1981) obtained similar findings. Using the Bem Sex Role Inventory (Bem, 1974), a measure of self-concept that asks women to rate themselves on adjectives widely considered to reflect femininity and masculinity, the mean femininity scores for women in four family statuses—never-married, married with children, married without children, and divorced with children—were virtually indistinguishable. The range on this instrument is 1 to 10, and the means for the four family status groups all clustered tightly around 5.7, with the highest being 5.9 and the lowest 5.6!

It might be argued that the women Teicholz studied were young and still had the option of changing their minds and therefore did not have to deal with the impact on their femininity of actually not having children. The women in the Barnett and Baruch study described above, however, were almost all past the point in their lives when having children was an open issue.

A second finding from the same study may be useful to therapists working with divorced women patients. Divorced women, it is widely believed, suffer a loss of self-esteem related to their sense of failure as women and wives. The divorced women in the study were all employed mothers and had been divorced for an average of 7 years. On the indices of well-being, these women scored very high. As a group, they had high levels of self-esteem and did not report many symptoms of anxiety or depression. Knowing that divorced mothers who are employed and who have been divorced for several years feel as positive about themselves as do their married counterparts ought to help therapists in supporting their women patients who are struggling with divorce and cannot imagine how they can put together a satisfying postdivorce life.

Such research findings can be particularly helpful to women agonizing over the risk to their "femininity" of making deviant choices. These findings are also useful for therapists who do not have enough personal experience with women in these various alternative patterns to draw upon. And many of us are dealing personally with these issues and may have a difficult time separating our concerns from those of our patients.

Most women who come into therapy with these concerns are acutely depressed and cannot imagine a personal future free of the anxiety they are currently experiencing. Commonly heard are such painful formulations as these: What will I do to fill the emptiness of my life? How can I possibly come home every night to a childless home? Knowing that women typically can move beyond these crises, create meaningful lives, and have a firm sense of their own femininity can help therapists, and in turn their patients, to develop a life-span perspective, focusing more on the resolution of the crises than on the crises *per se*.

BEING RESPONSIBLE

Perceiving that one needs to make choices, and confronting the risks involved in so doing, inevitably raises the question of responsibility. Traditionally, women did what they were "supposed" to do; they did not have to take responsibility for their lives. Happiness was marrying the right man and having children of whom you could be proud. Misery was having an alcoholic husband, or one who was an insufficient provider, or having children who were a disappointment. Whatever the outcome, women were passive victims of life's circumstances.

It is much harder today for women to avoid seeing themselves as responsible for the way their lives turn out. However, many adult women are ill prepared for feeling in control, for being able to take appropriate pride in choices that work out well and for assuming personal blame for those that do not. Not too long ago, even when economic necessity did not force a woman into the labor market, she could claim that she was working for her family—the college tuition bill was more than her husband could handle, the children needed money for extras. These claims were attractive because they lent social approval to her choice and left her free of personal responsibility. With their consciousnesses newly raised, adult women can no longer "get away" with such rationalizations. Moreover, such decisions as not to marry or not to have children do not easily lend themselves to self-sacrificial explanations.

Women also experience anxiety over the fear that the choices they are making are the "wrong" choices. A major psychological obstacle to making active choices is fear of taking responsibility for how one's life turns out. The women who puts off having children so that she does not jeopardize her career advancement may find that being vice-president of the company is not as rewarding as she thought it would be. And there is no one to blame. For the woman who took a new path and failed, it may be especially hard to hear "I told you so," particularly if this message comes from one's mother.

The vocabulary of right and wrong choices seems highly inappropriate. When the marriage that seemed so right 15 years ago is so wrong today, the notion of right and wrong needs scrutiny. The test of whether a decision is right cannot be how things turn out years later. Too much is in flux. Perhaps what is right needs to be defined in terms of what conforms best to one's truest feelings as one knows them at the time. This is not a comfortable definition. Traditional definitions of morality (the old familiar standbys—security, stability, commitment, loyalty, faithfulness) alone are not enough to sustain us. A hard look reveals that these old definitions of what is right didn't sustain us anyway, only we weren't willing to take a hard look. We weren't willing to question our faith in prescriptions.

While it is difficult to see oneself as actively choosing a life pattern for which one has no precedents and that has been and may still be stigmatized, there are substantial psychological gains to be had for so doing. Recent findings support the speculation that knowing yourself well enough to know what life pattern you want, and being in that pattern, contributes to feelings of well-being (Hoffman, 1976). If you are a nonemployed mother and prefer to be employed, your self-esteem is lower compared to your counterparts who prefer to be homemakers. Being in a pattern because someone else wants you to be in that pattern, or because you are afraid of what others might think if you were to make a change, turns out to exact a high price in a woman's feelings about herself. While such a woman may experience the comfort of not taking sole command of her life and of avoiding responsibility, there are no noticeable long-term rewards for that strategy.

In fact, recent data (Baruch, Barnett, and Rivers, 1983) indicate that feelings of well-being for a woman in the middle years are associated with her preferring to be in whatever life pattern she is in. Never-married women who prefer to be single are higher in well-being than never-married women who wish they were married. Employed women who would choose to remain employed even if they had enough money to live comfortably are higher in well-being than employed women who would rather be homemakers, and so on. Clearly, it is difficult to distinguish preference from adaptation and denial. Perhaps never-married women "really" prefer to be married but are denying that preference. Our interpretation, based on additional findings from the same study, is that denial is not an adequate explanation, although adaptation—increasing the goodness of fit of self and role—may be. Indeed, it appears as if the never-married women at the midpoint in their adult lives have organized a life-style that is rich and meaningful and in which the absence of marriage is not significant.

But as independent adult women we need to learn that there are no guarantees; in a sense, we are all involved in experiments in which we cannot predict the outcomes. All we can do is make honest choices, learn to take whatever consequences follow from those choices, and deal with the outcomes. Since the old formulas for women have failed miserably, newer ideas about finding a life pattern that fits one's realistic appraisal of what one needs is a better long-term bet. But it is still only a bet.

REFERENCES

Barnett, R. C., and Baruch, G. K. *Role strain, number of roles and psychological well-being.* Working paper of the Wellesley College Center for Research on Women, 1981.

Barnett, R. C., and Baruch, G. K. *On the psychological well-being of women in the mid-years.* Working paper of the Wellesley College Center for Research on Women, 1982.

Baruch, G. K., Barnett, R. C., & Rivers, C. *Lifeprints: New patterns of love and work for today's women.* New York: McGraw-Hill, 1983.

Bem, S. L. The measurement of psychological androgyny. *Journal of Consulting and Clinical Psychology,* 1974, *42,* 155–162.

Elder, G. H. Historical change in life patterns and personality. In P. Baltes and O. G. Brim, Jr. (Eds.), *Life-span development and behavior* (Vol. 2). New York: Academic Press, 1979.

Hagestad, G. O. Problems and promises in the social psychology of intergenerational relations. In R. W. Fogel, E. Hatfield, S. Kiesler, and J. March (Eds.), *Stability and change in the family.* New York: Academic Press, 1981.

Hagestad, G., Smyer, M., and Stierman, K. Parent–child relations in adulthood: The impact of divorce in middle age. In R. Cohen, S. Weissman, and B. Cohler (Eds.), *Parenthood as an adult experience.* New York: Guilford Press, 1982.

Hareven, T. K. The last stage: Adulthood and old age. *Daedalus,* 1976, *105,* 13–27.

Hoffman, L. M. Effects of maternal employment on the child: A review of the research. In A. G. Kaplan and J. P. Bean (Eds.), *Beyond sex role stereotypes: Readings toward a psychology of androgyny.* Boston: Little, Brown, 1976.

Inkeles, A. *What is sociology?* Englewood Cliffs, N.J.: Prentice-Hall, 1964.

Kagan, J. Acquisition and significance of sex typing and sex role identification. In M. L. Hoffman and L. W. Hoffman (Eds.), *Review of child development research* (Vol. 1). New York: Russell Sage, 1964.

Kohlberg, L. A cognitive-developmental analysis of children's sex-role concepts and attitudes. In E. Maccoby (Ed.), *The development of sex differences.* Stanford, Calif.: Stanford University Press, 1966.

Marecek, J., and Johnson, M. Gender and the process of therapy. In A. M. Brodsky and R. T. Hare-Mustin (Eds.), *Women and psychotherapy.* New York: Guilford Press, 1980.

McMahon, S. L. Women in marital transition. In A. M. Brodsky and R. T. Hare-Mustin (Eds.), *Women in psychotherapy*. New York: Guilford Press, 1980.
Notman, M. T., and Nadelson, C. C. The woman patient. In M. Notman and C. C. Nadelson (Eds.), *The woman patient*, Vol. 1. New York: Plenum, 1978.
Pearlin, L. Sex roles and depression. In N. Datan and L. H. Ginsberg (Eds.), *Life-span developmental psychology: Normative life crises*. New York: Academic Press, 1975.
Teicholtz, J. *Psychological correlates of voluntary childlessness in married women*. Paper presented at the meeting of the Eastern Psychological Association, Washington, D.C., 1978.

Chapter 16

Reflections and Perspectives on 'Therapeutic Issues for Today's Adult Women'

MALKAH T. NOTMAN

Women in their middle years are at varying points in their own life cycles. One women at 40 may be a grandmother, another may be having her first child. Women's lives are also not linear—that is, they do not progress in a predictable sequence; many roles, positions, and psychological states may occur in varying sequences. Although women are affected by their reproductive timetable, this is not the only major framework, and the interrelated components of biology, culture, and psychology have an enormous impact. Therefore, women who are in their "middle years" will bring a variety of therapeutic issues to attention. There is some similarity, however, in the threads that run through many of these issues, particularly if one focuses on the midlife aspects of the problems presented. In confronting the finiteness of life as one comes to perceive it in midlife, an assessment is made of where one is and where one might like to be. Choices that were made, choices that still can be made, and their consequences are considered and evaluated. For women these sometimes concern decisions about having children, sometimes about careers, marriages.

In the past few years, many women have come for consultation and help with problems about these choices, whatever paths they have taken. Barnett has written about some of the central concerns that today's adult women are confronting and that they have been bringing to therapists. She has attempted to suggest the impact of recent major

---

MALKAH T. NOTMAN • Tufts University, Boston, Massachusetts 02146.

social changes in women's roles on these issues. The emphasis on the need to take risks, the importance of assuming responsibility for one's own life, and the importance of choice are crucial. But choice exists on many levels and it is a complex issue with many dimensions, related both to external reality and to internal reality. A few of these complex issues will be addressed and then some clinical examples described that have a bearing on choices and their implications.

Although we are all struck with the enormous impact of social change on women's roles, it is sometimes impossible to separate those problems that are related to these social changes from those that seem to be "old wine in new bottles." For example, the particular manifestations of generational conflicts and value shifts in our current historical period reflect not only new possibilities for women's lives but also some of the inevitable consequences of generational discontinuity, competition, and conflict, as well as identifications.

There is also some question as to how far-reaching the changes in opportunities for women have been (see Alington and Troll, Chapter 7). There is no question as to the availability of reproductive control, at least for middle-class Caucasian women, and therefore, of opportunities for limiting family size, clearly a far-reaching social phenomenon with lasting consequences. The increase in the life-span also means that commitments, such as marital commitments, and expectations of the content of one's life are different. A life can have a number of sequential periods. Some women today talk about their lives as if they have conscious expectations of phases, one to be occupied by marriage and child-rearing, another in which aloneness may not be chosen but may nevertheless have to be confronted. Longevity also means that marital commitments of fidelity and exclusivity, which were intended to last a shorter lifetime than now exists, may be strained as partners develop with the increasing years (Bernard, 1978). These issues are also brought to therapists, sometimes precipitated by the role changes of one or the other partner. They are sometimes presented as questions or disappointments, sometimes as newly awakened wishes that are conflicted.

There is also confusion as to which phases should precede which, whether childbearing and child-rearing should precede establishment of a career, whether this sequence should be the reverse, or whether both can take place concomitantly with some new integration of work and family at a later phase. These questions are also brought into therapy. The possibility of even considering an approach involving a series of life phases is based on the new expectation of many productive and healthy years.

In other spheres, however, the actual impact of social changes does not seem quite as clear. Given the enormous increase of women in the work force, their advancement into positions of high status, economic achievement, and authority has lagged far behind (Scott, 1982). Informal experience and contact with a number of women also indicate that although they may function with varying degrees of freedom at work, once they leave work and return home to their families and friends, their expectations of how they "should" be and what is expected of them are very different and much more conventional, and they speak about leading "schizophrenic" lives.

There are limitations of choice, then, which derive from the realities of particular work conditons and social options. Limitations of choice also are internal; for some women, the determining realities, the exigencies of the demands others make on them, and the limits of their situation may make options much less free in reality than they appear to be.

Most women who are aspiring to carrers do indeed have life potentials that are very different from the expectations that their mothers confronted. There is considerable disparity between the choices made by women today and the lives of their mothers. Dr. Barnett (Chapter 15, this volume) portrays the mother as the inhibiting, awe-inspiring, and feared person whom the daughter may be afraid to confront and who may limit her movement in new directions; Barnett points out that some of this image may be the daugher's internal perception and not actually correct. Situations where the daughters expect maternal disapproval certainly are common. Many women do express their own conflicts in terms of fearing their mother's disapproval. Sometimes this appears to be similar to an issue defined in an old way by psychoanalytic theory, as due to oedipal competitive anxieties—that is, anxiety at doing better than one's mother. This may be an internal concern, remaining from old unresolved conflicts, as well as externally reenforced. Competition with one's mother and the desire to exceed her achievements are often fraught with guilt even when success is not measured in terms of personal career achievement but in other dimensions. Applegarth (1976) describes a syndrome in which daughters fulfill a narcissistic role for the mother. They fulfill the mother's ambitions, and the mother sees them as part of herself. A gifted girl, then, may refuse, consciously or unconsciously, to use her gifts, as a means of establishing separateness for herself or for the purposes of rebellion and revenge. This possibility needs to be considered in relation to difficulties and inhibitions that women have in moving ahead in work. This dynamic may complicate what is consciously perceived as a choice, or a lack of one.

People teaching at an advanced level, or working with women who are striving for demanding careers, have also begun to see a reversal in the traditional picture, namely, to see women pressured by parents, including mothers, to move ahead. This may not be motivated by quite the same narcissistic gratification as that of the mothers to whom Applegarth refers. A mother simply may wish that her daughter not miss opportunities that she herself was unable to fulfill, without seeing her as a narcissistic extension of herself. However, this pressure can nevertheless create problems relating to achievement for the daughter. It may be expressed as the reverse of Barnett's example of the mother who cannot understand why a woman might prefer to have an abortion and finish school. The mother sometimes would prefer for the daughter to finish school, while the daughter—for her own reasons, as we have indicated—may choose not to have the abortion.

Many women need approval from others, and their mothers figure importantly in this. However, it is also interesting to observe movement and change take place in the mother, since we are concerned with the spectrum of adult women in midlife. A woman in her mid-20s or in her 30s today may have a mother in her mid-50s. This woman is also in midlife and may have confronted life situations or internal changes that have also made for adaptations of her own.

A clinical example illustrates this.

> Mrs. E was 55 and had had no previous work experience when she went to work in a large firm. First she was a relatively unskilled file clerk, but she eventually became a managing secretary of a whole unit. She described her life over the past 10 years. She had had three daughters, was married to a fairly conventional man who was a skilled worked, and lived in a tightly knit neighborhood where she was very much part of the community of women—a devout churchgoer, a supporter of all school activities, and a dependable friend, mother, and wife. As her daughters grew older, she felt distant from them. She could not understand their preferences in clothes, such as choosing what seemed to her to be unconventional or too seductive or too "loud" kinds of dresses or pants. One of them was allied with a political group that took a stand against racial bais, a stand that was much more overt than the family's position had been. Another had been active in the antiwar protest movement. Then, unexpectedly, Mr. E was killed in a work-related accident. Mrs. E was overwhelmed, felt helpless, lost, bewildered for a time. She relied for a while on the support of her family but then realized that both for her own well-being and for financial reasons she would have to seek paid work. She had few marketable skills, so she went to secretarial school and then into the inner city to take the best of the jobs that were available to her. There she met a whole different group of women. She began to wear pants to work, particularly in the winter. She cut her hair, since she could not take the time for visits to the beauty parlor. She found she had to cut corners in housekeeping, was less interested in some of the homemaking activities she had shared with her friends earlier. In contact with people from very different backgrounds, she found her attitude changing. She said that although she missed her husband a great deal and felt very lonely, the activities that she found she needed most help with were those that involved physical strength. She found new friends and discovered she could do by herself most of the household things for which she had previously relied on her husband.

> She had begun to date but really did not feel optimistic about finding somebody that she might marry; she realized she valued some aspects of her independence and freedom. To her amazement, she found that she began to share more of her daughters' attitudes. Her understanding of their positions and beliefs increased, as did the closeness of their relationship. At the same time, her shared activities with her friends diminished of necessity, and although she felt warm toward them, there was less time to do things with them as her own patterns changed.

This is an example of a woman whose own circumstances brought about both more understanding through a change in life-style that became closer to that of her daughters. (These changes can happen also by the effects of interactions between people, not only by force of life circumstances.)

Other mothers, of course, may remain disapproving. For many women, however, the extent to which they are fearful of their mother's opinions, or the opinions of others close to them, represents their own conflicts about choices and decisions. Their own ambivalence may be projected outward, so it is the other person who is seen as disapproving, rather than oneself who is in conflict.

A choice may thus involve internal discrepancies and potential conflict, not only a risk in a new uncharted direction, perhaps with less protection than in the past. It also contains the potential for confusion and disappointment when one feels one has done the right thing but has not experienced fulfillment. To recognize these internal issues brings greater possibilities for resolution.

A number of women currently come for help because they have done what seems to be the "right" thing, in contemporary terms, yet do not feel it has worked well enough. They have worked hard, earned promotions, higher degrees, job advancements, positions with considerable status and sometimes with considerable financial rewards. Nevertheless, they feel some sense of incompleteness or lack of fulfillment.

At times, the conflict has to do with "femininity" and with childbearing. Women who have initially made the decision not to have children fear that they may regret it and may then decide to have children. However, there may be a different issue, a conflict involving what one has intellectually chosen to do yet feels emotionally is unresolved. For example, a woman who has internal conflicts about achievement and success may not feel comfortable in a successful position. There may be a conflict between internalized expectations and current roles, which is derived not only from the way one's mother grew up and the consequent expectations but from problems reconciling the costs and benefits of their choices. Some of these women are not aware of their internal conflict but develop symptoms, feel depressed, or are puzzled about their dissatisfaction.

There are complicated determinants of most choices. Sometimes the conscious reason is not entirely consistent with some of the less conscious functions of a choice. For example, one may make a choice toward academic success and fulfillment and find that the process carries with it the need to be competitive and aggressive. This not only raises issues of femininity, as Barnett indicates, but stirs up conflicts about aggression itself.

There has been a good deal of restriction placed upon girls in both their sexual and aggressive expression (Nadelson, Notman, Miller & Zilbach, 1982). Women may have particular conflicts around aggression that often produce problems with achievement. Men have difficulties concerning aggression that may be expressed in relation to work; however, they can have a somewhat different constellation in that in the rest of men's lives, aggressive expression is not so limited.

A woman's triumph may feel like surpassing and showing up her mother as weak, stupid, and "only a woman." The "unfeminine" aspect of being aggressive and competitive has been mentioned. It touches more on the larger issue of self-esteem, not just femininity.

The concept of *femininity* has been very confused. One may use the term descriptively, normatively, and in a variety of other ways. Barnett finds a woman's own concept of femininity closely connected with her feeling about her reproductive or marital status, and that is indeed often the way women see it. If one considers femininity in relation to self-esteem, a woman who does not feel "feminine," in whatever terms she defines it, has a lower opinion of herself than one who does, since feminine is what women are "supposed" to be. Thus, problems can develop in the discrepancies or contradictions between one's own view of oneself and the ideal. If an individual receives sufficient support for competence and mastery, she is likely to have less concern as to whether or not she is feminine, even if unmarried or not a mother.

For some women, however, a career itself may be defined inevitably as a masculine activity, rather than be assessed in terms of its fulfillment. The extent to which this is true despite conscious decisions to the contrary is sometimes astounding.

A woman premedical student, who had come to an interest in medicine after exploring a variety of other jobs and fields, and therefore felt she was making a mature and reasoned choice, found herself unable to complete the last two courses of her premedical requirements. After many starts and failures, she stopped and decided to look more deeply into the conflicts that must be contained in this behavior. She realized that she was consciously committed to the values and choice of a career in medicine, but when she came to the threshold of the commitment, thinking of the number of hours involved in the training and in the work, she could only see a man doing this and not a woman. Furthermore, she felt that she could not bring herself to exceed the accomplishments of her mother without paralyzing guilt. Her mother was moderately supportive of her studies, but she herself could not at this point resolve her ambivalence and accept the support. It took a good deal of sorting out of her past attitudes and expectations from her current ones before she could proceed.

Another woman, an accomplished professional, had been for several years in a fairly stable, not very demanding job. She decided that she was bored by this and would prefer another job that was becoming available, which had as part of its appeal the fact that there was a clear possibility of advancement and even a position of some prominence. She became extremely anxious. When this was explored she said, "It feels like I'm going public with my ambition." This competent woman had been able to function well with her apparently successful career until a new situation brought what seemed a more open acknowledgment of a competitive and aggressive aspect that she had not previously dealt with directly. She was then forced to confront the fact that she acted as if she felt that ambition was a "bad thing."

To return to the question of the definition of femininity as related to childbearing, this relationship was assumed for a long period, and as Barnett emphasizes, the potential separation of the two issues needs to be made. However, the wish for a child is not always accompanied by a wish for a traditional or a conventional life-style. It is a very complex wish and involves not only narcissistic aspects, such as perpetuating oneself, but also the wish to care for another human being, or some identification with one's mother, which need not be a complete identification with one's mother's life-style. The woman who decides against childbearing or finds herself in a position where she is unlikely to have children must confront a real loss if this has been an important goal for her. Although it is possible to find fulfillment in other directions, the loss and its meaning for that individual cannot be ignored.

In the same way, the woman who does not marry may find certain freedoms, but she may also face loneliness, which makes her vulnerable to depression. This is not only because of the consequences of choosing a deviant path. The time limits on reproduction—that is, the limited time during which women may bear children—are important in the whole context of women's lives. Anxiety may result if a woman has not had children, finds herself growing older, and feels the opportunity is passing her by.

Women live their reproductive lives in a more time-related framework than men. Menarche is an abrupt beginning of reproductive potential, and menopause is a relatively clear-cut ending, even though it has a less abrupt quality. In addition, the monthly reminder of the menstrual periods constitutes an "inner clock," which many women feel is very much a part of their self-concept. These limitations may heighten awareness and significance of the passage of time, the changes that come with aging, and the limits of what can be accomplished in other directions. Choices about children thus become pressing in a different way from that for men, although many other choices and developmental experiences are unrelated to the reproductive timetable.

A recurrent theme in Barnett's chapter concerns the benefits of freeing oneself from old patterns, unfulfilling relationships, and needs for support. The importance of developing the sense of self and of independence is stressed. Although these are indeed very important, and differ from traditional goals for women and traditional components of femininity, it would be a mistake then to equate maturity with aloneness or to equate maturity and autonomy with nonrelatedness. Affirmation comes in the context of relationships, whether traditional, therapeutic, or other. Women sometimes need help in restructuring their relationships rather than in leaving them; their strengths also lie in the capacity to adapt, to compromise, to help others to change so that one's own needs as well as other people's needs are more adequately met. Not only independence but assertions and fulfillment within relationships are important and also take some knowledge of what one wants and courage to go after it.

Similar problems exist in sorting out the attitudes of *others* (including parents) toward steps that take a woman into a more unconventional position from one's *own* feelings of regret, loss, or failure—feelings that may be projected onto critical outsiders.

It is particularly crucial in dealing with patients to separate one's own concerns and values from those of the patient. For a therapist, the agenda must be to try to understand the patient's goals rather than to judge the patient's situation in terms of one's goals. A clinical example illustrates this. Mrs. A came for a consultation because of increasing marital difficulties. These were of long standing. She was married to an engineer with a predominantly unresponsive personality with many compulsive defenses. He was, however, reliable and companionable, even though his range of affect seemed rather limited. They had two children who were adolescents. She recognized the limitations of her marriage and had gone back to school to a program that would permit her to develop her work in a new direction. She had been in therapy, and her therapist, sensing the inadequacy of the marriage, had strongly supported her leaving her husband. Mrs. A felt that she really was not prepared to make that decision. She discovered that the therapist had recently been divorced, and then felt uncomfortable discussing her own ambivalence with this therapist. She wondered whether, because the therapist had found this solution effective for herself, she was proposing it strongly for her patient without taking fully into account the patient's own balance of dependency, attachment, and discontent.

This important problem can be expressed in many directions; for example, the therapist may have a bias in favor of marriage, of divorce, of the value of childbearing, or other issues. It is important to maintain as much clarity as possible as to which choices are appropriate for the patient. Certainly, there are fewer automatic answers today; the automatic attempt to establish self-esteem and femininity by marriage and childbearing was very unsuccessful for many women in the past. Perhaps because of the greater availability of careers and the range of choices, women with a particular pattern of problems have been seen recently with greater frequency. Some examples follow.

One woman was a successful lawyer. She came because of dissatisfaction with her work and with her relationship with a young man who was also successfully climbing a career ladder toward success. Her central complaint was that he became irrationally angry, and she then felt demeaned. In the course of therapeutic work, memories emerged in which, during her mother's depression and hospitalization, she had spent time with her father, who in his alcoholic periods would shout at her, and whom she never felt she could reach. The successful career she had embarked upon was meant both to finally win his approval and also to identify with him. Her lover was in part also chosen for his resemblance to her father; her hope was that in quelling his outbursts, she could master the painful experiences of the past. In therapy she was able to sort out past goals and wishes from present possibilities to realize and, to some extent, give up her expectations of her father and her disappointment with her lover. She was able to pursue her work more for its own sake and find gratification in it, and then to choose another man. Disappointment that the career success had not made possible the fulfillment of a childhood wish had initially been experienced as disappointment with the career choice itself. In helping women deal with impediments to productive work and relationships, understanding of these latent meanings and agendas become important.

Another young woman was fairly successful in a business career in a larger organization. She had been the youngest of three children. Her two brothers were considerably older and she always felt that she had been an afterthought. Although admired for her prettiness, she was left alone for long periods of time and was often depressed and lonely as a child. Her parents were socially prominent, her father a successful lawyer. She married and found herself bitterly resenting her father's interest in her husband, a relationship from which she felt excluded. Her mother had had a period during which she too had been depressed, although not to the point of hospitalization, but had been remote, sad, preoccupied. This coincided with the illness of her own parents. The mother's depression took place when this young woman was about 9 or 10; she remembered that there would be long periods of being with her mother while she was uncommunicative and seemed not to notice much about her. She too had worked very hard to achieve and to please. The daughter was bitterly competitive and resentful and eventually separated from her husband, who seemed to offer nothing more than the reflected status and prestige of his success, but little warmth. Although in her mid-30s and functioning fully as an adult, she still was driven to fury by her father's inability or refusal to listen to her seriously.

Although one could go into considerable detail about the individual histories of these women, one part of the pattern seems to stand out. These are women who have had a mother who was either severely or moderately and chronically depressed, and who, whether employed or in a traditional housewife role, was emotionally unavailable to the girl growing up. The father was turned to for support and also identification, and there was a wish for the father's admiration, some closeness to him, or some sense of relatedness and attention. This became incorporated into a life pattern involving effort, achievement, and success, with at least one goal being to finally "make it" in forming the desired relationship.

One important aspect of this constellation is that the disappointment felt by these young women seemed on the surface to be due to the fact that the career for which they had worked so hard and had been successful in was not fulfilling its promise. The central wish they had was not expressed in terms of "femininity" or realizing the traditional role of mother or marriage, but had to do with a long-standing wish to achieve some special relationship to their fathers. We have known through the work of many child developmentalists, particularly in recent years, how important the father is for the development of the self-esteem of the girl and even for her sense of "femininity." In these cases, the fathers were especially important by contrast to the depressed and unavailable mothers. The success in the achieving and mastery aspects of these women's careers was considerable and real, as were the gratifications. However, the importance of the unfulfilled part of the wishes went unrecognized until further explored.

This syndrome appears to be occurring more frequently, and it raises questions about the effects of a mother's depression on a daughter's directions and identifications. In the cases cited, a choice that seemed to lead to fulfillment still had some components missing. Perhaps a family constellation of a mother who is depressed and a father who is clearly more successful. interesting, available to some degree—although not really making the girl feel valued and supported—may be a spur for her toward achievement. This spur can result in very considerable and genuine accomplishment on the part of the daughter, even if there is disappointment at not winning her father's approval or closeness. This discontent should not be seen as simply due to the problems of choosing a life-style that might be nontraditional; one must clearly understand the meanings of the relationships and strivings involved.

Another example is worth considering, that of a woman who is a successful physician. As a young girl, she had been shy. Her mother, a schoolteacher, seemed to be able to do anything—to run the family, cook, be an admired professional, and maintain a marriage. Her father was a scientist. She herself was bright in school but avoided all the areas in which her mother excelled. One day she hesitantly talked with her mother about her vague future plans. To her surprise, her mother supported an interest in medicine, saying she herself would have wanted to do this but had no talent for science. Her mother's admission of a weakness and, at the same time, her support seemed amazing to the girl. She felt less intimidated, explored the possibilities, and eventually went to medical school. At another point of indecision she sought counseling. The female therapist also felt it was an appropriate and possible goal, an important factor in her decision. Later, when she was in her 30s and worrying whether there was still time for childbearing, her mother said on a visit to her city, "Why not?" Eventually, not only did she become a mother but her career tended in an academic direction and she too became a teacher, completing an identification with her mother that had in some ways previously been conflicted because of her perception of her mother's greater strength, and her own competitiveness and ambition.

We may expect mothers to play an increasingly positive role in the lives, accomplishments, and well-being of their daughters, and therapists' attention to patterns of needs, fulfillments, and relationships of women certainly must occur in the context of full awareness of new life patterns, new solutions, and new options. These may help us find ways to support the strengthening of women's self-esteem without relying on outmoded views of appropriate behavior or "femininity."

REFERENCES

Applegarth, A. Some observations on work inhibitions in women. *Journal of the American Psychoanalytic Association*, 1976, 24, 251–268.
Bernard, J. *Perspectives on marriage*. Paper presented at the Radcliffe College Precentennial Conference on Perspectives on the Patterns of an Era, 1978.
Nadelson, C., Notman, M., Miller, J., and Zilbach, J. Aggression in women: Conceptual issues and clinical implications. In M. Notman and C. Nadelson (Eds.), *The woman patient* (Vol. 3). New York: Plenum Press, 1982.
Scott, J. The mechanization of women's work. *Scientific American*, 1982, 247, 167–187.

Chapter 17

Sexuality and the Middle-Aged Woman

Zella Luria and Robert G. Meade

Menopause: The Wrong Question

Government-funded research on sexual behavior is usually about one of two groups: adolescents or those over age 60. For the former group, the goal is to stop, or regulate, the behavior; for the older group, the aim is to document the potential lifelong availability of a God-given sexual gift, driven by the rule "Use it or lose it." As the proportion of older citizens in the population increases, their political clout sparks research on the conditions that maintain sexual behavior after age 60. Lost in the push (the aged) and pull (back the young) are the middle-aged, those roughly 40–60 years old.

Middle age, like other life stages, is not pure biology. Its onset and duration depend on self-image, life events, presumed life-span, and the interaction among these factors. Our notion of the life cycle may be critically related to particular milestones and to our reference groups. Gender, class, education, and occupation undoubtedly influence our views of middle age and life's course. Female sexuality is intimately related to a woman's life-cycle concepts.

Insistence on reproductive capacity as the key to women's sexuality flies in the face of available evidence. In Neugarten's study (1963) of 100 women aged 43–53, only one-sixth of the women thought that sexual relations became less important with menopause; the rest rated sex the same as before menopause, or even better now that pregnancy was

---

Zella Luria and Robert G. Meade • Psychology Department, Tufts University, Medford, Massachusetts 02155

impossible. There were no personality differences among premenopausal, menopausal, and postmenopausal women. In fact, only 4% of the women saw menopause as a principal concern. These middle-aged women feared losing their husbands, getting older, and cancer—not menopause. A volunteer "opportunity" sample of 484 women of mixed ages had similar results: no significant grief accompanying the passing of menses and reproduction (Boston Women's Health Book Collective, 1976). Rossi (1980) suggests that menopause is a private event but postmenopausal signs are public: "grey hair, wrinkles, dentures, drowsiness, age spots, thickening of the waistline, sagging of abdomen and breasts, and biofocal glasses."

Recent changes in women's sexual behavior belie the notion that female sexuality exists only as an adjunct to romantic love, yet we know remarkably little about the meanings of specific sexual acts in women's lives. The almost total absence of such information in our culture is unlikely to continue, however. Anthropological studies of other cultures are already providing us with knowledge that we lack about our own society (Ortner and Whitehead, 1981). What we do know about women's experience of being sexual in midlife depends on the women's age cohort, their marital status, and the measure of being sexual.

Middle-Aged Women in Kinsey's Time

Information about what middle-aged women's sex lives were like in the relatively recent past comes from the Kinsey, Pomeroy, Martin, and Gebhard volume on women (1953). Those data are based on small and selected samples. Middle-aged women are reluctant to talk about their sexual experiences; in Kinsey's day, they were even more so. However, without this basis for comparison with the past, current data on the middle-aged woman's sex life fall into a vacuum.

Kinsey's sample of middle-aged women came from the birth cohorts of 1880 to 1910. Those cohorts are not entirely homogeneous with respect to sexual histories. Women born after 1900 were likely to have had more premarital intercourse and more petting to orgasm than did the earlier cohorts. The liberal sexuality of the post-World War I world had a much greater impact on women born after 1900 than it did on those born before the turn of the century. In spite of these differences, some clear-cut findings emerged from the data of these mixed cohorts.

Married women had more frequent intercourse as well as other forms of sexual "outlets" (Kinsey's term) than women of the same age who were not married. Unmarried middle-aged women showed low levels of all forms of sexual activity, but no lower than younger unmarried women!

Among women who were born before 1900 and had never married (aged 50–69), one-third never had any overt sexual activity beyond simple petting; they experienced little sexual arousal during petting, and no orgasm ever. The other two-thirds of these never-married women had more sexual experience; 62% of them had had intercourse, 16% had had extensive homosexual relations. The rest had engaged in other forms of sexual behavior (Christenson and Johnson, 1973). While these relatively barren sexual histories may seem ascetic to modern readers, these women were not so unusual in their day. Theirs was a culture in which there were substantial numbers of unmarried women. Sex went with marriage or was an exchange made just before marriage. Most women had one sexual partner in their lives—their husband. Given that framework, the heterosexually active and the homosexually active groups are extremely interesting.

Overall, availability of a partner predicted how much sex a woman had. But even stably married women reported age-related changes in their sex lives. As a group, married women over 40 experienced a steady drop in incidence (do you ever . . . ?) of intercourse (Pfeiffer and Davis, 1972). Current knowledge bears out Kinsey's intuition about the cause of the decline; often, erectile difficulties lead husbands to discontinue sexual intercourse.

How often a middle-aged married woman experienced intercourse was related to her age and to her husband's age, too. But age and partner availability are not the only factors leading to declines in married sexual behavior. A striking decline in sexual activity occurs among young married pairs. A large urban sample of recently married young women, all under 30, showed a decline of about 25% in frequency of sexual intercourse as early as the first 4 years of marriage (Udry, 1980). These are especially important findings because they are based on longitudinal data, which are in short supply in the sexual behavior literature. Given that declines in sexual behavior can be found in both the middle-aged and the young, we must attend to the multiple sources other than age that feed into coital decision-making by couples.

Kinsey viewed the decline in frequency of intercourse as due to males. He saw the age-related testosterone decrement in men as the biological basis for the lower levels of sexual behavior seen with increasing age. The behavioral decline is doubtlessly real; it occurs in study after study (Kinsey, Pomeroy, and Martin, 1948; Kinsey *et al.*, 1953; Udry, 1980; Westoff, 1974). Age-related declines in both circulating testosterone levels and sexual behavior are characteristic of the male in all mammalian species studied. However, low hormone levels do not account in any simpleminded way for all of the behavioral decrements, at least in the human male, since the decrease in behavior antedates the hormonal decline. Hormone–behavior relationships are typically described with arrows (of causality) going from hormone to behavior. Yet evidence supports the arrow going in the other direction, too. Testosterone in men goes up following sexual behavior, at least in some studies (e.g., Kraemer, Becker, Brodie, Doering, Moos, and Hamburg, 1976). Our hunch is that habituation in marriage and competing family interests (especially children) help to lower the rate of sexual turn-ons (accounting for the early drop in marital coital frequencies). Diminished sexual behavior and slowly decreasing hormone levels conspire to further lower levels of sexual behavior in men. Testosterone levels in women are about 10% of those in men, and they do not decline with age. The role that testosterone plays in female libido is unknown. Recent work in stumptail macaque monkeys indicates that, at least in this species, sex steroids are not required for the maintenance of sexual attractiveness, receptivity, or proceptivity by females (Baum, Koos Slob, de Jong, and Westbrook, 1978).

About half of a small sample of middle-aged men and women, of Kinsey-study vintage, report a decrease in sexual interest and activity by age 45. By 55, 75–80% of the sample report declines. More women than men are aware of declines in sexual interest (Pfeiffer, Verwoerdt, and Davis, 1972).

For middle-aged women from the birth cohort 1900–1925, marital status alone predicted sexual enjoyment, sexual frequency, and sexual interest. Health, subjective or objective, was the predictor for men. But health did not account for the variance among women. A partner meant stability and the sanction of the law to these women (Pfeiffer and Davis, 1972). Is all this work a belabored discovery of the double standard? Studies of women aged 40–60 in the 1980s would reflect an ailing, but by no means dead, double standard. Again, one searches for the meanings of women's sexual acts.

What Causes the Age-Related Decline in Sexual Behavior?

For every married man who decided that his active sex life was over because of erectile problems, at least one woman has shared the cost. Recent research leads to the counsel to men that erectile dysfunction is less likely and appears later when men eat well and exercise to control high blood pressure and to maintain weight. Lots of early sexual practice also serves to forestall the onset of erectile difficulties (Martin, 1977). Given the dependence of the sacral-mediated erectile reflex on the vascular and peripheral neural systems, the current generation of regular joggers and exercise devotees may well be the group to watch in their middle and Medicare years. Pfeiffer and Davis's correlation of male good health and frequency of marital coitus fits well with Martin's findings. The sexual rule for men is: Stay well. For women, it is: Stay married. For both, the implicit rule is: Stay sexually active.

The search for the causes of the decline in marital sex with age interests endocrinologists, survey researchers, and developmental psychologists alike. Kinsey found that wives typically reported higher frequencies of intercourse than husbands. He reasoned that the actual frequencies seemed higher to wives because they were having more sex than they wanted. He thought that husbands were apt to underestimate the frequency of intercourse because they would have preferred a higher rate. Thirty years later, Hunt's (1974) admittedly selective sample suggests that husband–wife views on what constitutes "enough" have reached parity.

Using large-scale survey data on samples aged 44 and younger, Udry and Morris (1978) examined the relative contributions of males' and females' ages to the decline in the frequency of marital coitus. They calculated the mean decline in monthly coital frequency across successive 5-year age intervals. By holding the age of one spouse constant, they were able to examine the contribution of the age of the other spouse to the decline. That portion of the decline attributable to male age is smaller in each successive sample. The contribution of female age to the mean decline shows a complementary increase, starting low in 1965, picking up substantially in 1970, and again in 1974. This finding should not be interpreted as indicating that wives today are depressing the quantity of marital coitus more than they did in Kinsey's time. Today's young marrieds are having intercourse more often than did their counterparts in previous generations. Udry and Morris's data most likely reflect the increased role played by wives' sexual appetites or wishes in coital decisionmaking. Such coital decisions by women can be based on nonsexual reasons.

Degler (1980) provides an exciting array of reasons for the sexual choices of 19th-century women. The reasons given do not add up to a simple lack of sexual interest by women. There is independent evidence from medical books and from purity-movement documents that sexual relations were important to women. But it was to be a qualitatively different relationship: gentler, more slowly paced, affectional, and less frequent.

Degler's summary suggests that 19th-century women were using sex to change power relations in the Victorian family, to prevent recurrent pregnancies, and to provide sufficient postpartum abstention so that women could nurse children through the dangers of early childhood. Demographic statistics from the late 19th century suggest that these women succeeded in their nonsexual motives by sexual means. Of course, some men helped them, convinced by the arguments of the various purity movements and of their wives.

A Drop in Female Libido

On the basis of a sample of about 900 adults, aged 18 to 60, Eysenck (1976) reported that "the libido of older subjects [is] weaker than that of younger subjects." His measure of sexual libido is based on scores from 50 self-report scales that examine the degree of pleasure derived from sexual thought and action, as well as attitudes toward many sexual issues (i.e., polygamy, masturbation, prostitution). Eysenck (1976) holds that genetic/hormonal contributions drive the reported libido of males. Data on females appear to fit a cultural-pressures model instead. All told, however, the sources of female libido are yet to be convincingly specified.

Do Gay Women Show Age-Related Decline?

The primary source of information about social sexual behavior is data describing heterosexual acts. Thus, conclusions drawn about the behavior of one sex are, of necessity, confounded by the contribution of the other sex. Heterosexual acts bring together people who differ not only in genital morphology and brain/hormone organization but also in cultural socialization. What happens to sexual behavior with age when the sexual pair have not been socialized in different directions? Gay people have no other-sex partner who can account for age-related changes in sexuality. The largest study of gay men and women finds that sexual interest is not age-related for gay men, but that it is for gay white women (Bell and Weinberg, 1978). ("Interest" is based on two interview items concerning thinking about sex and the importance of sex to the respondent.) In fact, across all ages, gay white men report significantly higher sexual interest than do gay white women. This sex difference is also reflected in behavior patterns, with gay white males showing higher frequencies of sexual interactions than their gay female counterparts. Both gay men and gay women show declines in the frequencies of actual sexual encounters with age, however.

The difficulty in making any general predictions about female sexuality from the data on gay women is that gay women are far from homogeneous. Black gay women do not report lower sexual interest than do black gay men, nor do they show any age-related decline in sexual interest. They are not like their white gay counterparts in this respect. In addition, while black gay males show overall higher frequencies of sexual behavior than their white counterparts, this racial pattern does not exist among gay women. Results like this explain (but do not justify) why many researchers preferred single-sex studies.

Color and Sexual Subculture

Black and white cultures differ markedly in their acceptance of female sexuality (see Angelou, 1981, pp. 66–67). As white cultural proscriptions against female sexuality are relaxed, we may see patterns of sexual behavior among white women moving toward those associated with the behavior of black populations. Some shifts in sexual behavior among young women suggest that this may be so, i.e., earlier age at first coital experience, greater acceptance of premarital sex.

SEEKING OUT SEX: KINSEY TO ERICA JONG

What determined the likelihood of a middle-aged woman of Kinsey-sample vintage seeking out sexual relations? A woman's past orgasmic experience makes seeking further sexual opportunities more likely when she is postmarried (Christenson and Gagnon, 1965). This accords with more recent findings that, in married women, past sexual enjoyment was significantly correlated with sexual functioning in middle age (Pfeiffer and Davis, 1972). Past enjoyment alone predicts sexual functioning in middle age for women; for men, past sexual frequency, enjoyment, and interest predict sexual functioning in middle age. Sexual activity, once encountered and enjoyed by women (and men too), tends to continue. Good sex begets good sex later.

Even though they lacked easy access to sexual partners after their marriages ended, 37% of the postmarried women in the Christenson and Gagnon study reported having intercourse at age 50. At 55, 29% were doing so, and at 60, 12% were. By 65 and older, none reported coitus. At 55, the frequencies of intercourse were only two-thirds that of married women their age, but double that of sexually active never-married women (Christenson and Johnson, 1973). Given the birth cohort of these postmarried women, these results are striking evidence of the middle-aged woman's capacity to seek out and maintain sexual relations once she has already had steady sexual experience with a marital partner. But they also emphasize the fact that marital status goes with the highest incidences and frequencies of sexual intercourse. The married need negotiate less than any other subgroup in order to have sex. And their partners are built in.

Gebhard (1971) extended and refined the data cited above by interviewing divorced and widowed women in the sample. Interviews of 632 white women led him to conclude that, even with ages matched, divorced women are almost twice as likely as widowed women to have postmarital coitus (82% vs. 43%). Beyond age 50, this difference in sexual activity diminishes. At that point, a woman's age was a more salient factor in her sexual behavior than was the cause of the end of her marriage. Obviously, the way a marriage ends provides different sexual contexts for the divorced woman and for the widow. Although both situations surely involve loss, cultural stereotypes have the divorcee freely moving into an easygoing postmarried life-style, while the widow bravely shoulders her grief. How a marriage functioned affects its aftermath too: 8% of the widows had had extramarital relations during the marriage, while a third of the divorced women had had the experience, often during the last year of the marriage, the year of *de facto* divorce. Fewer widows than divorced women remarried—27% and 47%, respectively. Among many factors, the grief and the continuing attachment of the widow to her dead spouse delay her reentry into sexual relations.

Nonetheless, even in the Kinsey cohort, most women who are sexually active postmaritally (whether widowed or divorced) have more than one sexual partner. Once a woman reenters the sexual scene, she has acknowledged her motivation for sex—and, probably, marriage—and it is unlikely that her first partner will fulfill all her expectations. For most postmarried women, the sexual marketplace is much different from what it was in their premarital days. Entry into that new marketplace involves learning new gender-role values and new negotiation skills (Hunt, 1966). Having acquired these new skills, the postmarital woman who has one sexual partner is more likely to move on to another.

To what extent do postmarital women use masturbation as a compensation for decreased sexual intercourse? It would seem to be as close a physiological substitute as possible. Kinsey surely conceived of masturbation as an "outlet" of just that sort. Masters and Johnson (1966) provide data that support masturbation as being more orgasmically efficient than coitus. When postmarried women are age-matched with married women, a markedly higher incidence of masturbation occurs among the former—almost double at age 50, 1 ½ times greater at 55 (Christenson and Johnson, 1973). All the masturbation episodes of the postmarried women do not add up to the frequencies of coitus plus masturbation of their married counterparts of like age.

Reading these studies, one is impelled to ask what masturbation stands for in relation to coitus among women. We wonder if a woman researcher would have conceived of sexual behaviors as "outlets," with masturbation and coitus as simple variants of sexual expression. That concept carries with it the image of a well of undifferentiated sexual energy waiting to be discharged—a concept not unfamiliar to Freudian theory. It is dubious whether women experience their sexual needs or wishes in this way. In truth, Kinsey, and Freud too, were well aware of the psychological differences in the experiences of masturbation and coitus. The difference between the two experiences seems to us to be potentially greater among women than among men because of gender-role differences. Coitus is a relational act and masturbation is not (except in fantasy). The female gender scripts embeds sexual acts in personal, emotional relationships. The "zipless fuck" violates that script; it titillates, but is finally doomed by its woman author (Jong, 1973).

SEXUAL MOTIVATION, AROUSAL, AND GENDER SCRIPTS

Current efforts to legitimize female masturbation contribute to the sexual development of women who often lack feelings of sexual entitlement (Barbach, 1975). The relational context of sex in the female gender script leads to a predominantly incentive theory view of female sexuality. An available social sexual object helps to produce sexual drive. Such sexuality is not driven by deprivation (as much of male sex drive in thought to be) (Luria and Rose, 1979). Incentive theory does not fit the masturbation data on women, however. Again, we need to know more about what masturbation means to women.

Arousal Is Simpler for Males

There may be some biological reasons that make more probable the separation of sexual arousal from relational issues in males than in females. The penis is a well-engineered biofeedback device. In addition to providing pubescent males with information about where their minds/genitals are, it permits the ready labeling of discrete objects and events as sexual turn-ons. Obviously, females have the potential for such biofeedback of their arousal state, but it is more subtle and requires more learning. Unlike the male, the female requires prior sexual experience to identify arousal. Geer and Morokoff (1974) find clear physiological evidence of vaginal vasocongestion in women shown arousing stimuli. But the sexually inexperienced women in the sample do not report arousal; the sexually experienced women do. Even among orgasmic, sexually experienced women, the correlation between subjective arousal and the most reliable physiological indicator of arousal (vaginal color change due to vasocongestion) is lower and less sure than it is for men (Steinman, Wincze, Sakheim, Barlow, and Maussakalian, 1981). Nature has arranged the penis to be visible and handy. While both males and females learn the culturally defined classes of events and persons to whom one may respond sexually, females must also learn to discriminate subtle changes in their own state of sexual arousal. Pubertal increases in testosterone in males assure many visible erections, hence many opportunities to learn sequences of behavior that lead to pleasurable outcomes. Males who do not discover ejaculation through conscious effort are initiated by nocturnal emissions. No equivalent exists for the pubescent female's orgasm. Female nocturnal orgasm, if it is experienced, tends to occur later in life, among the sexually experienced.

Penetration Makes a Difference

Sexual intercourse is an act that violates female body space, like violent acts. Acts that pierce body space—i.e., force feeding, prizefighting, inoculations—are typically regulated by authorities. While societies regulate sexual acts in all cultures, females must also monitor any potentially violent acts against them. This issue will occur only in societies where females are victims of such violent acts, especially forcible rape. The sorting out of violence and sex requires some knowledge of the space violator. Our surmise would be that this alone would assure women's concern with relationships. Even nonhuman females do not mate randomly. Obviously, one could construct a world that would severely mute the sex difference in awareness of arousal and concern with relationships. With respect to the latter, there is some evidence of merging of the two gender scripts—with males moving closer to the female script—among the educated young (Finger, 1975). It is conceivable that, in a world with no double standard, women would have more opportunities to learn about sexual arousal, especially through the removal of mislabelings and misattributions of female arousal (Barbach, 1975). But there is no Rousseau-esque world where male and female sexuality are the same in the "natural" state. Even in cultures where sexual pleasure is equally expected (and realized) by males and females, teaching about how to make love is tailored to each sex separately (Marshall, 1971).

UPDATING KINSEY: THE 1970s AND EARLY 1980s

Kinsey's pioneering work made it easier for researchers following him to study sexual behavior. However, current studies have a narrower focus than did Kinsey's work. Nowhere do we find a recent study with the same breadth of population sampled and behaviors surveyed. Very few studies permit the luxury of Kinsey's comparisons across birth cohorts. Kinsey's work virtually ended the era of studies with very long data-collection periods and with mounds of data on each individual studied. Funding agency policies assured the demise of such high-risk enterprises. Instead, we have more sharply-focused studies with smaller samples and fewer measures. The group least likely to be studied is the middle-aged.

The studies described so far are based on earlier cohorts than those that furnish our current popular view of middle age. Alice Rossi (1980) has described the special conditions encountered by the cohort born during the years 1920–1932: a lowered birthrate during the late 1920s, which made for a small birth cohort; the experience of the Great Depression in adolescence or younger; participation in World War II and/or the Korean War; the postwar economic boom, complete with significant and stable financial rewards (especially in comparison with those of their parents).

Rossi describes life for many women of this cohort: the pioneering and isolating settlement of suburbia, large families, and rising incomes. These families were members of that "lucky generation who came closer than any other to the ideal of American domesticity: a nice suburban home; a breadwinner husband and a homemaker wife; dedication to childrearing; and status gained from a high level of consumption of housing, automobiles, appliances and other consumer goods" (Masnick and Bane, 1980, pp. 1–2). Ironically, the net outcome of this is a squeeze on income when three, four, or five children reach adolescence and college age. In many cases, family income cannot keep pace with education costs and felt consumer needs.

The gap between expenses and income has largely been filled by middle-aged, married women's entry into paid work. The working mother changed family life-styles as much as, if not more than, the escape to the suburbs. It has also had the effect of making work of special importance to the sense of self-worth of many middle-aged women (Baruch and Barnett, 1981). Middle age is their time for themselves.

More Sex and More Variety

Because the Playboy Foundation wanted an early 1970s study to compare with Kinsey's two volumes, Hunt (1974) included middle-aged respondents in his "replication." While his sample is flawed, it is valuable because it surveys many sexual behaviors and it includes people's feelings. When median weekly frequency of marital intercourse was studied, Hunt found increases for every age category compared to Kinsey's. Thus, middle-aged married couples in the 1970s were having more sex together than earlier cohorts at a similar time in their lives.

Since the extent of sexual functioning in middle age is highly dependent on early experience and enjoyment of sex, the trend toward more marital sex is hardly surprising. Remember, the middle-aged generation of Hunt's study was the young generation studied by Kinsey *et al.* Kinsey found consistent differences between the younger and older subsets of the female sample, always with greater sexual freedom among the young. (That is still true in every Western country studied today.) Fully 20% more of Kinsey's young married women were having orgasms than were their older counterparts. The young experienced more nudity, variation in coital positions, and variety in foreplay. Younger married women were more likely than older married women to experience stimulation from oral–genital, manual–genital, and mouth–breast contacts.

Given this increase in the variety of coital techniques and types of foreplay used, it requires no great leap of imagination to infer that marital sex among the more recent birth cohort was generally more pleasurable and hence would be practiced more often. Inferences about the relative contributions of the husbands and the wives to the increase in frequency are somewhat more speculative. In comparing the Kinsey data with his own, Hunt consistently found that, in both sexual attitudes and behavior, the magnitude of liberalization was greater for females than for males. (Females were farther away than males from ceiling on most measures. Thus, they had more room for increases.) Hunt argues that the social emancipation of women of this generation removed many cultural inhibitions surrounding sexuality. This, in turn, led to a general increase in wives' desire for marital coitus.

Hunt assumes that part of the new freedom for women is the freedom to tell their partners their sexual wishes. Lest the reader be reassured that modern women readily communicate their sexual wishes to their partners, Hite (1976) notes that two out of three women in a feminist sample find it difficult indeed. This is not so when a male communicates to a female (Pietropinto and Simenauer, 1977). Pietropinto and Simenauer found that although men insist that they want their lovers to communicate their sexual desires, women believe that men don't want to know their wishes.

While we have no data that directly support the assertion that it is wives who are responsible for the general increase in the frequency of marital coitus, a recent study seems to support that conclusion. Large-scale National Fertility Surveys of married couples showed, at all ages, an increase in average 4-week coital frequency in 1970 as compared to 1965—up 2.46 for women under 25, up 2.06 for women 25–34, and up .43 for women 35–44 (Westoff, 1974). The rate of increase is lower for the older than for the younger women, but at all ages Westoff found increased frequencies. This sexualization of all ages is considered a major sociological event. Some investigators are dubious that the trend will continue (Udry and Morris, 1978), but that the sexualizing events have occurred is universally acknowledged. Westoff (1974) saw some of the trend as due to a subset of educated women with "modern" gender views. Later work changed his mind (see p. 389).

The influence of marital status on middle-aged sexuality is less clear-cut for the post-World War I birth cohort than for the previous one. Its limitations notwithstanding, the Kinsey study did provide comparable information on married, postmarried, and never-married men and women in convenient 5-year age intervals across the adult life-span. No directly comparable data exist for the more recent cohort. The only current information we have on sexual behavior among postmarried women is that of Hunt. His survey of postmarrieds is limited to the divorced and never-married; unfortunately, the samples are too small to permit reasonable analysis by age. For the purpose of cross-cohort comparisons, the closest match to Hunt's data on divorced women is the divorced subset of the Gebhard sample, a comparison across 30 years. These women were all under age 55 at the time of the interview. Hunt found that 90% of the divorced women in his sample were coitally active, compared to Gebhard's 70%. Among the coitally active women in the Hunt study, the median weekly frequency of coitus is twice per week as compared to Gebhard's report of a mean frequency of slightly over once per week. Women in both studies reported high rates of orgasm and satisfaction with postmarital coitus. A majority of divorced women in the Gebhard sample reported that they had more orgasms in postmarital than in marital sex. While Hunt provides no directly comparable data, his sample reported that their postmarital sex was generally more liberated than their marital sex had been, and over 90% of the women rated postmarital coitus as very or mostly pleasurable. But we can't be sure that the samples are comparable across the 30 years.

Hunt supplies no information about never-married middle-aged women; in fact, only 5% of the 1970s population of women had never married. Hunt's never-married are all under age 35. The only current information that we have on middle-aged single women comes from a recent study of 60 women, aged 35 to 65 years (Lowenstein, Block, Campion, Epstein, Gale, and Salvatore, 1981). The criterion for being single in this "snowball" sample was that the women defined themselves as single, rather than viewing lack of a partner as transitional. In actual fact, only 38 of the women had never married; the balance were widowed, divorced, or separated. None of these women had children under 18 living at home. The sample overrepresented highly educated and professional women. Of the 38 never-married women, 1 provided no data concerning sexuality, and 22 (60%) reported that they had never engaged in coitus. The frequency of coital (or other) activity among the remaining 15 women is not reported. For the group as a whole, current sexual gratification bore no relation to life satisfaction. (This finding is replicated in a *Consumer Reports* study, cited just below.) Approximately half of Lowenstein's women expressed no sexual needs. The provocative contents of this study make one wish to know more. What about masturbation? Is sex really a take-it-or-leave-it matter for women without stable male partners? Are sexual partners important only when women have them?

In a recent, as yet unpublished, survey of 1845 middle- and upper-class women readers over age 50, the magazine *Consumer Reports* finds 91%% of the women expressing some degree of interest in sex and 84% coitally active. In a sample in which almost one-third of the women are never-married, widowed, or divorced, 84% represents a high incidence of sexual activity. Selective sampling may increase the figures for sexual interest somewhat since the sample is solidly middle class and highly educated (Corby and Brecher, 1984). Nonetheless, it is of interest that any class of women over 50 is found with such high coital incidences, given the rest of the literature. On the other hand, incidence figures always follow the rule "A swallow makes a spring." It takes only one coital act to be counted among the coitally active. The story of the coital decline with age shows up first in frequency statistics and is subsequently corroborated by lowered incidence figures.

Masturbation

Current data describing masturbatory patterns among middle-aged women are nonexistent. Hite's book (1976) is not organized so that one can extract reliable data by age. Hunt reports that, by their late 20s and early 30s, over 80% of single women and 70% of married women are masturbating. No one has ever shown that females stop masturbating once they have begun, Freud's "On the Anatomical Distinction between the Sexes" notwithstanding. Even if one assumes that Hunt's figures are inflated by his selected sample, these figures suggest an increase in the incidence of masturbation among women since the time of Kinsey, when one-half of single and one-third of married women reported that they masturbated. Women have found their genitals, even though culture and morphology made it somewhat difficult for them to do so.

Wholesale modifications of sexuality during middle age are relatively rare, even during the recent sexualization of our society. For most people, their sexual self-concept ripens during the earlier, more formative periods of preadolescence, adolescence, and young adulthood. Pfeiffer and Davis cite the high correlation between levels of sexual functioning in young adulthood and in middle age. Important factors characterizing one's personality tend to display relatively consistent patterns throughout adult life. Pfeiffer and Davis call this "continuity of life-style." Most of the middle-aged women that Hunt interviewed reported that while the "sexual revolution" of the 1960s had liberalized their attitudes, their marital sexual patterns were too well established to undergo much change. Some expressed regret. Middle-aged women differ from young women not only in biology but also in the different scripts they learned for sexual experience and initiation. Among divorced women (middle-aged and younger) some reschooling in the new sexuality occurs. Many of the middle-aged women in the Rubin (1979) study reported that their marital sex had improved over time, but some bemoaned their inability to be sexually liberated like the younger generation—"too many years of repression and too many lessions learned too well."

The Baby Boom in Middle Age

Any extrapolation from the Kinsey data to the middle age of the women born from 1945 to 1960 (the baby boom) would be an error. The Kinsey sample was a mixture of cohorts, viewed by Kinsey as pre- and post-1900 births. Kinsey documented the sexual revolution that came with the adolescents of the post-World War I world, those born 1900 and after. One part of that post-World War I birth cohort is the 1920–1932 group described by Rossi. That post-1920 birth cohort produced the children who are the upcoming middle-aged of 1985 and thereafter. The post-World War II cohort, called the baby boom, grew up with economic prosperity, many jobs, high consumption, extended education, widespread travel, and high occupational aspirations. They hit their 20s at the time of shifting cultural views of the double standard, premarital sex, and oral sex.

While the 1960s represent the period of shifting sexual views, the 1970s represent the period of changed sexual behavior (Reiss, 1972). Although some women still marry as virgins, the norm has shifted toward "premarital intercourse with love." In many Western countries (France, Germany, United States), the sexual experience that women once acquired first in marriage is now far more likely to be gained premaritally. The changes include (a) relatively speedy climbing of the scaled steps from the French kiss to intercourse, (b) becoming reliably orgasmic in oral sex and/or intercourse before marriage, (c) greater acceptance of initiation of sexual invitations by women, (d) greater availability and use of reliable contraception by women, (e) greater probability of having more than one premarital sexual partner, (f) having premarital sex in stable relationships more frequently, hence having more sexual practice premaritally.

Predicting the Sexual Future

All of these factors lead to the prediction that, on average, women of the baby boom cohort are going to have more sex and more orgasms than their grandmothers did. Since the predictors of continued incidence of sex and frequency of sex are previous experience and enjoyment of sex, the baby boom cohort should be a relatively sexually active group in middle age. Permissive and abundant sex in a woman's teens and 20s should predict more sex later.

What happens when one goes beyond the correlational data just cited and asks: What are the concurrent social factors most likely to influence the sexuality of the next generation of middle-aged women? We see three main factors exerting a change: greater social acceptance of women as sexual beings throughout life; the growing absence of stable male sexual partners for many women, due to high rates of divorce and the shorter life expectancy of males than females; and women's changing role in the paid work force. Predicting how these factors will affect the sexuality of middle-aged women is a matter of data and conjecture.

We would expect that the middle-aged woman will be seen as asexual far less often than she is today. Better health and longer life-spans should help to convince older people that sexuality is a life-span process. But middle age, with its skewed sex ratio, means that more women than men will be without stable sex partners. Current data on young women suggest that there will continue to be lesser salience of genital sex for women in comparison with relational aspects of sex. This lesser salience in a context of significant proportions of male-absent, late-middle-age households will probably continue to depress the social sexual activity of women for reasons that will be as valid in the future as they were in the past: the absence of a stable sexual partner with whom a woman has a relationship.

As the base rate for early female masturbation goes up (as it has), a safe prediction is that tomorrow's divorced, widowed, or never-married middle-aged women will enjoy solitary sex more often than did her older sister or mother in like circumstances. It is unlikely to be a simple substitution for social sex. Short- or long-term sexual relationships outside of legal marriages are already on the increase—a trend likely to continue. Our society has begun to accept the Scandinavian model of cohabitation as an aspect of courtship. The Swedes came to that model from a rural history where cohabitation tested a woman's fertility: we have come to the model as a test of interpersonal/sexual compatibility. Such a test is as important for the middle-aged woman as it is for her younger counterpart.

Extramarital sex will frequently be in the context of transition out of marriage into new sexual and/or marital arrangements. Demographers see the future life-span being divided into more married and unmarried sequences than has been customary heretofore. Social sexual sequences will probably show the same on/off timing, with social sex on for a period of time, then off.

Among middle-aged women of the recent past, an extramarital affair was predicted by marital unhappiness. This isn't as true for women now beginning to push middle age; they are somewhat more likely to be seeking variety. These are younger women with more premarital sexual experience than middle-aged women of the past had. Their appestats, experience, sexual values, and knowledge of scripts for sexual solicitation may be higher.

Influence of Labor Force Participation on Sexuality

How will being in the paid labor force affect women's sexual lives? Masnick and Bane (1981) describe three revolutions—already realized or potential—in women's work patterns. The first, a dramatic increase in participation in the paid labor force by women, especially married women, has already occurred. The second revolution, in the nature of women's attachment to the labor force, is just under way. The shift is toward full-time, permanent attachment to the labor force. Government projections show about 80% of the women aged 35 and over remaining stably in the labor force by 1990. Part, but not all, of the steady attachment to the labor force is caused by increasing numbers of women with college education. As women invest more in preparing for careers, they are less willing to stay out of the labor force. Married women who are permanently and full time in the labor market differ from both women who do not work and women who work part time or sporadically. Women and their families who come to expect wives' earnings regularly and predictably are likely to change in economic and noneconomic ways: Wives' incomes will be required in the family budget; the amount of time devoted to responsibilities related to home and family is likely to change; pressure not to bear children is likely to be higher than we have seen in the post-World War II period; and where children are born, they are likely to be few and to be born when mothers are older. As we write, Massachusetts has reported a record high proportion of first births to women over 30. The strategy of entering the labor market after an early birth typically founders when the husband's higher earning ability sets up the traditional role pattern, ending with a wife at home, rather than in the labor market (LaRassa and LaRassa, 1981).

Masnick and Bane (1981) surmise that a quiet third revolution may be starting because of women's increasing relative contribution to family income. Working women under 24 in two-worker families are providing a somewhat larger portion of family income than did older women. Although the number of two-worker families in which women earn more than men is still low (< 10%), it is well known that women's earnings often bring their families' incomes over the poverty line. The obvious mutual protection against unemployment in two-earner households is also well known. Should earnings approach parity, real shifts in power can be expected, and power in negotiating sex may move sexual activity up or down.

Not only are more women working, but for increasing numbers of them—married and unmarried—working represents a way of life. The picture of the breadwinner husband with a homemaker wife who periodically drops in and out of the paid work force to provide the family with "luxuries" is being rapidly replaced by a scenario in which it takes two full-time salaries to achieve even a minimal desired level of material comfort. For most families, breadwinning now requires the full-time efforts of two people outside the home. A new revolution—akin to the Industrial Revolution—is taking women of all ages into the labor market. It is emptying homes of women, just as the Industrial Revolution pulled workers out of the countryside and into the cities.

Only among women who never marry will these changes have little effect. Without the economic advantage of a working husband, these women have traditionally engaged in lifelong work (their career span averaging 45 years). Widowed, separated, and divorced women have also been overrepresented in long-term attachment to the labor force when compared to women in general. Loss or absence of a stably present working partner represents not only loss of companionship and, of course, social sex, but also loss of income (Cherlin, 1981). All of these losses are important, but at least partial substitutes for male companionship and sex are available; substitutes for the kind of money that men earn are the most difficult to come by.

In past generations, commitment to family-building, loyalty to one man, and an elastic commitment to the labor market characterized women's lives. Women's occupational training was once likened to a mattress: something to fall back on. Women's first commitment was to family; men's first commitment was to work.

While both men and women today report that their greatest gratifications come from family ties (Gurin, Veroff, and Feld, 1960), some major pushes and pulls are coming from the world of work. These pushes and pulls do not stop at the bedroom door. Women who marry late, who have entered the labor force well before marriage, and who know that they will remain in the labor force throughout marriage are likely to experience themselves as more equal partners in marriage than did their mothers and grandmothers. In matters sexual, this may mean that the presumed sexual rate-setting prerogative of the male will be muted, in cohabitation as well as in marriage.

It is an open question whether stably working women will negotiate sexual activity in marriage up or down. A West German survey found working women reporting that they are so tired after work that marital sex is less often desired by them than by nonworking women (John Gagnon, personal communication, 1979). The Udry and Morris (1978) survey data show nonworking wives having intercourse more often than working wives. Estimates of coital frequency have recently been called into question as a measure. Follow-ups of continuously married women revealed that coital frequencies were "unlikely to be associated with socioeconomic, demographic, or even attitudinal variables" (Trussell and Westoff, 1980, p. 249). Social scientists are rarely treated to such a thorough housecleaning of all classes of their most trusted variables. Only reliable contraception or sterilization has dependable effects on coital frequency.

More women of the future will probably spend part of their adult lives without spouses. This does not mean that they will never marry. They will probably marry more often, but they will also divorce more frequently. Thus, for many adult women, life patterns will include periods with spouses and periods without. Permanent attachment to the work force might make divorce a somewhat less traumatic event than it has been in the past, when the inevitable losses of divorce were confounded by the economic and emotional dilemma of the displaced homemaker. The fatigue and lack of time engendered by full-time work, especially in the case of single mothers, may place even more constraints on the sex lives of postmarried women than on these of their married counterparts. Single parents (often with teenaged children) must shoulder the same responsibilities that were shared by two people when they were married. For a woman with no live-in, stable sexual partner, sex requires more negotiation, time, and effort, as well as social skills and economic resources. Some women will consider the effort worthwhile; others will join the take-it-or-leave-it group.

Exposure to the paid work world may promote the maintenance of social skills that are useful in the sexual marketplace when women reenter it after marriage. Additionally, the shared work world of men and women gives more women independent access to a pool of potentially available sexual and marriage partners.

Any attempt to predict what sexuality will be like among tomorrow's middle-aged women is filled with hazard. Adult women do not constitute a homogeneous group. If marriage continues to be the popular choice it has been since World War II (with 95% of Americans marrying at some time in their lives), then one set of predictions would fit the large married group. There, the major issue would be: To what extent do the variables that predicted sexual behavior in middle-age in the past apply to this new group?

If current divorce trends do not attenuate radically, middle-aged women will constitute many subgroups: long-term marrieds (10 or more years), short-term or long-term remarrieds, divorced or widowed but not remarrieds, and never-marrieds. We have not even tried to make predictions about gay women because of the paucity of life-cycle data on gay women (even Bell and Weinberg provide few data on older gay women). While many of the same forces that operate on heterosexual women also operate on gays, there are special problems related to marriage and divorce that gay women do not share with straight women. These are problems related to changing sex ratios in middle and old age, and to the different views held by straight *men* and gay *women* about youth, age, and sexual attractiveness. Data on remarriage underline the salience of age in the heterosexual marketplace.

NEW FAMILIES, SEX, AND THE MIDDLE-AGED WOMAN

The lower rates of remarriage by women compared to men are age-graded: Divorced women aged 35–44 remarry at 75% the rates of their former husbands; divorced women 45–54 remarry at 62% of their former husbands' rates. For all women over 44, the remarriage ratio of divorced women to divorced men is 56:100. The 1980 U.S. census counts 8,870,000 divorced or separated women versus 5,915,000 men of that status. The female:male ratio for widowhood is even more ominous—245:100. The latter figure reflects both the earlier age of male versus female death, plus the custom of women marrying men older than themselves (Cherlin, 1981). On average, men die 7–8 years younger than do women; on average, first marriages find women 2–3 years younger than their mates. This makes a substantial period of widowhood highly likely for most women. Where middle-aged men divorce and remarry, their second wives are, on average, 9 to 10 years younger than they are. These women will be widowed for an even longer time than first wives, if they do not remarry.

Some factors will affect the sexuality of all three groups: never-marrieds, marrieds, and postmarrieds. These include widespread acceptance of nonmarital sexuality, widespread knowledge of female capacity to enjoy sex, and increased permission for the expression of female sexuality, as reflected in bestsellers from *The Total Woman* to *The Joy of Sex*.

Beyond that, the sexual patterns of the three groups are likely to differ. The single factor that made the most difference in the past for middle-aged women was availability of a sexual partner. A major reason for that effect in the past came from operation of the double standard. Attenuation of that standard has meant that more divorced, widowed, and never-married women of all ages are sharing quarters, and sex, with men of all statuses, marital and nonmarital. While the popular literature (Hunt, 1966) on the formerly married suggests fast entry and exit from sexual relationships, we know of no solid study of the nature and course of such relationships where female age is followed as a variable. Remarriage rates by age suggest that the scene of the formerly married is anything but age-blind.

When marriage meant breadwinning for men and child-rearing for women, the age relations of husbands and wives made good sense. A man better equipped to earn (more experience at work, an established trade or profession) traded his earning capacity for sexual favors, family and personal care, and fertility in a woman. In the years of the Feminine Mystique, the ideology behind that division of labor persisted, but some of the objective conditons that had supported the trade-off were changing. Maximum fertility was no longer so highly valued; women's education was no longer so different from that of men; family care became less onerous as the incidence of life-threatening diseases in children decreased; and sex was no longer something that women reluctantly "gave" men—rather, it had become a feminine pleasure. Betty Friedan's (1963) rage caught on because she challenged the already obsolete trade-off that kept women dependent.

Today, women trade attractiveness for the advantages of marriage. The social psychological literature makes it clear that physical attractiveness is the single most powerful variable determining men's choices in the dating and sexual scene. For women, that would be a careless luxury. Women look for men who do well in life. (Woody Allen catches the difference in *The Front* when he tells one woman in a resort hotel that he is a writer, and another woman that he is a dentist. Only the latter woman finds him attractive.)

If divorce becomes more common and more men must share their earnings with earlier families, the earning capacity of the middle-aged woman may expand the choices available to her. Some remarriages by men occur because their new wives have earning capacity, i.e., "I could only marry a woman who earns a lot." Men who wish to work at jobs with financial uncertainty (e.g., writing, art, politics) may seek out partners who can share the economic risk. Trade-offs such as this imply that some women will be able to shed the old division of gender roles, which dictated that the husband be older, a better earner, and more powerful than the wife. Such roles work against middle-aged women.

Regardless of strategies, there are fewer men than women. Humans start life with more male than female conceptions, more male than female births, but by middle age, the higher vulnerability of males to accidents and disease leaves more females than males. What are middle-aged women to do if they want sexual relationships? So long as we are not a polygynous society, it is clear that some women will not have husbands during their middle years. The number of possible solutions is finite: (1) Women can marry younger men; (2) women can have sexual relationships stably or sporadically with married men; (3) women can have relationships with men who are between marriages; (4) more than one woman can have sexual relationships with the same man; (5) women can have homosexual relationships on a stable or a sporadic basis.

All of the above five alternatives are occurring. The alternative that we have not cited is that suggested by the Lowenstein sample: Opt out of sexual relationships altogether. It is possible that the take-it-or-leave-it position is an adaptation to a sex ratio that is unfavorable to middle-aged women. No man or woman ever died of sexual deprivation. It is our hunch, however, that young women sexualized during the 1960s and 1970s will not lightly give up sexual relationships. It is possible that the five alternatives cited above will be chosen more often. A recent sampling of just three 1982 issues of *Cosmopolitan* leads us to believe that the outrage that some of today's older women express toward the alternatives cited above may not be true in the future, given the wide-ranging social sexualization occurring in popular magazines for younger women. In August, *Cosmopolitan* told their readers how to be a mistress to a married man while being independent. It also offered advice on how to have sex at conventions and how to marry older men. The September issue contained a complete (and quite explicit) "guide to lovelier (lustier) sex," while in October, readers were offered some insights into lesbianism and a lyrical, well-written essay on fellatio.

Almost all of the alternatives violate some of our gender rules. Some violate widely held beliefs. We all "know" that men can be turned on only by youth, that families will be destroyed by extramarital liaisons, and that people are not able to perform homosexually if they are heterosexual in orientation. We can all think of instances that challenge each of these beliefs, too. Our purpose in citing these beliefs is to show what barriers exist to middle-aged women implementing any of the above choices. It is our guess that there will be some surprises in the future.

Once upon a time, the third alternative—sex with a man between marriages—was unthinkable because "good" women stayed away from divorced men. Today, this alternative gives no offense. There will be fewer men than women in the unmarried pool. Moreover, these men will remarry down in age. It may well be that the middle-aged woman's sexual life will often be a matter of temporary liaisons with men *en route* to marriage with younger women. In considering all these alternatives, we do not recommend any in particular. An examination of the alternatives may make it easier to understand the women in Lowenstein's sample who opt out of the search for sex.

Despite our optimistic predictions concerning the sexual pleasure of the next group of middle-aged, the baby boom cohort, caution is in order. More of the next group of middle-aged women will work than ever before. Work and other responsibilities, especially family responsibilities, compete with sex for time. Life with a stable sexual partner is filled with more than sexual feelings and goals. Gagnon (1982) suggests that couples may have to decide how important sex is to them in comparison with other goals; tired people don't have a lot of sex whether they are older married couples or young medical students. People who value careers over personal commitments are likely to defer sex. Couples who are married for long periods are more likely to develop activities that compete with their sexual time. Gagnon believes that the decrease in frequencies of sexual intercourse seen in married couples reflects this competition for time, rather than a biological decrease. The explanation may well be a combination of biological and social factors.

Being in the labor force may produce competition for time but it may also render a woman a more interesting partner. She knows more about the world of paid work and brings home the wisdom, the mores, the peopled quality of her workplace. To the extent that this "new" input is a turn-on, sex may become more—rather than less—interesting in a dual-job or dual-career family.

Similarly, new postdivorce couples would be expected to start their sexual relations with higher rates of coitus, if only because they haven't accumulated competing demands for time together. In all couples, children present enormous competing needs. Rubin (1979) reports that some of the women that she interviewed were hypersensitive to the nearby presence of children during intercourse. The women reported that their partners were unconcerned.

Marital sex has built-in gratifications as well as problems. Sex is there upon request in marriage. The forms of request are personally worked out, from the direct to the indirect; they are the couple's forms. Marital sex lacks some of the elements of the nonmarital sexual search. Once one is married, the partner has said "yes" to sex. While partners can be tired, they cannot routinely say "no" without violating the marital contract. Eliciting a "yes" during early erotic attraction carries a sexual confirmation of self that marital sex probably loses after the first few years. We believe that this factor operates to reduce the frequency of marital sex over time.

Tomorrow's middle-aged women have had their sexual appestats set higher than did previous generations. They are likely to have enjoyed their early sex and to expect to enjoy their latter, middle-aged sex. The context for their sexual lives will determine how much sex they have, as well as how they feel about that sex. Married sex is regular, relatively frequent, but goes down with age. Middle-aged women who had positive starts to their sex lives are likely to experience higher coital frequencies and higher orgasmic rates in marriage than did earlier generations. Smaller families will produce less competition for time, but paid work will increase competition for time. Where the interaction comes out probably depends on the couples' valuation of sex. Movement in and out of marriage is associated with less stable sexual relationships, but with more partners. Middle-aged women are likely to have a difficult time (as compared with younger women) in the postmarried sexual milieu as they are less frequently chosen from among sexual partners for the middle-aged man's marital intimacy. While marital sexual intimacy is not the only form of sustained sexual intimacy, it is the most common form that commits men to stable sex.

The never-married middle-aged group will probably bear little resemblance to the Kinsey group with those characteristics. These women will be sexually experienced in youth and are likely to remain sexually active in some form during middle age, much more so than previous generations in their situations. The defining characteristic of this group of women is their decision to postpone marriage, to give higher priority to paid work and education and lower priority to childbearing. In past generations, some opprobrium attached to women neither marrying nor bearing children. This group of women is likely to have greater acceptance; they will be less likely seen as asexual. Their stability in the labor force may make them economically advantaged, too.

The Framework for Sexuality: A Search for Meanings

Any statement about any group's sexuality based on a single culture requires some qualification. The cross-cultural story underlines the view of male sexuality as more often urgent and of female sexuality as more "discretionary" (Ford and Beach, 1951). However, our anthropological colleagues tell us that there are some cultures where that definition of sexual appetite is not accepted. Mangaian women (and men) seek out sex. Tshambuli women want sex more than do Tshambuli men (Mead, 1935). Some cultural arrangements sanction older husbands taking male sexual partners while no sexual arrangements are made for wives who have had their complement of babies, a presumption that men "need" sex and women (at least older women) don't. A culture's conceptions about sexuality are not independent of the general *Weltanschauung* held by that culture. Sexuality requires some such framework to make sense within a culture (Davenport, 1977).

In our society, men and women share a decline in sexual performance with age. Couples who are stably paired show a slow decline with age, perhaps reflecting the danger of routine, the ultimate anaphrodisiac. "He's turned on by our bed, not me; he only touches me in bed," says the intimacy-seeking 40-year-old wife. Few couples can afford restorative sex in hotel rooms away from children. Family experiences other than having sex take on greater legitimacy since they exclude fewer family members. Nonsexual issues drive decisions in the sexual area.

The view that men are sex-driven without wifely provocation surely is opposite to that which motivated the writing of *The Total Woman* (Morgan, 1973). The syndicated newspaper columnist, Abigail Van Buren, tried to find out, in her own way, whether or not women over 50 liked sex (Van Buren, 1981). She asked older readers of her "Dear Abby" column. Half of her respondents wanted out; one wrote, "Even a hooker gets to retire." The other half invented tricks, à la Marabelle Morgan, to entice their sexually dormant husbands. While the *Consumer Reports* survey required answering a long questionnaire, Dear Abby required only that her readers write a short note. Moreover, Dear Abby's respondents probably represent a wider sample of middle-aged women.

Dear Abby's survey results raise many questions. National magazines, e.g., *McCall's*, run columns quoting psychiatrists on sex, love, commitment, and intimacy. *McCall's* is flooded with letters from troubled women responding to the helping and self-help nature of the articles. Women readers ask how to get husbands to interact, pay attention, express affection. Their letters reflect a world in which many men feel that it is enough if they support their families economically. The women search for affection, sex, and intimacy. Sex is often the only—and infrequent—intimacy, and many women feel that coitus is less sexual outside of a broader context of expressed affection.

We have stayed fairly close to the few existing sets of survey data on the sexuality of women in middle age. The big question for the soon-to-be-middle-aged centers around how the two gender scripts will fuse and change. What will be most interesting and hardest to predict is how those changes will be experienced by tomorrow's middle-aged women. The only certainty is that the range of their sexual choices will be greater than it was for their mothers and grandmothers. We wonder whether the choices will satisfy the heightened expectations of the upcoming middle-aged cohort.

References

Angelou, M. *The heart of a woman.* New York: Random House, 1981.
Baum, M. J., Koos Slob, A., de Jong, F. H., and Westbrook, D. L. Persistence of sexual behavior in ovariectomized stumptail macaques following dexamethasone treatment or adrenalectomy. *Hormones and Behavior,* 1978, *2,* 323–347.
Barbach, L. *For yourself: The fulfillment of female sexuality.* Garden City, N.Y.: Doubleday, 1975.
Baruch, G. K., and Barnett, R. Who has multiple role strain? The "woman in the middle" revisited. Paper presented at the Meeting of the Gerontological Society, Toronto, 1981.
Bell, A. P., and Weinberg, M. S. *Homosexuality: A study of diversity among men and women.* New York: Simon & Schuster, 1978.
Boston Women's Health Book Collective. *Our bodies, ourselves.* (2nd ed.). New York: Simon & Schuster, 1976. Pp. 327–336.
Cherlin, A. J. *Marriage, divorce, remarriage.* Cambridge, Mass.: Harvard University Press, 1981.
Christenson, C. V., and Gagnon, J. H. Sexual behavior in a group of older women. *Journal of Gerontology,* 1965, *20,* 351–356.
Christenson, C. V., and Johnson, A. B. Sexual patterns in a group of older never-married women. *Journal of Geriatric Psychiatry,* 1973, *6,* 80–98.
Corby, N., and Brecher, E. *Love, sex, aging.* Mt. Vernon, N.Y.: Consumers Union, 1984.
Davenport, W. H. Sex in cross-cultural perspective. In F. A. Beach, *Human sexuality in four perspectives.* Baltimore: Johns Hopkins University Press, 1977.
Degler, C. *At odds.* New York: Oxford University Press, 1980.
Eysenck, H. J. *Sex and personality.* Austin: University of Texas Press, 1976.
Finger, F. W. Changes in sex practices and beliefs of male college students over 30 years. *Journal of Sex Research,* 1975, *11,* 304–317.
Ford, C. S., and Beach, F. A. *Patterns of sexual behavior.* New York: Harper & Row, 1951.
Friedan, B. *The feminine mystique.* New York: Dell, 1963.
Gagnon, J. Are you really too tired for sex? *Working Mother,* 1982, January, 53–55.
Gebhard, P. Postmarital coitus among widows and divorcees. In P. Bohannan (Ed.), *Divorce and after.* Garden City, N.Y.: Doubleday, 1971.
Geer, J., Morokoff, P., and Greenwood, P. Sexual arousal in women. The development of a measurement device for vaginal blood volume. *Archives of Sexual Behavior,* 1974, *3,* 559–564.
Gurin, G., Veroff, J., and Feld, S. *Americans view their mental health.* New York: Basic Books, 1960.
Hite, S. *The Hite report.* New York: Macmillan, 1976.
Hunt, M. *The world of the formerly married.* New York: McGraw-Hill, 1966.
Hunt, M. *Sexual behavior in the 1970's.* Chicago: Playboy Press, 1974.
Jong, E. *Fear of flying.* New York: New American Library, 1973.
Kinsey, A. C., Pomeroy, W. B., and Martin, C. E. *Sexual behavior in the human male.* Philadelphia: Saunders, 1948.
Kinsey, A. C., Pomeroy, W. B., Martin, C. E., and Gebhard, P. *Sexual behavior in the human female.* Philadelphia: Saunders, 1953.
Kraemer, H. C., Becker, H. B., Brodie, H. K. H., Doering, C. H. Moos, R. H., and Hamburg, D. A. Orgasmic frequency and plasma testosterone levels in normal human males. *Archives of Sexual Behavior,* 1976, *5,* 125–132.
LaRassa, R., and LaRassa, M. M. *Transition to parenthood: How infants change families.* Beverly Hills: Sage, 1981.

Loewenstein, S. F., Bloch, N. E., Campion, J., Epstein, J. S., Gale, P., and Salvatore, M. A study of satisfactions and stresses of single women in midlife. *Sex Roles*, 1981, *11*, 1127–1141.

Luria, Z., and Rose, M. D. *The psychology of human sexuality*. New York: Wiley, 1979.

Marshall, D. S. Sexual behavior in Mangaia. In D. S. Marshall and R. C. Suggs (Eds.), *Human sexual behavior*. Englewood Cliffs, N.J.: Prentice-Hall, 1971.

Martin, C. E. Sexual activity in the aging male. In J. Money and H. Musaph (Eds.), *Handbook of sexology*. Elsevier/North Holland Biomedical Press, 1977.

Masnick, G., and Bane, M. J. *The nation's families: 1960–1990*. Boston: Auburn House, 1981.

Masters, W. H. and Johnson, V. *Human sexual response*. Boston: Little, Brown, 1966.

Mead, M. *Sex and temperament in three primitive societies*. New York: Morrow, 1935.

Morgan, M. *The total woman*. Old Tappan, N.J.: F. H. Rovell, 1973.

Neugarten, B. L. Women's attitudes towards the menopause. *Vita Humana*, 1963, *6*, 140–146.

Ortner, S., and Whitehead, H. *Sexual meanings*. Cambridge, England: Cambridge University Press, 1981.

Pfeiffer, E., and Davis, G. C. Determinants of sexual behavior in middle and old age. *Journal of the American Geriatric Society*, 1972, *20*, 151–188.

Pfeiffer, E., Verwoerdt, A., and Davis, G. C. Sexual behavior in middle life. *American Journal of Psychiatry*, 1972, *128*, 1262–1267.

Pietropinto, A., and Simenauer, J. *Beyond the male myth*. New York: New York Times Books, 1977.

Reiss, I. L. Premarital sexuality: Past, present, and future. In I. L. Reiss (Ed.), *Readings on the family system*. New York: Hall, 1972.

Rossi, A. Lifespan theories and women's lives. *Signs*, 1980, *6*, 4–32.

Rubin, L. *Women of a certain age*. New York: Harper & Row, 1979.

Steinman, D. L., Wincze, J. P., Sakheim, D. K., Barlow, D. H., and Maussakalian, M. A comparison of male and female patterns of sexual arousal. *Archives of Sexual Behavior*, 1981, *10*, 529–547.

Trussell, J. and Westoff, C. F. Contraceptive practice and trends in coital frequency. *Family Planning Perspectives*, 1980, *12*, 246–249.

Udry, J. R. Changes in the frequency of marital intercourse from panel data. *Archives of Sexual Behavior*, 1980, *9*, 319–325.

Udry, J. R., and Morris, N. M. Relative contribution of male and female age to the frequency of marital intercourse. *Social Biology*, 1978, *25*, 128–134.

Van Buren, A. *The best of Dear Abby*. Kansas City, Kansas: Andrews McMeel, 1981.

Veroff, J., and Feld, S. *Marriage and work in America*. New York: Van Nostrand, 1970.

Westoff, C. F. Coital frequency and contraception. *Family Planning Perspectives*, 1974, *6*, 136–141.

Index

Academic institutions, programs for women in, 157–158
Accidents, mortality rates from, 280
Adult child–parent relationship, 221–241
Adult education
  barriers to learning in, 326–331, 332–333
  cognitive development and, 320–322
  heterogeneity in, 317–318
  learning capacity and, 317–320
  motivation for learning in, 323–326, 332–333
  participation in, 158–159, 315–317
  psychological adjustment in, 333–335
  role involvement and, 322–323
Affirmative action programs, 255
Age, chronological
  as factor in occurrence of breast cancer, 290
  learning capacity and, 318–320
  psychological well-being and, 140–141
  and sexual behavior, 373–376
Age-grading, 33–34, 318
Arthritis, 245
Asthma. *See* Respiratory diseases
Attenuation, correction for, 41–42
Autonomy, in adult family relationships, 207, 217

Basic duality, as stage of cognitive development, 321
Berkeley Growth Study, 11, 141
Black women
  behavioral science and, 247–249
  coping patterns of, 257–258
  divorce and remarriage among, 249
  economic status of, 254–255

Black women (*cont.*)
  education and financial security among, 246
  employment among, 254–255
  as heads-of-household, 247–248
  intrafamilial relationships of, 252–253
  literary portrayal of, 249–251
  marital relationships of, 253–254
  participation in Women's Movement by, 256–257
  political representation of, 246
  socioeconomic variations among, 246, 259
Breast
  fibrocystic disease of, and malignant neoplasms, 290
  malignant neoplasms of
    detection, 291
    estrogen and, 286
    mortality rates, 279, 280, 281, 283, 290
    treatment, 291–292
Bronchitis. *See* Respiratory diseases

Cancer. *See* Neoplasms, malignant
Cardiovascular diseases
  mortality rates, 279, 280, 283, 294
  Type-A behavior and, 289
Cerebrovascular diseases
  mortality rates, 279–280, 283
  Type-A behavior and, 289
Cervix uteri, malignant neoplasms in
  detection, 292
  mortality rates, 279, 280, 281, 283
Change
  assessment of, 38–39
  multidimensionality of, 47–51

399

Change (cont.)
  qualitative, 48–51
  quantitative, 47–48
  reliability versus, 39–40
  life span approach, 33–39
Chemical substances, as occupational hazards, 293
Chemotherapy, in treatment of breast cancer, 291
Cirrhosis, mortality rates from, 280
Cognitive education, hierarchical stages of, 320–323
Colleges. See Academic institutions
Commitment, as stage of cognitive development, 321
Consistency, as form of measurement reliability, 39
Continuity, maintenance of, in adult family relationships, 207
Convents, as source of scholarly excellence for women, 156–157
Corpus uteri
  malignant neoplasms of
    estrogen and, 285, 286, 292
    mortality rates, 279, 280, 281, 283
Crises, work-related, 293
Cross-age validation, 45
Cross-sectional designs, in life-span developmental research, 52–54, 58–59
Crystallized intelligence, contrasted with fluid intelligence, 318

Daughterhood. See Family relationships; Motherhood; Parent–child relationship
Dependency
  in adult-family relationships, 207, 208–211
  contrasted with equity, 216
Depression, among black women, 258
  "empty-nest" syndrome, 35, 141–142
Development
  definition of, 32–33
  life-span, 32–33
  research issues concerning, 37–62
Diabetes
  as health concern of black women, 245
  mortality rates, 280
Diethylstilbestrol (DES), 278, 286
Disability insurance, 127. See also Old Age Survivor's Disability and Health Insurance; Retirement benefits; Social Security
Discrimination
  in education, 150–151; 156–159
  in employment, 85–86, 91–92, 93–113, 159, 172, 254–255
  in occupational health issues, 293–294
  racial, 254–255, 280
  See also Employment; Financial well-being; Poverty
Divorce and remarriage, 249, 271

Education
  as factor in hierarchical arrangement of social roles, 195, 196, 197
  and financial security, 246
  sexual equality in, 150–159
Employment
  and adult child–elderly parent relationship, 225, 228, 237–240
  among black women, 254–255
  and demographic changes affecting midlife women, 279
  racially discriminatory patterns in, 255
  role conflict and, 93–101
  and sexual behavior, 387–390
  sexual equality in, 159–169
  as source of psychological well-being, 144–147
  See also Discrimination; Financial well-being; Poverty
Endometrium: See Corpus uteri
Environment
  as factor in learning capacity, 320
  as factor in occurrence of breast cancer, 290
Equal opportunity programs, 255
Equality, sexual, social change and, 155–172
Equity
  contrasted with dependency, 216
  maintenance of, in adult family relationships, 207, 211–216
Equivalence, as form of measurement reliability, 39
Erectile dysfunction, as factor in decreased sexual activity, 373, 374
Estrogen
  and breast cancer, 286
  in control and prevention of osteoporosis, 278

Estrogen (cont.)
  in oral contraceptives, 278
  in treatment of menopausal symptoms, 278, 284–286
  and uterine cancer, 285
Experience, as determinant in influences controlling development, 33
Explanatory research, 61–62

Family life cycle, 113–117, 228
Family relationships, 206, 207–214
  of black women, 252–253
  employment and, 186–200
  equities and inequities in, 215–217
  impact on psychological well-being, 149–152
  intergenerational development and, 169–170
  of middle-class Americans, compared with other societies, 270–272
  and participation in educational programs, 327–329
  See also Motherhood; Parent–child relationship
Financial well-being
  of black women, 254–255
  education and, 88–89, 246, 316
  marriage and, 117–118, 148
  motherhood and, 118–119
  public policy and, 84, 124–128
  sex differentials in, 84–91, 120, 159–172
  social roles and, 195, 196, 197
  See also Discrimination; Employment; Poverty
Fluid intelligence, contrasted with crystallized intelligence, 318

Harassment, sexual, 107
Health care
  biomedical model of, 277–278
  menopause and, 277, 278, 282, 294, 295, 296
  sex bias in, 282
  social change and, 277–278, 279
Heart disease. See Cardiovascular diseases
Heredity
  as determinant in influences controlling development, 33
  as factor in occurrence of breast cancer, 290
History-graded influences, 34, 318–319, 320

Homicide, mortality rates from, 280
Homogeneity, as form of measurement reliability, 39, 41
Homosexuality
  and age-related decrease in sexual activity, 376–377
  as means of fulfilling need for body contact, 269
  among subjects in Kinsey study, 373
Hot flashes, 285, 287
Hypertension, 245, 296

Income. See Financial well-being
Infectious diseases, and life expectancy, 279
Influenza. See Respiratory diseases
Insomnia, as symptom associated with menopause, 287
Instrumentation
  as threat to validity of cross-sectional design, 54
  as threat to validity of longitudinal design, 54
Integration-differentiation-reintegration hypothesis (of intellectual development), 50
Interrater agreement, as form of measurement reliability, 39

Kidney diseases, mortality rates from, 280, 281

"Late bloomer syndrome," 170–172
Learning, barriers to
  dispositional, 326, 330–331
  institutional, 326, 329–330
  situational, 326, 327–329
Learning, motivation, 324
Learning capacity
  environment and, 320
  relationship chronological age to, 318–320
Life expectancy, 279
Life-span developmental approach, 31–68
Literature, portrayal of middle-aged women in, 69–79
Longitudinal design, in life-span developmental approach, 54–56, 58–59
Lumpectomy, 291

Mammography, 291
Marriage
  and multiple roles of midlife women, 85, 117

Marriage (*cont.*)
  professional status and, 167
  as source of psychological well-being, 147–149
Mastectomy, radical, 291
Masturbation, 269, 378, 384–385, 386
Maternal mortality, and life expectancy, 279
Measurement
  reliability of, in life-span development approach, 39
  validity of, 43–46
Menarche, 15, 303, 365
Menopause
  biological aspects of, 284–288
  definitions of, 284
  effect on sexual behavior, 371–372
  estrogen and, 278, 284–286
  as health care issue, 277, 278, 282, 283–290, 294, 295, 296
  and psychological well-being, 141–142, 288, 303–311
  symptoms, 287–288
Menopause Collective (Cambridge, Massachusetts), 277, 295
Midlife crisis, 142–144
Motherhood
  employment and, 85–124, 167
  financial well-being and, 118–119
  and intergenerational development, 168–169
  and poverty, 118–119
  professional status and, 167
  psychological well-being and, 149–150
  and relationships with adult family members, 203–220; 221–241; 361–369
  and social-role commitments, 177–200
  See also Family relationships; Parent–child relationship
Motivation
  in adult education, 323–326, 332–333
  as factor in achievement, 170–171
Multidirectionality, as characteristic of developmental change in adulthood, 33
Multiplicity, as stage of cognitive development, 321
Multiplicity prelegitimate, as stage of cognitive development, 321

National Ambulatory Medical Care Study (NAMCS), 281
National Women's Health Network, 277, 295
Neoplasms, benign, mortality rates from, 280
Neoplasms, malignant
  of breast
    detection and treatment, 291
    mortality rates, 279, 280, 281
  of *cervix uteri*
    detection, 292
    incidence, 292
    mortality rates, 279, 280, 281
  of *corpus uteri*
    estrogen and, 285, 286
    mortality rates, 279, 280, 281
Nephritis. *See* Kidney diseases
Nephrosis. *See* Kidney diseases

Oakland Growth Study, 11
Occupational health, 283, 293–294
Occupational stress, 293
Old age, Survivor's, Disability, and Health Insurance (OASDHI) program, 124–125, 127
  See also Disability insurance; Retirement benefits; Social Security
Oral contraceptives, 278, 289
Osteoporosis, 278, 296

Papanicolaou (Pap) test, 292
Parent abuse, 204
Parent–child relationship, 27, 203–218, 221–241, 343–345, 349, 368–369
  among blacks, 247–249
  divorce and, 348
  employment and, 29, 111, 167–170, 225, 228, 235–240
  among middle-class, compared with other societies, 265, 267, 268
  impact on social well-being, 149–151
  See also Family relationships; Motherhood
Parental relationships, and psychological well-being, 150–151
Peer relationships, and psychological well-being, 150
Personality change, as factor in achievement, 171–172
Pneumonia. *See* Respiratory diseases

Poverty
  as factor contributing to dependency, 210
  as factor in problems of black women, 245, 254–255, 258
  marital status and, 86–87, 117
  and medical care, 245, 280–281
  motherhood and, 118–119
  public policy and, 84, 124–128
  sex differentials in, 85–86
  See also Financial well-being
Power, as factor in sex roles, 109
Progesterone, in treatment of menopausal symptoms, 286
Psychological need
  for body contact, 263, 264
  for reproduction, 263, 268
  for stimulation, 264
  for support, 267
  to predict events, 268
Psychological well-being
  chronological age and, 140–141
  comparative sex studies, 139–140
  definition of, 135–138
  during "empty nest" stage, 141–142
  employment and, 144–147
  marriage and, 147–149
  menopause and, 141–142, 288, 303–311
  multiple roles and, 151–152
  parental relationships and, 150–151
  parenthood and, 149–150
  peer relationships and, 150
  quality of life and, 136–139
  sibling relationships and, 150
  sources of, 144–153

Quality of life, and psychological well-being, 136–139

Radcliffe College study, 24–25, 26, 27
Relativism, as stage of cognitive development, 321
Reliability
  change versus, 39
  stability versus, 40–41
  validity of measurement and, 42
Religious rituals, as source of social stimulation, 264–265
Respiratory diseases, mortality rates from, 280

Retirement benefits, 126
  See also Disability insurance; Old Age, Survivor's, Disability, and Health Insurance (OASDHI) program
Role conflict
  and cardiovascular diseases, 107
  as consequence of competition, 187
  defined, 177
  and employment, 93–102
  methods of coping with, 102–104, 178–183
  reduction of, 95–101
  role partners and, 105–108
Role distance, as means of reducing role conflict, 101
Role importance, multiple classification analysis of, 190–192
Role involvement, and adult education, 322–323
Role overload, 177
Role–person strain, 178
Role strain,
  description and definitions, 177–178
  means of coping with, 178–183
Roles, social
  changes in, 155–172, 162–165, 177–200, 278–279
  combination of, and psychological well-being, 151–152
  delegation of
  sex structuring of, 108–110, 111

Septicemia, mortality rates from, 280
Sequential research designs, 57–60
Sex roles,
  legal aspects of, 110
  sex role socialization, 90, 91, 92
Sexual behavior
  arousal and motivation in, 379–380
  cervical cancer and, 292
  chronological age and, 373–376
  employment and, 387–390
  future predictions concerning, 386
  among homosexuals, 376–377
  menopause and, 371–372
  research and studies on, 371–395
Sexual harassment, 107
Sibling relationships, and psychological well-being, 150
Sleeping patterns, cross cultural study of, 263–264

Social change
  equality and, 155–172
  and health care, 277–278, 279
Social Security, 124, 125, 127, 128
  See also Disability insurance; Old Age, Survivor's, Disability, and Health Insurance (OASDHI) program; Retirement benefits
Socialization
  anticipatory, 22, 23
  sex-role, 90, 91, 92
Stability
  as index of individual change, 48
  reliability versus, 40–41
Statistical regression, as threat to validity of longitudinal design, 56
Stimulation, as psychological need, 262, 264–265, 266
Structural validity, 45–46
Suicide, mortality rates, 280
Support, as psychological need, 262

Taxonomy of life events, 21, 22
Testosterone, effect on sexual behavior, 373–374
Therapeutic issues
  acknowledgment of sexuality, 351–352
  anxiety and insecurity, 346–349
  decision-making, 343–346, 359–369
  femininity, 349–351

Thermography, 291
Transitions, as motivating factor in adult learning, 324–326
Type-A behavior, association with cardiovascular and cerebrovascular diseases, 291
Uterus. See Corpus uteri

Vaginal dryness, as symptom associated with menopause, 285, 287
Vaginal vasocongestion, 379
Validation, cross-age, 45
Validity, age-related, 43–45, 46
Variability, as characteristic of developmental changes in adulthood, 33

Wages
  of black women, 255
  as factor in hierarchical arrangement of social roles, 195, 196
  sex differentials in, 90, 91
  See also Financial well-being
Well-being, psychological. See Psychological well-being
Widowhood
  and economic well-being, 86, 87, 125
  and parent–child relationship, 207, 210, 222–223
  as part of family life cycle, 113, 115
  and sexual behavior, 378, 390